A FUTURE
OF
CONSEQUENCE

A FUTURE

OF

CONSEQUENCE

THE MANAGER'S ROLE
IN HEALTH SERVICES

Gary L. Filerman, Ph.D.
Editor

A WITT ASSOCIATES INC.
CONTRIBUTION TO THE HEALTH ADMINISTRATION
PROFESSION

A Future of Consequence: The Manager's Role in Health Services
edited by Gary L. Filerman

This book has been published with the support of Witt Associates Inc. and
was produced by Princeton University Press.

ISBN 0-910591-07-5

Library of Congress Catalog Card Number 89-80548

Association of University Programs
   in Health Administration
1911 North Fort Myer Drive
Suite 503
Arlington, Virginia 22209
(703) 524-5500

Witt Associates Inc.
1211 West 22nd Street
Oak Brook, Illinois 60521
(312) 574-5070

ORGANIZATION OF THE BOOK

INTRODUCTION
John S. Lloyd   ix

PART I   EDUCATION

1   Toward a Future of Consequence: The Education of a Health Service
     Administrator
     Gary L. Filerman, Ph.D.   3

PART II   INSTITUTIONAL SERVICES

2   The General Hospital: Managing for Stability in a Changing
     Environment
     Daniel A. Kane, Dr.P.H.   31

3   Multihospital Systems: Applying Corporate Structures and Strategies
     to Health Services
     S. Douglas Smith and Phyllis M. Virgil   54

4   Rural Hospitals: Big Impact in Small Communities
     David J. Robertson   76

5   The Nursing Home: Where Management Shapes the Quality of Life
     Miner L. Brown and John R. Kress   99

6   Mental Health Services: The System and Its Management Move to
     the Mainstream
     Aaron Liberman, Ph.D.   112

PART III   NONINSTITUTIONAL SERVICES

7   Managed Care: Administering Emerging Comprehensive Care
     Systems
     Gail L. Warden   129

8   Home Health Services: New Technologies, New Organizations, New
     Growth
     Louis Katz   147

9 Medical Group Practice: Working with Physicians
   F. Kenneth Ackerman, Jr. 160

   PART IV   THE INFRASTRUCTURE OF HEALTH SERVICES

10 Health Insurance: Managing a Vast and Complex Industry to Serve
    the Individual
    David H. Klein 175

11 Health Management Consulting: Solving Problems and Providing
    Advice
    John S. Lloyd, with the assistance of Karen M. Kelly 186

12 Education and Health Services Research: Giving Future Direction to
    Administrative Education
    *Samuel Levey, Ph.D., with the assistance of James Hill, Ph.D., and
    Daniel Russell, Ph.D. 198*

13 Foundations: Promoting Change Through Giving
    Robert A. DeVries 214

14 Professional Associations: A Powerful Influence on People and
    Institutions
    Jean-Claude Martin 222

    PART V   PUBLIC SECTOR

15 Canadian Government: Making the Most of the Public Investment
    Ambrose M. Hearn 239

16 Government in the U.S.: Managing for Policy and Political
    Accountability
    Malcolm Randall 248

17 International Health: Responding to the Global Challenge
    Willy De Geyndt, Ph.D. 281

    PART VI   CAREER DEVELOPMENT

18 Physicians in Administration: Working at the Medicine and
    Management Interface
    John T. Ashley, M.D. 291

19 Nurses in Health Administration: From Bedside to Boardroom
Ellen W. Gutstadt 301

20 Career Entry and Career Development
John S. Lloyd 314

INTRODUCTION

There is no more challenging career arena today than health care. The industry has grown and changed so dramatically in the past few years that the only prediction safe to make is: More change. No one can foresee now what the health care industry will look like in 10 years. What used to be regarded as a backwater has become a most highly charged dynamic environment.

All of this change requires management, of course. The exciting possibilities will only be realized by organizations that have excellent executive talent to guide them through the sometimes difficult path of progress. The people who lead this health care industry into the 21st century will need to be wise and adaptable and visionary. Does that sound like you? If so, you have come to the right place.

This book, developed by the AUPHA in cooperation with Witt Associates, is designed to offer you a panoramic view of the health care industry, and to lay out the wide variety of options you may wish to consider as you narrow your choice of management career interests.

Make the most of this extraordinary opportunity. It has been a very satisfying experience to assist in bringing it to you.

—John S. Lloyd
President
Witt Associates Inc.

PART I

EDUCATION

1

TOWARD A FUTURE OF CONSEQUENCE: THE EDUCATION OF A HEALTH SERVICE ADMINISTRATOR

GARY L. FILERMAN, Ph.D.

" **A** s I walked up to the entrance, I realized that my knees were knocking." My long-time colleague was describing his first day in a new position in a new city. The friend who shared his experience with me was not a neophyte. It was an unusual admission but very understandable. He had not been planning a job change but when asked to consider the new position, he looked it over thoroughly and accepted the new challenge. It was his third move in the 11 years since he had received a master's degree in health services administration and it was his first appointment as a hospital chief executive officer.

I was told this story by a well-known and respected health service executive. He went on to explain that he had realized from the outset that the hospital would have to change in many ways if it were going to maintain its traditionally strong leadership role in community health. He would have to give the organization a new vision and get everyone behind it, even though most people thought things were all right the way they were. "It was very

---

Gary L. Filerman holds a master's degree in health administration from the University of Minnesota. He earned a bachelor's degree with multiple majors, master of arts, and doctor of philosophy degree from the same university. Dr. Filerman is president of AUPHA—the Association of University Programs in Health Administration. He is editor of *The Journal of Health Administration Education*.

complicated, very high risk, and very consequential for the community. I knew before starting," he said, "that I was the most dispensable person in the organization and that if I were not very skillful in working with people, I would fail and the hospital would lose valuable time."

Reflecting on the contribution of professional education to his career, he said that it gave him "an appreciation of the complexity of leadership, taught me to be comfortable with change, and to understand my limitations." That comment did a lot to explain both his professional success and the knocking knees. Even when stepping into a senior position and having good experience, he recognized that he would have to keep on learning and growing if he were to succeed.

Health services administration encompasses the most complex and consequential management responsibility in modern society. It is a profession in which one individual can have a direct influence on the quality of life in the community. The health services administrator does not personally prevent or cure illness, but plays the key role in providing an environment in which those who do can reach the highest potential of their professional skills. The administrator is also responsible for assuring that the public has access to appropriate high quality services. Neither are possible unless the organization is financially strong, forward looking, and responsive to its community. These, too, are the administrator's responsibilities. It is hard to imagine a more consequential management responsibility.

No one wants to use health services but when we do need them, we want easy access to services in which we have confidence. In fact, most people do not pay much attention to the role of health services in their community until they are needed. The impact of health service organizations on prevention is particularly hard to identify because often it goes on behind the scenes. Public agencies such as state, provincial, city, and county public health departments work closely with doctors, hospitals, and other service providers to identify and stop potential threats before many people are involved. The most well known examples are problems with food supply, water provision, and sewage disposal. There are constant efforts to prevent sickness by managing the increasing threat to the environment from radioactive materials and industrial wastes, and by reducing workplace hazards. The control of communicable diseases, most dramatically AIDS (acquired immune deficiency syndrome), falls in the traditional domain of public health services. There is a direct relationship between reducing such threats to the public's health and providing medical care—the more successful prevention services are, the more resources there will be available to cure the illnesses which cannot be prevented.

The promotion of wellness is also a part of health services. Many years ago it was demonstrated that a healthy environment and life style have more impact on the individual's health status than do all the efforts of hospitals and doctors. In the past 15 years, there have been major strides in understanding the linkage between specific factors such as weight, diet, exercise, smoking, and drinking and the causation of disease. Whereas disease prevention strategies fend off threats, wellness strategies are aimed at getting people to take deliberate actions which will enhance their long-term health status.

Screening programs in offices, factories, schools, and unions help identify high risk individuals who will particularly benefit from effective wellness programs. Educational programs inform the public about everything from the value of high fiber diets to the negative impact on unborn babies of mothers using drugs. Employers provide exercise rooms and cafeteria diet counseling because they know these actions will help reduce sick days and increase employee morale. Wellness counseling services of many kinds have proliferated as freestanding entities and in conjunction with other health services. There is a great deal of interest in finding new ways to organize and promote wellness programs which will be attractive to the public and cost effective.

A substantial portion of health services can be more appropriately called "sickness services." The distinction is useful because it helps clarify the missions of individual practitioners, institutions, organizations, and services. There has been a tradition of separation between those services with a health mission (prevention and wellness promotion) and those services with a sickness mission (curing or rehabilitation). That separation is rapidly disappearing.

The most visible symbol of sickness services is the community hospital. Every chamber of commerce effort to promote the community includes references to the availability of quality medical care and hospitals, and often to their size. The implication is that the presence of a successful hospital means that qualified doctors and other health services are readily available. Conversely, the closing of a hospital, particularly when it is the only one in the community, is often seen as an economic and social disaster. The implications are that doctors will not be accessible, that urgent needs will not be met effectively, and for many communities, that the local economy is in deep trouble. Obviously, the hospital is a highly valued social institution.

While hospitals are organized primarily to manage episodes of acute illness, chronic disease care is generally rendered in nursing homes or at home. Most nursing home patients are elderly but the number of younger people requiring long-term care is increasing. Patients at home are served by an increasing number of home health agencies, which may provide specific therapies or comprehensive care. Hospices, either freestanding or hospital based, are also well established as a part of the service system.

There are other medical care institutions that have traditionally been organized primarily for the purpose of providing sickness services. Physicians, podiatrists, and other providers often create group practices, which may be called clinics. Some have become large enough to support their own hospitals. There are many ambulatory surgery centers ("surgicenters") where an increasing variety of relatively simple surgical procedures are performed on an outpatient basis. Urgent care centers offer routine care to the public, which is much like what is provided by a family doctor but on a walk-in basis. Publicly supported neighborhood health centers make comprehensive care available to communities which are underserved by private practitioners. These proliferating service organizations may or may not be linked to hospitals or to each other.

There is a complex system of public agencies and private organizations which finance, own, manage, or regulate preventive, wellness, and sickness services. The most visible are the public and private systems for paying the bill. They include federal, state, and provincial programs (e.g., Medicare); insurance plans which reimburse for costs; and prepaid, comprehensive care systems which provide all needed services in return for a fixed monthly premium. Within the private sector there are both for-profit and nonprofit systems for paying for services. New ways of organizing services and payment mechanisms are constantly evolving.

Patterns of ownership are also dynamic. Traditionally hospitals, nursing homes, clinics, and home health services were owned by independent nonprofit boards of directors, public agencies, private individuals, or small corporations. Now many are moving into larger organizations which include church systems, investor-owned chains, and voluntary networks to share services. Many are regional; some span the country. There have been many mergers of institutions to achieve economies of scale, and in the United States, to gain competitive advantages. Behind any familiar health service there is now likely to be an elaborate corporate structure, many times headquartered in another city.

Health services are highly regulated. Most regulation is conducted by public agencies but private and voluntary organizations are also important regulators. Every level of government gets involved in assuring the safety of health services, thereby maintaining a large professional bureaucracy. Regulators are also the conveyors of the public's often conflicting desires to have all of the appropriate services available, and to control the cost of providing them. Public policy generally relies on a system of private organizations to assess and improve the quality of care in health services, a system which is therefore voluntary only in theory. All of these structures and organizations are integral to the provision of prevention, wellness, and sickness services.

All health services are under pressure to contain costs. However, both public and professional values commit us to make health, and especially medical services, available to everyone as a matter of right. Not just medical services, but we hold to the belief they should be the best. The price of the best keeps going up, driven by expensive new technologies, an aging population, and perhaps most important, by public expectations. All of the sources of payment—individuals, employers, governments, insurance schemes, and charity—are caught between having limited means and virtually unlimited expectations for access to quality health services.

One response has been the development of new ways to organize services to achieve efficiencies. The efficiencies are professional as well as managerial and economic. Merging preventive and wellness programs within curative organizations such as hospitals reduces the utilization of services, and thereby cost, through prevention and early sickness detection. This is the goal of health maintenance organizations (HMOs) and other kinds of managed care plans. Hospitals have been expanding their mission to include wellness services, which moves the hospital toward becoming a truly comprehensive health care center. When doctors move into groups they promote continuity of care as well as achieving more effective use of expensive staff and equipment. Cost containment is a driving force behind the organizational change which is affecting all kinds of health services.

Another response to the cost squeeze has been for employers to get involved in efforts to control health care costs. Employers, along with the government, pay most of the steadily increasing cost of health insurance and must ultimately pass these costs on to the consumer. Many observers believe that one negative impact of health insurance is that insured individuals do not feel much of the direct impact of using health services and would, in fact, be more hesitant to use the services if they did. Others argue that the purpose of health insurance is to remove the expense barrier to services at the earliest possible moment and that any delay because of costs leads to advanced illness and higher long-term expense. In many communities, employers have formed business coalitions to work together on health benefits cost-containment strategies. Increasingly, as the impact of cost containment is felt, their concerns are directed to quality and access issues.

Every health service organization embodies such conflicting goals, values, forces, and policies. Issues of ethical organizational behavior will become more serious as resource limitations become more apparent. For example, the increasing number of aged who benefit from very complex technologies, and chronically ill young people who are kept alive by expensive new treatments, claim resources which could be invested in wellness activities aimed at children. In some rural communities the underutilized hospital is a significant employer, pitting the need to achieve medical efficiency against the community's economic vitality. Within all institutions, the roles of certain health professions will be threatened with dramatic change or even obsolescence as new technologies evolve, raising the dilemma of which is the most important.

These developments and others focus attention on the role of the decision makers. There used to be a separation between clinical decision makers and administrative decision makers. But the changes, problems, and challenges are no longer clearly on one side of the line or the other, because every financial decision has clinical implications and vice versa. Clinicians and administrators are learning each other's languages. They are working together to resolve the problems for which they share responsibility. Clinicians, particularly doctors and nurses, are participating in decision processes which require solid management skills such as data management and finance. Administrators, in the same decision processes, must be capable of assessing the impact of resource allocation choices on the health status of the community or the quality of care implications of new technology. Together they are operating in a legal and public regulations goldfish bowl where every decision will be scrutinized by someone. No wonder my friend's knees were knocking.

The professional health services administrator contributes organizational leadership and managerial skills to this complex, challenging, and exciting environment. Leadership is the process of defining the organization's mission, setting goals, and getting everyone behind them. All of the health professions have missions of their own, which are essential to the organization's goals. Leadership is required to overcome the tendency of each profession or department to be independent, and to show how their activities affect everyone else and how they contribute to the success of the total organization.

What distinguishes leaders in health care administration from other managers is an understanding of how the health of people is affected by organizational behavior and a readiness to do what is necessary to protect and improve health as the organization's highest priority. The public expects to receive the highest possible quality of services, provided by appropriately qualified personnel, using state-of-the-art equipment and supplies, applied in a safe environment. The professional administrator conveys these expectations to everyone in the organization, and is ultimately held accountable for the results. To keep the organization responsive, the leader in health services administration must sometimes articulate values and advance strategies which challenge important interests within the organization. Doing so, and keeping the job, requires communication skills and tact, which are the essence of professional leadership.

On the basis of having watched many administrators come, rise, and go throughout all kinds of health services, I can, with some confidence, describe the skills necessary for effective health services administrative leadership. No one person has all of the ideal strengths and characteristics, so the most important skill is in assessing yourself objectively. If that can be done honestly you are likely to seek complementary strengths in your colleagues through employment and development. This will lead to recognition for management team building, rather than to an image of going beyond your personal capacity, which has contributed to the downfall of many administrators.

The second skill is in listening. That sounds simple, but in health care institutions there is a tendency to attempt to establish authority by demonstrating how much you know. The result can be the opposite, which can be a very expensive lesson. If administrators do not listen carefully small problems often become big ones. Many people judge the quality of administrators by how well they are perceived to listen.

Negotiation also ranks high on my list of skills. Often there are not only conflicting pressures, but there are no right answers. The administrator must be skilled at negotiation, through which he keeps everyone together and focused on the organization's mission in spite of their own differing priorities and agendas.

The critical technical skills all revolve around the need to understand, integrate, and communicate quantitative information. Central managerial control responsibilities are access to services, the quality of those services, and the utilization of resources. That control is implemented through data systems which generate complicated information. The effective administrator can identify what information is really needed, if it is being provided, and if not, why not. Then the information must be interpreted to identify problems, clarify options, and implement solutions. Because all of these steps are accomplished through other people, the administrator must also develop skills in communicating quantitative information.

Health service administrators work with many community audiences to keep them informed, to expand the organization's market, to develop political and financial support, and to assess needs. Over time, this interaction through management gradually reshapes organizational mission, which must be dynamic to respond to a changing environment. The process of environmental scanning is systematic and requires constant effort. The administrator is looked to by everyone in the organization to be well informed about developments in the community, health sciences, education, government, and economics which will affect the organization. Developing a communications network, keeping informed, integrating and interpreting information is an immensely rewarding dimension of health administration leadership. The effective administrator continually grows through working at keeping well informed.

Is value conveyance a skill? I think so. The emphasis upon hard data and accountability may appear to produce a kind of value-free management. On the contrary, it mandates that administrators convey the organizational value system into the decision-making process. It is to be hoped that the mission of the organization addresses values. It is management that operationalizes values, and that is a skill. In fact, I think it is at the very core of the professional health service administrator's contribution and the reason why the role is valued by society.

Reading about the health services system and the contributions of professional administrators is a good way to begin exploring your potential interest in this field. The next step is to talk directly with men and women who are in key administrative positions in a variety of health organizations. They are usually very willing to discuss their personal experiences and their outlook for the future. In fact, there is a strong tradition of welcoming young people into the profession, which extends beyond just talking to mentoring. Mentoring is the process of taking an active interest in someone who is exploring or growing into the field. It often includes providing advice and helping with planning relevant job experience and professional education.

Experience in a health service organization can be a highly valuable way of exploring this career. First, it will give you the real flavor of the health services environment. That may be very exciting or it may convince you that it is not the kind of a place where you want to spend the rest of your professional life. Second, practical experience is a source of learning about the culture and vocabulary which will be useful as you move through a professional education program. And it may provide useful contacts which will help with later job placements and, not unimportantly, with recommendations for admission to selective educational programs. These advantages will be gained in almost any full- or part-time job. It is smart to let the senior administrators of the organization know that you are considering a career in health services administration. That will open doors for you regardless of the specific job that you are holding.

A degree in health services administration is the best preparation for a career in the field. Employers and the other health professionals know what education and skills a recognized professional degree represents. Their positive experience is reflected in the continual vertical and horizontal expansion of opportunities for graduates of programs in health services administration. Vertical expansion includes the growing expectation that key managers at all levels in complex organizations such as hospitals will have professional degrees, instead of only a few top-level executives. Expanding employment opportunity vertically means that program graduates are being recruited by a constantly expanding variety of service, finance, regulatory, planning, and coordinating organizations.

The most important reason for seeking a professional health services administration degree is the assurance that your education is appropriate to your aspirations. It is essential that you invest your educational time and money well. If the program meets recognized quality standards, a prospective student can be assured that it has been designed to provide a combination of behavioral, administrative, and health sciences which is optimal preparation for career-long growth. The faculty are constantly studying health services and have a good understanding of what is required for effective managerial practice. The college or university has established relationships with health services organizations which assure exposure to practicing administrators, access to guided field experiences, and assistance in job placement.

There are both bachelor's and master's degrees in health services administration which are designed for entry into management practice. There have been a few experiments with associate degree programs, but there is a strong consensus among educators and practitioners that they did not provide adequate or appropriate preparation. The doctoral degree programs are intended primarily as preparation for careers in teaching, research, and policy development, although a few of the graduates have moved into management.

Bachelor's degree programs have developed in recent years in response to the expanding market for professionally educated individuals and the movement toward more career-oriented undergraduate education. They are offered in private liberal arts colleges, comprehensive state universities, and in research universities. Several are based in departments which also offer graduate degrees. They are both full and part time. The programs are based in a variety of university settings, among which are schools of allied or community health, business administration, interdisciplinary studies, nursing, public health, and others. With few exceptions, they award the bachelor of science degree.

The mark of quality and professional recognition of baccalaurate degrees in health services administration is full membership in the Association of University Programs in Health Administration (AUPHA). Full membership in the consortium of programs is earned by successfully meeting criteria that are established by faculty members. Programs maintain their membership through periodic reviews by panels of peers. The process assures prospective students and employers that the program's curriculum, faculty, and performance expectations are of high quality. Full membership also identifies those faculties which have committed themselves to working together toward constant improvement of their educational capacity and competence. Programs which are developing and are working toward full membership may be associate members of AUPHA. This is a good indication of progress toward full membership recognition.

AUPHA membership is a useful guide for the prospective student contemplating the variety of institutions, settings, and degrees that are available. All of the recognized bachelor degree programs include four elements; general and liberal education, management science and practice, health services administration, and field experience. There is a strong commitment to education in the liberal arts fundamentals which are essential to citizenship and personal growth, including economics, mathematics, political science, psychology, and sociology. The management sciences include accounting, managerial ethics, applied psychology, business law, management information systems, and statistics. The relative weight given to each topic will differ among colleges and universities.

Health services administration content in recognized programs will include attention to the individual, social, and environmental determinants of health and disease, epidemiology, health services delivery systems, health planning, health finance, health applications of organizational and management theory, the roles of clinicians, and health services law. A supervised field experience integrates the theoretical coursework with the real world of health services administration.

Baccalaureate programs have attracted a variety of students following many different career paths. A substantial number come directly into college from high school and begin their health services administration concentration as juniors. Others have completed degrees in a health profession such as nursing, physical therapy, or laboratory technology and are preparing for managerial roles within the clinical field. A few of the students have previous bachelor's degrees in non-health related areas. The age distribution can be described as bimodal, reflecting the mix of younger students and those who have considerable work experience.

The principal mission of undergraduate programs is preparation to enter management practice. Of course, students who aspire to go on to graduate degrees are encouraged to do so and it has been estimated that about 10 percent do go on to advanced education in health service administration or in a related field. There is no evidence that completion of an undergraduate health services administration major provides a competitive advantage or disadvantage for admission to the selective graduate programs. Some graduate programs prefer students who have completed a strong general education program, rather than one designed to equip them to enter the profession. Other graduate programs welcome bachelor's program graduates.

Many baccalaureate degree holders go into middle management positions in hospitals. They may serve as unit managers who coordinate all of the services and personnel on large nursing units. Some are beginning their careers as department heads with assignments in central services, materials management, purchasing, security, admissions, information systems, planning, marketing, or in the business office. It is important to note that in many large institutions each of these functions may involve more personnel and a larger budget than an entire average-sized hospital. Other graduates have been accepting positions in the top management of nursing homes, ambulatory care programs, neighborhood health centers, community mental health centers, emergency services, hospices, and group practices. There are also expanding opportunities in regulatory agencies, associations, insurance programs, HMOs, and in the industry which provides supplies, equipment, and services to health care organizations.

Most undergraduate institutions or undergraduate divisions of large universities draw the majority of their students from nearby communities or from within the state and province in which they are located. Job placement patterns are similarly circumscribed. The recruitment and placement patterns of health services administration programs tend to follow those of the parent institution.

What if you decide to seek a graduate degree and want to prepare optimally as an undergraduate? The first rule is to start deliberate preparation as early as possible in your undergraduate career. Most graduate programs require a few specific courses as prerequisites for admission. It is a good idea to identify them by reading the catalogs of the programs to which you might eventually apply. Introductory courses in accounting, economics, and statistics are the most frequently required prerequisites.

My own philosophy is that the undergraduate years are your best chance to explore the world through education. It is the time to indulge your curiosity by aggressively exploiting the resources of the university, especially by using electives to move outside of your major. It may be tempting to take more courses in prerequisite areas to impress a graduate admissions committee. There will be time for more of that in graduate school, but that is not the time to come back to humanities, history, or philosophy of science. This path will contribute to a more satisfying professional life in the long run. Many baccalaureate programs in health administration are designed to encourage general education.

The most commonly used criterion for admission to a graduate program is the undergraduate grade point average. Most faculty members, despite questioning the relevance of grades as a predictor of professional success, continue to look at grades first. Grades remain a major consideration even when an applicant has been out of school for several years. Grades reflect self-discipline and may relate to one's ability to handle some of the challenging quantitative content that is essential for modern health services administration.

Undergraduate major or previous professional education is also important, and is considered quite differently among the selective programs. Overall, undergraduate liberal arts majors prevail among successful applicants, with business majors the next highest. Graduate faculties seem to prefer students with the broadest possible educational backgrounds. The program is less likely to have to repeat introductory material on the social sciences for such students. The business undergraduate is most likely to have the background required for admission to the programs affiliated with business schools and awarding the MBA degree in health administration.

Regardless of the undergraduate major, most programs favor a strong background in quantitative skills. Quantitative knowledge can be gained in calculus, statistics, advanced mathematics, operations research, finance, economics, psychology, and other areas. The trend toward increased quantitative content in the graduate programs reflects the administrator's responsibilities for establishing organizational indicators of quality, implementing financial controls, and interpreting their results to various audiences.

Nonacademic life is also relevant to preparation for a graduate or undergraduate program. If you are a full-time student, summer employment should be in a health care organization. A particularly effective strategy is to move around from summer to summer, working in a nursing home one year and perhaps for an insurance company the next. If you are working full time and are going to school part time, consider a move to the kind of organization in which you hope to start your management career.

Participation in academic and community affairs, or both, is also useful preparation for professional life. Campus political, academic, and service organizations are always looking for people to share leadership responsibilities. They provide unique opportunities to develop public speaking, writing, and group leadership skills. Faculty advisers can be an excellent source of graduate school recommendations. Community activities which provide similar advantages are church groups, service organizations, and political parties. Many leading health services administrators attribute their comfort with the responsibilities of leadership to early experience in student government and similar activities.

I have noted that many individuals with allied health credentials are taking bachelor's degrees in health services administration. In most cases, their objective is managerial leadership within their field. There is also a trend for physicians, dentists, pharmacists, and nurses with bachelor's degrees to seek graduate education in health services administration. This is a predictable development reflecting the dramatic changes in health services organization.

Physicians in particular see new administrative roles developing in managed care programs, group practices, and in hospital positions for which clinical background is essential. Typical positions are HMO medical director, hospital vice president for clinical affairs, or medical director of a group practice clinic. The administrative dimensions of these roles are very complex, particularly as they pertain to the assessment of quality of care and leadership in quality improvement. There is no relevant content in medical education. A graduate degree in health services administration will provide the necessary skills and, in some cases, the curriculum can be shaped to accommodate the clinician's interests.

One problem, however, is that many physicians are not well positioned to pursue a graduate degree in health administration. They are unlikely to have taken the requisite undergraduate courses. If that describes your situation, it is important to take the time to take the courses rather than attempt to negotiate around them. The background is essential and the content is necessary to compete successfully with students who are generally better prepared. These courses will give you a sense of comfort with managerial (aggregate) as opposed to clinical (individual) data. The clinician with a recognized health services administration degree will have both a personal and professional advantage over those who learn administration by apprenticeship or through a succession of short courses.

Many dentists and pharmacists are moving to health services administration as a career change. The current economics of both fields are constraining their traditional career opportunities. Health services administration can be a logical new direction, but the same admonition about appropriate background applies. That is, take the frequently required prerequisites and get ready to compete for admission and grades with students who have solid quantitative skills.

For nurses, health services administration degrees offer a special challenge. There is increasing recognition that nursing perspectives and skills are the very essence of most health services. As other professions become more specialized and more high technology invades most settings, it is the

TABLE 1: Health Services Administration Graduate Degrees

Master of Health Administration	M.H.A.
Master of Hospital and Health Administration	M.H.H.A.
Master of Health Services Administration	M.H.S.A.
Master of Health Sciences in Health Administration	M.H.Sc.
Master of Business Administration	M.B.A.
Master of Business Administration (Health Administration)	M.B.A.(H.A.)
Master of Business Administration (Health Care Management)	M.B.A.(H.C.M.)
Master of Management	M.M.
Master of Public Health	M.P.H.
Master of Professional Studies	M.P.S.
Master of Science in Health Administration	M.S.H.A.
Master of Science in Health Services Planning and Administration	M.Sc.
Master of Science in Public Health	M.S.P.H.
Master of Science in Health Systems Management	M.S.
Master of Health Sciences	M.H.S.
Master of Public Administration	M.P.A.
Master of Arts	M.A.

nurse who remains the consistent caregiver to the total patient and is the advocate for the patient within the organization. Yet nursing itself needs more effective advocates in the councils of management and many nurses are seeking the skills to provide that leadership. A degree in health services administration provides skills and knowledge which will enrich the management capacity of nurses. It is gaining increased acceptance as appropriate for careers in nursing administrative leadership.

A master's degree in health services administration is the most widely recognized credential for a career as a health services administrator. It is a unique degree, not only because of its content but also because it is the rare case where several degree designations are equal in professional stature. The variety of degree designations is the source of some confusion, but it also reflects an important strength of the field (see Table 1).

All of the degrees listed are professionally equal. Most are offered by programs that are accredited. Others are offered by programs that aspire to accreditation. It is the accreditation of the health services administration program which assures the potential student and prospective employer that the program provides the core of knowledge that the health services administration profession considers essential. The differences among the degrees are largely in what the program offers beyond that essential knowledge framework.

One interesting development is the proliferation of programs offering two degrees, which are in response to student and employer interest in broader proficiencies. When a program normally results in students receiving two degrees, they are called "dual." If two schools are involved, such as public health and business administration, it is generally called a "joint" degree. However, the terminology is not standard among universities. In either case, it essentially means getting two degrees instead of one. A few programs offer only two degrees. In other cases, the second degree is available as an option requiring an additional year. The idea is to get the advantages of both. The currently available combinations are MPH/MBA, MHA/MBA, MHSA/MBA, MPH/MPPM, MHS/MBA and MS/MBA. There are also some opportunities to combine degrees in health services administration with degrees in law, medicine, or social work.

It is important to know why there is such a diversity of degrees since it does complicate program selection and, in small ways, professional identity. One reason is the history of the profession. Health services administration grew out of two separate but closely related fields, hospital administration and medical care administration. Before the two kinds of programs merged a few years ago, they had separate identities and in fact coexisted within some universities.

The medical care administration programs were based in schools of public health and, of course, granted the degree authorized by those schools (MPH, MSPH, and so on). Hospital administration programs were based in schools of public health, public administration, business schools, and other settings. Their founders emphasized management, behavioral science, public health, or hospital management as the core of knowledge and sought out schools that were most hospitable to that content. The degree was usually whatever the school offered or the MHA. In the early years there was consensus on the mission but not on the educational means. Some programs have retained their historic identities.

The second factor reflects the size of the programs. In terms of number of full-time faculty, they are the size of most academic departments. If the programs were as large as schools of medicine, nursing, or business administration it might be possible to establish a single degree across all institutions. However, small units embedded within larger schools are in many cases permitted only to offer the parent school's degree. In the case of schools of public affairs, business administration, and public health, the health services administration program's curriculum is generally designed around the school's core curriculum or core of knowledge as required of all students in the school.

The third reason is a source of strength to the field. Persuasive arguments can be made for emphasizing the perspectives of general management, public health, public administration, or behavioral sciences as most important to health administration practice. When you consider the scope of the issues, problems, challenges, and responsibilities faced by the health services ad-

TABLE 2: The Accrediting Commission on Education for Health Services Administration

Participating Organizations
American College of Health Care Administrators (ACHCA)
American College of Healthcare Executives (ACHE)
American College of Medical Group Administrators (ACMGA)
American Hospital Association (AHA)
American Public Health Association (APHA)
Canadian College of Health Service Executives (CCHSE)
Canadian Hospital Association (CHA)
Association of University Programs in Health Administration (AUPHA)
Association of Mental Health Administrators (AMHA) (Consulting Member)

ministrator, it is clearly important to employ the most open and creative approach to management. There is no one perspective that gives the correct answer to every situation and there is no one model that is applicable to all health service organizations. The public benefits when the leadership of this vital social service brings a variety of perspectives to problem solving. An orthodoxy, or firm belief in one perspective on approaches to issues and solutions, would foster inflexibility and inhibit the adaptability that is essential to foster quality health services.

The health services administration accrediting process encourages diversity, setting parameters without enforcing rigid standardization. This is difficult to maintain, because many institutions expect accreditation to be rigid and prescriptive. The Accrediting Commission on Education for Health Services Administration (ACEHSA) is broadly representative of both academic and administrative practice. The commission has criteria (not standards) that assure content in health, behavioral science, and management science. It is also important to note that the commission stresses the need for graduates to have strong analytic skills in information science, finance, and quantitative methods, in other words, manager's skills applied to health services. That emphasis remains firmly based in the commitment and culture of the healing mission (see Table 2).

Schools of medicine, public health, business administration, and public administration also have schoolwide accreditation which is important to maintaining overall quality. It is not the same as or equal to accreditation by ACEHSA. Schoolwide accreditation does not embody the expertise or the perspectives of the health services administration field. ACEHSA and the schoolwide accrediting bodies cooperate to achieve their common quality assurance objectives. To avoid overlapping, their efforts are coordinated by the Council on Postsecondary Accreditation (COPA), which represents colleges and universities.

There may be valid reasons why a program is not accredited by ACEHSA. In some circumstances, you can be reasonably confident that their degree will eventually have accredited status. New programs may not seek ACEHSA accreditation until they have graduated a class, which may be two or three years after the program starts. A program may lose its accreditation because of a problem which is being resolved, creating a temporary accreditation lapse. It is important to investigate why a program is not ACEHSA accredited. If a graduate program of any type (part time or full time) has no commitment to achieve the peer recognition embodied in health services administration accreditation, there is a valid basis for concern.

Canadians are less familiar with accreditation than are their colleagues south of the border. Voluntary academic accreditation by nongovernmental organizations is a peculiarly American phenomenon. Health services administration is among the few professions for which accreditation is relevent in the Canadian context. There has always been close affinity and collaboration between U.S. and Canadian health service leaders and educators who are continually learning from each other. Educational design and content in health services administration programs is similar, allowing, of course, for the significant differences in health services entitlement and financing. Accredited Canadian degrees are recognized in the United States and vice versa. Canadian professional organizations participate fully in ACEHSA.

Ideally, graduate professional education would be completed through a full-time program which usually requires two years to complete. I say ideally since it facilitates full immersion in the stimulating intellectual, professional, and social dimensions that surround most of the programs. There are often interesting professional visitors and research projects that present opportunities for student involvement. And of course, informal interaction with fellow students and faculty adds considerably to the richness of the educational experience.

However, many potential health services administration graduate students do not have the option of going to school full time for two years. About half of all health services administration graduate students in all programs (both accredited and nonaccredited) are part time. This is a relatively recent development, reflecting trends in graduate education generally. Increasing educational costs, decreasing student aid resources, and a changing age profile are pressing higher education to increase access through modified educational delivery systems (much like health services!). Health services administration education is changing too.

A third pattern of graduate education has begun to emerge. It is usually called "nontraditional" because of two characteristics. The first is that the programs do not depend upon traditional classroom teaching. The content may be mailed to the student or even communicated by computer to an individual working alone at a remote location. The second characteristic is that the student may receive some academic credit for demonstrated competence or knowledge acquired by any means, including experience. Some of the programs combine traditional and nontraditional approaches by offering classes in cities that are remote from the campus and employing local faculty. The nontraditional programs are appealing because they are convenient and recognize experience. Several ACEHSA accredited graduate programs and programs that aspire to accreditation are involved in these creative, high quality nontraditional programs.

Anyone contemplating enrolling in a nontraditional program should investigate it carefully to be certain that the program is designed and controlled by competent professional health services administration educators and that the program emanates from an educational base with appropriate professional experience. The program should be subject to quality review by full-time faculty who are teaching health services administration. In my judgment, regional accreditation of the university or college which sponsors the program is not adequate to assure the quality of the program in health services administration. Nontraditional programs are eligible for ACEHSA accreditation. Some careful reading of the catalog and questioning of the program coordinators are essential to assure yourself of investing in a venture which has academic and professional creditability.

If you do have the option of considering several selective graduate programs, where do you begin? The first rule is to not narrow your horizons by focusing on programs based in one kind of school or on programs offering one of the recognized degrees. Look carefully at the curricula of several of the programs and it will be clear that differences in health services content between programs in settings such as public health, graduate schools, business administration, and so on are often more apparent than real.

Second, be wary of making decisions on the strength of reputation alone. Academic reputation follows reality, but often by a long time. An individual who graduated ten or even five years ago from what was then considered a fine program may know little about the same program today. Programs are strong for different reasons and program strengths change over time. For example, a program that enjoys a positive reputation for a strong orientation to multihospital systems may lose the faculty member who has that interest, but add a leader in insurance applications to managed care. The change in program emphasis may go unrecognized by those in the field of practice for several years. Some programs have decided to focus on one or more sectors of the industry such as long-term care and, as a result, may not have an effective placement network in other sectors such as hospitals. Thus, reputation may vary among sectors of the field.

Another key to program selection is to distinguish the reputation of the program from the reputation of the university. Some of the best professional education opportunities in the field are offered by programs which are based in universities with middle-level visibility and stature. Some more famous universities have not developed strong health administration programs. I think it is an expensive mistake to opt for university over program stature, because the field does know the difference. Ultimately, you will too.

All these considerations lead us back to the previous point about how to invest your educational time and money well. First obtain a copy of AUPHA's directory of education, which includes descriptions of both undergraduate and graduate programs as well as other important information. The directory, published every other year, is the standard guide to professional education. Write for the catalogs of the programs that may be of interest. Read them carefully to determine the strengths of the faculties and how the curricula respond to your interests and to identify the programs' dominant philosophies.

What should the applicant look for? First, a challenging environment, one that encourages the student to probe deeply into the subjects covered and the issues of the day. Evidence of this desirable characteristic is close contact with the faculty, both in seminars and through supervision of written and field work. The conscientious student wants a rigorous graduate program encouraging the type of thorough analysis that will be expected of the professional in the field. Are the faculty members who are well known as writers and consultants actually working with and available to the students? Have faculty members achieved the university's senior rank that measures scholarship? Do faculty members conduct research and publish the results? What are the research interests of program faculty? Ask whether faculty conduct doctoral-level education—a good indicator of an intellectually active environment.

Participation by faculty in continuing education of practicing health services administrators indicates academic immersion in real world problems. But the most important determinant of the program's scope can be measured by what the program hopes its graduates will contribute, what they will be doing in their careers. Programs should be willing to tell you about their alumni. What graduates of ten years ago are doing is interesting but it is more important to know about the experience of the graduates of last year and the year before as they entered the job market.

Programs' objectives also differ. Some concentrate on the senior administrative role in general acute hospitals, or on multihospital systems. Others concentrate upon strategic planning, epidemiology, marketing, or finance. Others try to avoid such specificity in order to provide the broadest possible overview of the total health system. Some programs offer the opportunity to select tracks or concentrations in such functional specialties as marketing, human resources management, finance, gerontology, health economics, and so on. Several offer health sector options in long-term care, mental health services, managed care programs, health insurance, international health care and so on.

To understand and cope with the complex challenges of health services delivery, health services administration draws upon the knowledge and skills of many disciplines. How much access does the student have to other disciplines? Few programs possess all the resources necessary to fulfill all academic requirements through their own faculty. Are there opportunities to take courses in subjects in which the student may develop a special interest? What if the courses are offered in another part of the university? Many programs offer opportunities to take electives, but the actual degree of freedom differs substantially. Some programs offer few or no electives because of the heavy demands of the core content in health services administration and the requirements of the core curriculum for the degree, or both. Investigation will provide insight into the program's organization, resources, and educational philosophy.

Most educators and practitioners agree that both undergraduate and graduate programs ought to include a substantial exposure to the real world. A period of observation and work in any health care program or facility helps the student grasp the relevance of coursework. As a result, almost every program has a required field experience component; however, programs differ markedly in the way they handle this portion of the curriculum.

The term residency is widely used to describe the most substantial required field work component, during which the student carries the title administrative resident. Residencies required for the degree may be as short as 3 months (the summer between two academic years) or as long as 12 months. Some graduate programs consist of one academic year of course work and a 12-month residency in a health services program or facility. Others require three semesters of course work and a 5- or 6-month residency. There are other patterns as well.

Most programs requiring the residency also require the student to be enrolled and to pay tuition for its duration. At the same time the student receives a stipend from the residency health care institution or program. Programs require all students in residency to spend the period doing similar activities, although they may be scattered across the country in different kinds of health services organizations. Most programs have established ties with a few carefully selected administrators of health services delivery organizations with whom the students spend the residency periods. These administrators are called preceptors and may have university faculty appointments as professional leaders with interests in education. The student studies the preceptor as well as the organization.

Preceptor selection and faculty supervision of the residency are a measure of graduate program quality. It is very important to look for programs that treat required residencies, whatever the length, as an integral part of the program and pay close attention to the quality of the student experience. Residents should be visited by a faculty member, progress reports sent to and reviewed by the university personnel, and preceptor participation in preceptor conferences should be required.

An increasing number of programs do not require a residency on the premise that the students should devote all of their time to formal class work. This approach assumes that the graduate will have many opportunities to learn about the world of work and to progress gradually through guided management development. The academic programs that do not have formal residency requirements may encourage students to work in the health care field during the summers. This is particularly true when the student has had no previous health care experience.

Every year more graduates start out on a one- or two-year advanced fellowship. The fellowships resemble the management development programs in many large corporations. They are not formally related to the university. Good career planning for an inexperienced individual should always include a fellowship for transition into the market. Graduates who have had experience in the field have less need for, and perhaps less patience with a fellowship; however, many have found it to be an invaluable experience.

After learning about the characteristics of programs, the next step is to establish the necessary admission test scores. There is no single standard test that is used by all programs. Not all programs require tests but all pay attention to available scores, especially when the grade point average is a source of doubt. The most frequently used tests are the Graduate Record Examination (GRE), Graduate Management Admission Test (GMAT), and the Miller Analogies Test (MAT). It is definitely worthwhile to take both the GRE and GMAT and, perhaps, the MAT for good measure. Foreign nationals applying to U.S. programs must complete the Test of English as a Foreign Language (TOEFL). Although there is controversy over whether the tests accurately predict academic performance, a good score definitely impresses most admission committees. Large colleges and universities have testing centers where one can take such examinations. However, some are administered only on certain dates that can be months away, so it is incumbent upon the potential applicant to start early.

With your research completed and test scores available, it is time for a decision on applications. Every year excellent applicants are turned away from their choice of programs because they failed to follow the most sagacious application strategy. It is wise to start early in the fall of the senior year of college, since applications should be submitted that December or, at the latest, in January of the year in which you plan to enter graduate school. The most selective programs will have filled their fall classes by February or March. Some programs admit students both in midyear and the fall but a majority have a single starting date.

After timing, the next most important strategy is to keep your options open. Competition among programs differs markedly and all programs experience changes in their pool of applicants from year to year. Some programs accept as few as 15 students a year and others accept more than 50. Some of the older, better-known programs receive as many as 12 applications for every opening, while newer, equally good programs may have a ratio of 2 to 1. An applicant with a good record may not get into one program while easily gaining admission to another. It is a good idea to apply to as many programs as you can.

Some admission committees begin their work by selecting individuals to be interviewed. If they do not, it is good to insist on having interviews with at least your first and second choice of programs. Visit the program at a time when students are present and ask to meet both first and second year students. Also, insist on talking with the program director and, perhaps, with other key faculty members. A meeting with a nonteaching administrative aide will be helpful but it is not sufficient. Come prepared with questions to make it a two-way interview. Some programs have alumni around the country who interview applicants as part of their selection process. That may not contribute much to your selection process because alumni cannot provide the insights that faculty members can.

Selective programs are not all looking for the same characteristics. Of course as a minimum, all look for solid evidence of ability to perform graduate work, but when 100 good people apply for 25 places, other factors come into play. A common one is mix, based upon the assumption that students learn from each other and that different student backgrounds make for an exciting learning environment. Thus, an admissions committee may look for some students with experience and others without, given a minimal grade point average.

There are no easy answers to the problem of steadily increasing costs of education. Overall, the price of higher education has been increasing faster than inflation and expectations are that the trend will continue indefinitely. The increases affect all students, whether they are in public or private institutions, and whether they are studying part time or full time. At the same time, the number and purchasing power of governmental scholarships and loans of all kinds have decreased. The changing economics of education is gradually limiting the options for more and more students.

The programs' catalogs provide some basic financial information, starting with costs. If you know that your resources will not meet the costs of those programs to which you wish to apply, I suggest that you apply anyway. Once you have been admitted, the program has an interest in helping you overcome the financial barrier. The faculty will have knowledge of scholarships, loans, and employment opportunities or some combination thereof which may work for you. The key is to try to assemble a package of support resources rather than to rely on a single source of student aid.

For full-time students and, indeed, for some part-time students, debt management is the name of the game. The challenge is to find the most favorable loan conditions. The cost of interest is not the only consideration, although it is usually the most important. The ideal loan package allows you to withdraw funds gradually as they are needed. Depending on the administrative fees, it may be less expensive in the long run to take out several small loans over a period of time. Consolidating loans so that there is a single payment due each month is desirable. All of this requires good planning. There are some excellent guidebooks and planning worksheets published by banks and these are available through campus student aid offices.

All students in U.S. AUPHA member programs are eligible for the AUPHA/Chase Manhattan Bank, N.A., Education Funding Options. The AUPHA/Chase program makes readily available federally guaranteed loans up to the limit of an individual's eligibility. There are several other loan options included in the AUPHA/Chase program. Graduate students also qualify for federal health professions HEAL loans. The American College of Healthcare Executives' Foster McGaw Loan Fund is available to student affiliates in accredited programs. Many of the programs have their own loan funds that have been provided by alumni. When exploring these options, keep in mind the importance of loan consolidation, so you do not end up with several payments each month.

Scholarships are available much less frequently. The most accessible are federal government traineeships in the United States and provincial bursaries in Canada. The traineeships are awarded only by ACEHSA-accredited programs and by schools of public health. ACEHSA-accredited AUPHA graduate member programs award Foster McGaw Scholarships. Minority group students may qualify for the Albert W. Dent Scholarship of the

ACHE. Many programs have some scholarship funds contributed by alumni. All student aid inquiries should be directed first to the program director.

If you graduate confident that you are adequately prepared for a successful career, a degree in health services administration will be more of an impediment than an advantage. The degree is the beginning. It should be clear by now that a considerable proportion of the information you learn about health services while in school will become obsolete very quickly. Health conditions are changing and health care organizations are evolving at a rapid pace. No one can predict the direction of public policy or health care organization with a high degree of certainty, nor can educators confidently describe what senior administrative positions in health care organizations are going to look like a few years from now.

The most consistent quality of health care administration practice is change. Your educational program will have served you well if you anticipate being in the center of a changing organization, occupying a changing position, and managing ambiguous decision-making processes. That will either be daunting or it will present you with an exciting challenge for personal growth.

Professionalism demands personal growth. The public and your colleagues in the organization will be looking to you to set the tone for coping with change. Everyone would be more comfortable if one could succeed on the strengths of yesterday's accomplishments and yesterday's learning. That will not equip you adequately or provide the basis for positioning your colleagues to manage the future proactively.

Professional education is a foundation. You will have effectively exploited the opportunity if you come away with knowledge of fundamentals that will serve you well over time, an ethical framework that will help you face difficult decisions, and a propensity to learn. Professional education can give you no greater gift than an understanding of the direct relationship between continued growth through learning and a future of consequence in the administration of health services.

SOURCES OF FURTHER INFORMATION

Admission Testing
(SAT) Scholastic Aptitude Test
The College Board ATP, CN 6200
Princeton, NJ 08541
(ACT) American College Testing Program
P.O. Box 168

2201 North Dodge Street
Iowa City, IA 52243

(GRE) Graduate Record Exam
ETS—GRE
CN 6000
Princeton, NJ 08541–6000

(GMAT)
ETS—GMAT
CN 6000
Princeton, NJ 08541–6000

(MAT)
Psychological Corporation
555 Academic Court
San Antonio, TX 78204–0952

(TOEFL)
Test of English as a Foreign Language
ETS
Princeton, NJ 08540

Student Loan Information
AUPHA/Chase Manhattan, N.A., Education Funding Options
Association of University Programs in Health Administration
1911 North Fort Myer Drive
Suite 503
Arlington, VA 22209

McGaw Fund and Dent Fund
American College of Healthcare Executives
840 North Lake Shore Drive
Chicago, IL 60611

The List of Accredited Graduate Programs
(ACEHSA)
Accrediting Commission on Education for Health Services Administration
1911 North Fort Myer Drive
Suite 503
Arlington, VA 22209

The Directory of Undergraduate and Graduate Programs
(AUPHA)
Association of University Programs in Health Administration
1911 North Fort Myer Drive

Suite 503
Arlington, VA 22209

Professional Societies
The American College of Healthcare Executives
840 North Lake Shore Drive
Chicago, IL 60611

The American Hospital Association
840 North Lake Shore Drive
Chicago, IL 60611

The American Public Health Association
1015–18th Street, N.W.
Washington, D.C. 20005

The American College of Health Care Administrators
325 South Patrick Street
Alexandria, VA 22314

The American College of Medical Group Administrators
1355 South Colorado Boulevard
Denver, CO 80222

The Association of Mental Health Administrators
840 North Lake Shore Drive
Chicago, IL 60611

Canadian College of Health Service Executives
17 York Street, Suite 201
Ottawa, Ontario K1N 5S7
Canada

Canadian Public Health Association
1335 Carling Avenue, Suite 210
Ottawa, Ontario K12 8N8
Canada

Canadian Hospital Association
17 York Street, Suite 100
Ottawa, Ontario K1N 9S6
Canada

PART II

INSTITUTIONAL SERVICES

2

THE GENERAL HOSPITAL: MANAGING FOR STABILITY IN A CHANGING ENVIRONMENT

DANIEL A. KANE, Dr.P.H.

The derivation of the word hospital is in the word "hospes" meaning host or guest [1]. Today's hospitals have as their historical antecedent the medieval hospitals of England. Early hospices in England developed as a roadside shelter for travelers [2]. Hospices founded between 925 and 1170 A.D. were operated for the most as part of monasteries. Between 1270 and 1470 A.D. a decline in travel led to a gradual transition of hospices to places that cared for vagrants, chronic invalids, and the infirm [3]. The first hospital in the United States was founded in 1658 [4].

Voluntary, nonprofit hospitals are eleemosynary corporations, corporations organized for charitable purposes [5]. The fact that we refer to voluntary hospitals as nonprofit institutions should not be interpreted to mean that these hospitals do not or cannot earn a surplus but rather that any surplus earned may not inure to the benefit of the trustees.

In 1986 there were 3,262 short-term, nongovernment, not-for-profit general hospitals in the United States (see Table 1) [6]. A short-term hospital is one in which the average length of stay of patients is under 30 days, or 50 percent of all patients are admitted to a unit in which the average length of stay is less than 30 days. A general hospital is one in which at minimum medical and surgical care is provided. General hospitals often provide one

Daniel A. Kane is president, Montefiore Hospital, Pittsburgh, PA. He received an M.S. in hospital administration from Columbia University and a B.B.A. in public administration from the City University of New York. He also holds a Dr.P.H. from the University of Pittsburgh.

TABLE 1: Short-term, Nongovernment, Not-For-Profit General Hospitals
1986

BED SIZE	NUMBER OF HOSPITALS	BEDS	ADMISSIONS
less than 99	1,101	62,857	1,847,951
100–299	1,351	248,080	8,593,104
300–499	556	212,621	7,545,006
500 over	253	173,405	5,890,217
Total	3,262	696,963	23,876,278

SOURCE: Hospital Statistics—1986 (Chicago: American Hospital Association, 1987) Table 2A, pp. 6–7. Reprinted with permission.

TABLE 2: Short-term, Nongovernment, Not-For-Profit Psychiatric
and Other Hospitals
1986

BED SIZE	NUMBER OF HOSPITALS	BEDS	ADMISSIONS
less than 99	110	6,108	99,331
100–299	45	6,806	255,386
300–499	5	1,688	54,084
500 over	2	1,128	18,638
Total	162	15,730	427,439

SOURCE: Hospital Statistics—1986 (Chicago: American Hospital Association, 1987) Table 2A, pp. 6–7. Reprinted with permission.

or more of the following services: acute medical-surgical care, obstetrics, pediatrics, psychiatry, substance abuse, and rehabilitation. There were 162 short-term specialty hospitals in the United States in 1986, including 78 children's hospitals (see Table 2) [7].

Short-term, not-for-profit general hospitals are often classified by sponsorship or ownership. While most hospitals in this group are nonsectarian community hospitals founded by groups of citizens from the community at large, others were organized by religious and fraternal groups. As of 1985 there were 614 Catholic hospitals in the United States with just under 164,000 beds [8]. Catholic hospitals are either owned by a religious order such as the Sisters of Mercy or Franciscan Sisters of the Poor or by a local diocese. A major focus of the mission of Catholic hospitals is service to the poor and medically indigent and fulfillment of the ethical and moral teachings of the Catholic Church.

The Protestant Hospital Association numbered 200 hospitals as members as of 1986 [9]. Among the Protestant denominations sponsoring hospitals are the United Church of Christ and the Seventh Day Adventists. Unlike Catholic hospitals, the degree of ownership of hospital assets and control exercised by the church varies greatly. In many cases Protestant hospitals have a loose relationship with a denominational group primarily derived from historical association. There are Protestant hospitals, however, with highly defined relationships covering ownership of assets and governance of the institution. The degree to which the mission of Protestant hospitals is directly affected by religious affiliation also varies greatly.

There were 35 Jewish hospitals in the United States as of 1987 [10]. Unlike Catholic and Protestant hospitals, Jewish hospitals are not nor have they ever been controlled or directly sponsored by religious organizations. Most Jewish hospitals were organized in the late 18th and early 19th centuries to meet the needs of newly arriving immigrants and the Jewish poor. Among other reasons for the development of Jewish hospitals was the need for a facility in which Jewish dietary laws and other religious practices could be observed and a place for Jewish physicians to train and practice. Unlike Catholic and some Protestant hospitals, where it is common for the church or religious order to own and operate more than one hospital, all of the Jewish hospitals operate independently [11].

There are also a small number of hospitals that are sponsored by fraternal organizations—the 20 Shriners hospitals for children located throughout the United States are a prominent example.

Another way of classifying hospitals is by teaching or nonteaching status. Almost all hospitals are involved in education in one form or another from health education for patients and the public, in-service education for staff, in-hospital health professions education, to affiliation with health professions schools. However, the term teaching hospital is more specifically applied to the approximately 450 hospitals that have an affiliation with a medical school and are involved in undergraduate and graduate medical education [12]. A substantial part of undergraduate medical education takes place within the walls of a teaching hospital. In the third year of medical education students are taught physical diagnosis and other basic clinical skills within teaching hospitals and a major part of the fourth year of medical education involves elective assignments within teaching hospitals.

Upon graduation from medical school, in order to be eligible to be licensed to practice medicine in any of the 50 states, a graduate must complete one year of graduate training. That year after graduation, once commonly referred to as internship, is now known as the first year of graduate medical education or residency. Certification by medical specialty boards requires a minimum of three years of graduate medical education.

Hospitals can also be differentiated by the level of care that they provide. Smaller community hospitals tend to provide primary and secondary levels of medical care. At the other end of the spectrum are the teaching hospitals which, in addition to primary and secondary care, provide highly specialized tertiary care services such as kidney dialysis, open-heart surgery, cardiac catheterization, coronary angioplasty, and transplantation, to name a few examples. Falling somewhere in between are larger community hospitals that for the most part concentrate on the provision of primary and secondary services but not infrequently have one or more highly specialized tertiary care services.

The traditional emphasis of hospitals in our society was on the diagnosis and treatment of disease. Today hospitals realize that their responsibility is more broad. The mission of a contemporary hospital would include prevention, treatment, and rehabilitation; health education programs, screening programs for cancer, and other diseases, are almost as commonplace as operating rooms and cardiac care units. Substance abuse, geriatric, and cardiac rehabilitation programs are now also on the menu of services offered.

The broader role that hospitals are playing in today's society is most appropriate. Many communities have but one hospital. They are often among the largest employers, and have a physical and organizational presence that distinguishes them from other institutions in the community. Many of these characteristics can even be found in multihospital communities. It is therefore only natural for people to turn to a hospital for assistance in meeting a broad range of health care needs and it is fitting for the hospital to respond.

Hospitals are undergoing rapid change as a result of changes in Medicare reimbursement, growth in prepaid health plans, and other factors. Hospitals formerly were paid reimbursable costs for each day of care received by a Medicare patient. Under the new diagnosis-related group (DRG) reimbursement model, hospitals receive a fixed payment determined by the patient's diagnosis regardless of how long the patient remains in the hospital or the scope of services provided.

From mid–1986 to 1987, the number of prepaid health plans or health maintenance organizations (HMOs) increased 30 percent from 480 to 626 [13]. The number of enrollees increased 23 percent to 25.8 million from 21 million [14]. HMOs make money by keeping enrollees out of the hospital by substituting ambulatory care for inpatient care. HMOs also negotiate significant discounts from hospitals whenever possible.

The effect of these factors and independent changes in patterns of medical practice have led to a decrease in hospital admissions in recent years [15]. Hospitals have responded by mothballing unnecessary beds and reducing staff. They have significantly expanded ambulatory care programs, developed new services, and sought out business opportunities in health related areas such as clinical laboratories and home health services. Hospitals have also become much more aggressive in marketing their services [16].

Individual freestanding hospitals are by far the single largest component of our hospital system. Total health expenditures increased from $116 billion in 1974 to $387 billion in 1984. During that same period, expenditures for all hospital care increased from $45 billion to $180 billion [17].

In recent years the traditional hospital corporate structure has been altered to reflect the changing role of hospitals. As hospitals have become involved in nontraditional lines of business focused on market share and profitability, the need to form taxable corporate entities to encompass these activities has emerged. A typical corporate restructuring creates a nonprofit holding company to control the hospital corporation, a nonprofit foundation, the primary function of which is fund raising and administration of endowment funds, and one or more new taxable business corporations. (Figure 1 illustrates a traditional corporate structure while Figure 2 illustrates a restructuring.)

HOSPITAL ORGANIZATION

Society has long viewed hospitals as service organizations. However, they actually have characteristics of both service and manufacturing organizations. The service characteristics of the hospital organization are obvious. The patient care process is highly individualized with the care provided developed around the patient's specific needs. Physicians admit patients, after which all of the hospitals resources are directed at implementing the care plan. But within most hospitals is a laundry that processes hundreds of thousands of pounds of laundry per year and a highly automated laboratory that tests large volumes of blood and other body fluids. The average hospital produces and serves more meals on any given day than the largest of restaurants might produce and serve in a month. Thus, in economic terms, one could view the hospital as a place in which the factors of production are brought together to provide prevention, treatment, and rehabilitation services on a large scale.

To have a hospital run effectively requires dedicated well-trained employees, effective operating systems and controls, necessary supplies and equipment, adequate facilities, physicians, and of course, patients. Nurses, pharmacists, technicians, housekeepers, food service workers, laundry employees, and maintenance people, are only some of the employees required. Each must be oriented and trained and the operating departments must have the supplies necessary to carry out their tasks. Surgical instruments,

FIGURE 1: West Allis Memorial Hospital Organizational Chart

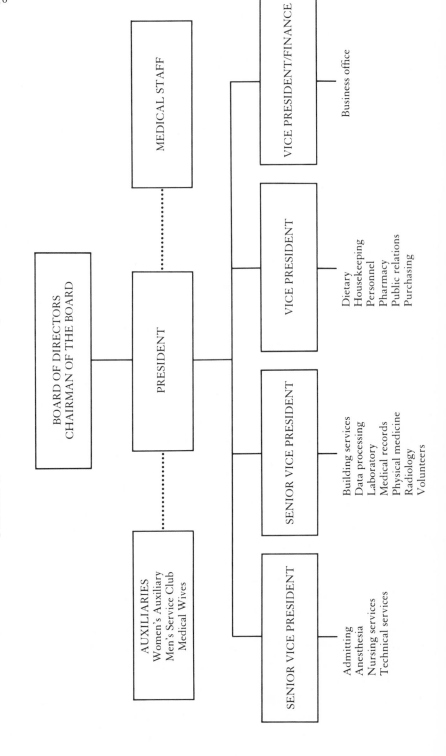

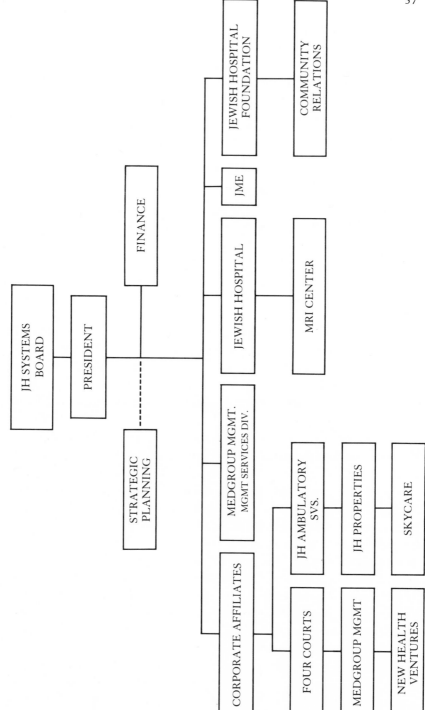

FIGURE 2:   JH Systems, Inc. Organizational Chart

electrocardiographic machines and myriads of other equipment and supplies, including pharmaceuticals, blood, food, light bulbs, and x-ray tubes are required and there are thousands upon thousands of other items used on a daily basis in the operation of a hospital.

Rooms must be cleaned and beds must be changed. Patients must be admitted and discharged. Bills must be submitted to patients and third party payers. Patients must be transported to departments and food must be transported to patients. If patients are being transported to x-ray at the same time that food is being placed at their bedside, something is wrong. No one would be very happy if a patient was placed on the operating table but the instruments required by the surgeon had not been prepared. The function of the formal organization is to make it all work through planning, budgeting, staffing, organizing, directing, coordinating, and evaluating.

THE GOVERNING BOARD

The governing board operates the hospital in trust for the community and has a fiduciary responsibility to protect the assets and to see to it that the hospital is managed in a prudent manner. The trustee's responsibility encompasses every facet of the operation, but most important, ensuring that the institution provides high quality medical care. The size of hospital govering boards varies widely. Trustees are usually selected from among the leadership of the community. Lawyers, bankers, merchants, and business people tend to predominate.

Trustees are elected in one of two ways. In many instances governing boards are self-perpetuating and the trustees are responsible for their own election and re-election. In other cases, a membership association elects trustees from among residents of the community. The size and composition of membership associations vary widely but they are commonly made up of individuals who have contributed more than a given dollar amount to the hospital annually or are elected by a self-perpetuating membership group. Boards typically meet between four times a year and monthly. The frequency often depends upon the size of the board and whether or not there is an executive committee exercising the responsibility of the board between regular meetings. Boards are divided into committees, the most common of which are planning, finance, audit, investment, joint conference, personnel, quality assurance, and building.

What is the role of the governing board? First and foremost, trustees must define the hospital's mission. Why does the hospital exist? Who is it intended to serve? An example of a mission statement follows:

The Miriam Hospital, Providence, Rhode Island
Mission and Goals Statement

Through the Jewish traditions of scholarship and charity, the Board of Trustees commits the Miriam Hospital to advancing the art and science of medicine through clinical excellence. The central mission is superlative patient care conducted in an environment of education and scholarly inquiry into the nature, cause, prevention and treatment of disease. Community outreach and restoration of health are integral components of this mission.

The Miriam Hospital is committed to developing excellence in health care delivery commensurate with the highest standards. Primary, secondary and selected tertiary levels of care that meet the needs of the community will be provided in both inpatient and outpatient settings to adolescents and adults, with particular attention directed to the special needs of the elderly.

As a major affiliate of the Brown University Program in Medicine, The Miriam Hospital will strengthen and maintain its relationship with the University. Selected academic programs of excellent quality and national stature will be developed to complement, enhance and contribute to the Brown University Program in Medicine. Additional programs will be established as necessary to attain those standards of care required to fulfill the stated goals of The Miriam Hospital.

While maintaining the central mission of superlative patient care, the Hospital will be administered with a high degree of fiscal accountability and awareness of available resources.

Research programs which are consistent with its patient care mission and responsibility as a teaching hospital with a University faculty will be fostered by The Miriam Hospital.

The Miriam Hospital is mindful of its historical relationship to its staff and will continue to ensure opportunities for the practice of medicine and surgery to qualified practitioners. Staffing plans will be regularly evaluated to affirm that staffing is consistent with the needs and goals of the hospital.

It is the goal of The Miriam Hospital to provide the highest quality nursing care through a contemporary nursing organization. The nursing staff and leadership will work to maintain national recognition as exemplified by its high degree of professionalism and qualitative performance. It will carry out this goal and provide quality care in a personal, compassionate and caring environment.

The Miriam Hospital will continue to maintain a fair and equitable position in employee salary, wage, and benefits programs; insure sound, safe working conditions for all employees and staff; and recruit persons without regard to age, sex, race, religion or national origin.

To facilitate better utilization of resources, the hospital will encourage and cultivate mutually beneficial relationships among other health care and educational facilities. The relationship will allow other area health care and educational institutions the opportunities to share expertise and skill needed to provide excellence in patient care.

The Miriam Hospital will maintain leadership of the hospital through a trusteeship representing the community. This leadership will continue to guide and direct the hospital toward achievement of its mission.

The close and special relationship enjoyed by The Miriam Hospital and the Jewish community will be maintained and enhanced recognizing that this relationship is an important feature of the hospital's history.

It is the responsibility of the governing board to work with the chief executive officer in the development of a strategic plan and to approve the annual operating plan and capital budgets.

One of the most important responsibilities of the governing board is to evaluate the performance of the chief executive officer (CEO) and develop a competitive compensation program. Life cycle changes, that is, resignation, retirement, disability or death, and performance problems will involve the governing board in the recruitment of a new CEO. The board should provide the CEO with a broad delegation of authority and, through the chairman of the board and committee chairmen, hold the CEO accountable for accomplishing the goals and objectives set forth in the strategic plan and annual operating plan and budget. A good CEO knows how to work effectively with the board and typically reports to the chairman of the governing board. The chief executive officer should keep the board chairman abreast of important issues and the chairman must allocate sufficient time to hospital affairs to hold the CEO accountable and to provide the support that the CEO and board committee chairmen will need.

An important function of the board chairman is to see that the board has the right mix of members. An ideal trustee is a person who is capable of making an intellectual and financial contribution to the hospital, and there are individuals who are capable of doing both. It is important, however, that the capacity to give is not the sole criterion since there are individuals who may only be able to contribute financially to a modest extent but who are extremely intelligent and can give the time to serve effectively on the governing board. It is also important for the board members to have a broad mix of backgrounds. Having all attorneys or businessmen is not as helpful as a balance between attorneys, accountants, bankers, industrialists, retailers, clergy, physicians, housewives, academics, and real estate developers. Careful selection of members will provide CEOs with a wealth of expertise that they can call upon when advice is needed in approaching and solving specific problems or issues. The mix of board members should be tailored to the needs of the hospital and not solely the demographics of a community.

THE MEDICAL STAFF

Every hospital has a medical staff organization composed of all of the physicians who practice at the hospital. The medical staff is a self-governing organization with bylaws, rules, and regulations. While the governing board is ultimately responsible for the quality of medical care, that responsibility is exercised through the medical staff. The governing board must approve the medical staff's bylaws, rules, and regulations and all applicants to the medical staff. One of the major responsibilities of the chief executive officer is to serve as a liaison with the medical staff.

The duties and responsibilities of the medical staff are carried out through the work of committees, typically including, but not limited to, a medical executive committee and committees on quality assurance, patient care, pharmacy and therapeutics, infection and utilization review.

In many community hospitals the medical staff is made up completely of physicians who are in private practice. In contrast, teaching hospitals characteristically have a combination of physicians in private practice and full-time salaried physicians who are employed by the hospital. The full-time physicians, in addition to operating teaching and research programs, usually have major administrative responsibilities. In some university hospitals the entire staff is salaried. In teaching hospitals in which there are full-time salaried chiefs responsible for the major professional departments, the chiefs report to the chief executive officer in much the same way as other senior managers.

AUXILIARIES

Many hospitals have auxiliaries, which are groups of individuals in the community, usually women, which raise funds and undertake other activities in behalf of the hospital. Auxiliaries are self-governing organizations with their own bylaws, rules, and regulations. Like the medical staff, their bylaws are subject to approval by the hospital's governing body. In addition to the specific tasks typically undertaken such as operating the coffee shop, gift shop, and sponsoring fund raisers, the auxiliary plays a major role in communicating the hospital story to the community. A skilled chief executive officer recognizes their importance and works with the auxiliary to enhance its role.

THE CHIEF EXECUTIVE OFFICER

Some people would say that the role of the board is to formulate policy while the role of the chief executive officer is to implement policy. The truth of the matter is that policy formulation and policy implementation can be viewed as two ends of a continuum. Toward the center of the continuum, the differentiation between policymaking and implementation can be blurred. A CEO must be intimately involved in the development of policy. In fact, more often than not, the CEO will be the primary initiator of policy. When bringing issues to the board, the CEO should thoroughly define the issue, describe alternative approaches or solutions and recommend a course of action. The CEO who defines a problem and asks the board what it would like to do is falling short of the mark. No matter how well the relationship between the board and CEO is defined in writing or through abstract discussions, role differentiation will be defined on a day-to-day basis as the CEO and board interact. CEOs must carefully guard their prerogatives, since authority that is ceded is not easily reclaimed.

What is the role of the hospital chief executive officer? One of the most important responsibilities is planning. Whether or not the CEO functions as the planner, or charges a senior staff member with the responsibility, the planning leadership must emanate from the CEO. The process often results in a written plan. While most people focus on the plan as the end product, the process itself can be equally important. Planning is a dynamic continuing process. It is the responsibility of the CEO to develop and install a systematic and ongoing planning structure and process. The structure should include a multidisciplinary planning committee within the governing board, the designation of individuals to be responsible for planning as a primary management responsibility, and the allocation of resources to support the planning function. An effective planning process should include periodic assessments of the environment locally, as well as on a state and national level.

A CEO should see to it that the hospital has a strategic plan covering a period of three to five years. The strategic plan should be updated annually and should be accompanied by an annual operating plan. The strategic plan should encompass an environmental assessment, a delineation and evaluation of alternative strategies, specific goals and objectives to be accomplished, the time frame for the goals and objectives to be accomplished, and the resources that will be required for implementation. Evaluation is often the stepchild of planning and a well conceived strategic plan should provide a specific framework for evaluating the efficacy of the strategies that are to be implemented as well as effectiveness in implementing the plan.

Another major role of the CEO is in the area of policy development. The CEO's role in policy development should be as a leader and manager. The CEO obviously cannot be involved in the development of every policy but the CEO will provide leadership and a framework for the development of policy. The CEO will also manage the policymaking process, determining through grants of authority which positions in the organization have responsibility for specific policy areas and determining the process for policy development and approval.

The key point is that the CEO must provide leadership and direction in the policymaking process and define who has authority to formulate specific areas of management policy. The granting of authority between the governing board and CEO and between the CEO and others in the organization varies widely among organizations. The variation can sometimes be explained by size since in a small hospital where the CEO has one assistant grants of authority would be handled far differently than in a large hospital in which a CEO has six assistants. Personal preference on the part of either the governing board or CEO or both will also explain some variance between hospitals.

Policy development occurs at multiple levels in the organization. As an example, a hospital's policy about free care or charity would flow from the hospital's mission and strategic plan and might be determined by the governing board upon recommendation of the CEO and finance committee. The CEO in turn might look to the chief financial officer and other members of management in recommending policy on this issue to the governing board. A policy on visiting hours on the other hand, might be one which normally would be approved by the chief executive officer and not the governing board. Not all policy issues require the direct approval or involvement of the CEO. As an example, a policy about how often various areas of the hospital are cleaned might be made by the director of the housekeeping department and the vice president for support services or equivalent person.

The CEO has the authority and responsibility for implementation of policy. The size of the organization, the CEO's span of control, and the quality of the management team should be the primary determinants of how authority and responsibility are delegated for the implementation of policy. Once again, administrative style and personal preference will play a significant role.

The *sine qua non* of delegation is accountability. Just as the governing board should hold CEOs accountable for fulfilling their responsibilities, so CEOs must hold accountable those to whom authority and responsibility are delegated. While that sounds relatively easy, it may be quite difficult. Accountability will vary with the ability of the managers and with the administrative style of the individuals involved. A skilled CEO should be able to determine how to get the most out of managers. Some managers function best in a highly structured environment with specific grants of authority, frequent direction, and close accountability. Others can be given an assignment in very general terms and will know exactly what to do, including when to consult the CEO. Holding managers of this type too closely accountable will impede their ability to function and result in job dissatisfaction.

Before CEOs can plan, develop, or implement policy, they must develop an organization structure. Obviously, except in the case of a new hospital, a hospital will have a structure and one of the first activities of a new CEO after an appropriate period of observation, is to make appropriate changes in the organization. The CEO must develop a table of organization that is appropriate to the organization's size and other characteristics. The major administrative functions are planning, finance, operations, and marketing. Within the operating organization are professional services such as nursing; pharmacy; physical, occupational and speech therapy; social service; and food services. The nonprofessional or hotel services include but are not limited to laundry, housekeeping, materials management, communications, central supply, security, and plant operations. (See Figures 3 and 4.)

The CEO's responsibility for developing an annual operating plan and budget was identified earlier. On an annual basis, managers must develop assumptions to project the operating environment of the hospital. Among the assumptions should be the number of admissions, patient days, average length of stay, new programs, the impact of changes in government and other third-party reimbursement policies, program changes, and changes in the physical plant. These assumptions are transmitted to the operating departments for guidance in formulating their operating plans and budgets. After these plans are reviewed by the department manager and appropriate administrative person, they are aggregated. The CEO and the senior managers will have to reconcile conflicting priorities and demands for resources to formulate an acceptable budget. Once approved by the board, the operating plan and budget become a framework for program development and resource allocation during the coming year. The goals and objectives that make up the operating plan of individual departments are then utilized in evaluating the effectiveness of that department in contributing to the hospital's overall operating results.

FIGURE 3: The Miriam Hospital Table of Organization—I

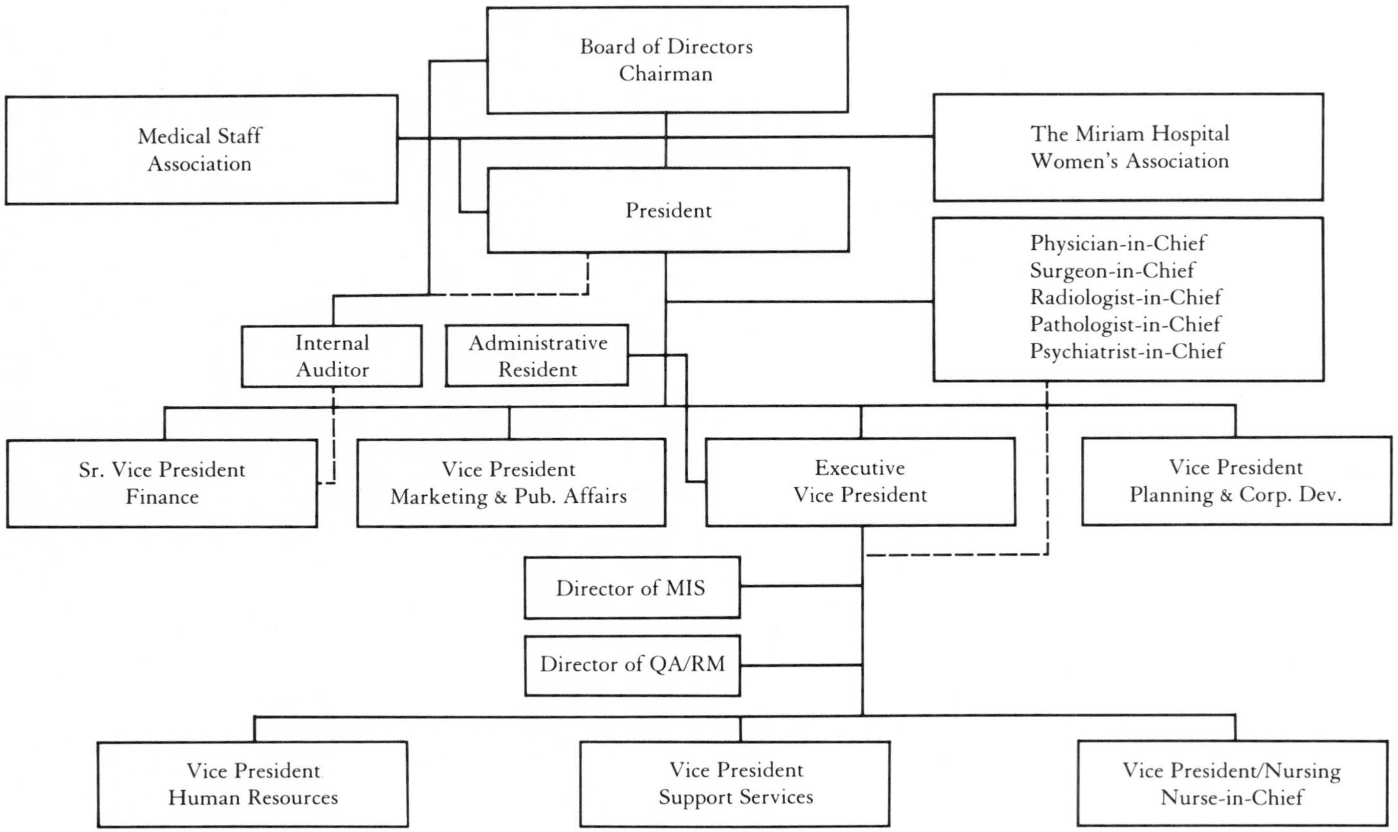

Medical Staff Association

Board of Directors Chairman

President

The Miriam Hospital Women's Association

Physician-in-Chief
Surgeon-in-Chief
Radiologist-in-Chief
Pathologist-in-Chief
Psychiatrist-in-Chief

Vice President Planning & Corp. Dev.

Internal Auditor

Administrative Resident

Sr. Vice President Finance

Vice President Marketing & Pub. Affairs

Executive Vice President

Director of MIS

Director of QA/RM

Vice President Human Resources

Vice President Support Services

Vice President/Nursing Nurse-in-Chief

FIGURE 4: The Miriam Hospital Table of Organization—II

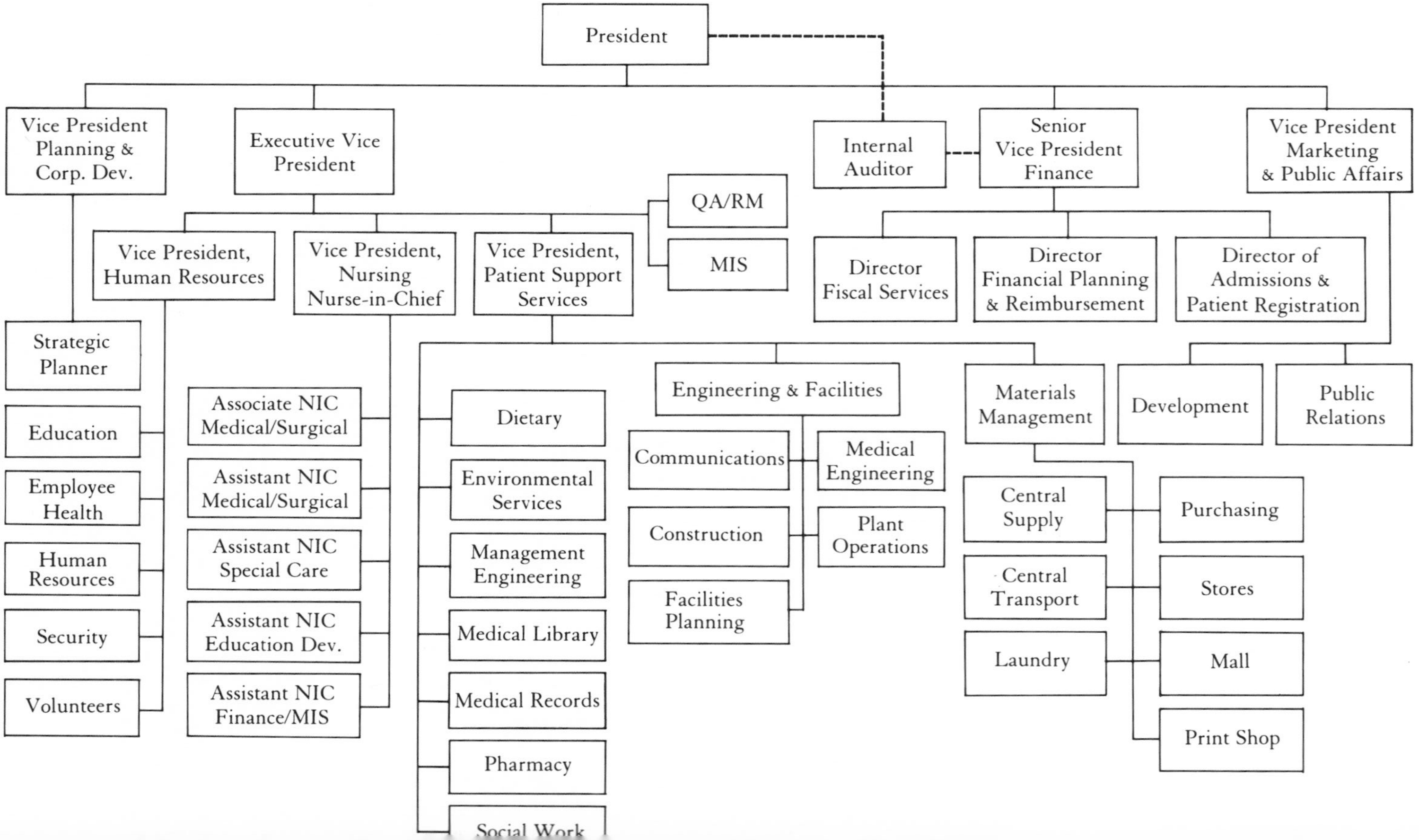

In addition to major responsibility for the operations, the CEO has responsibility for the relationship of the hospital and a wide variety of governmental and community agencies. Hospitals are among the more regulated organizations in our economy, and the CEO will be required to interact with the federal, state, and local regulatory agencies. The CEO will also be responsible for relationships with quasi-regulatory organizations such as the Joint Commission on Accreditation of Healthcare Organizations and other accrediting agencies. The CEO should participate in trade association activities particularly at the state and local level. Today very few patients pay their hospital bills directly and the CEO will be involved in negotiating with nongovernmental third-party payers including Blue Cross, other commercial insurance companies, and health maintenance organizations and preferred provider organizations. It would be very difficult to provide all of the health and social services required in the community, and the hospital should coordinate services with other hospitals and health and social services agencies. Interinstitutional planning and program coordination is a major responsibility of the CEO.

As a charitable organization a hospital has the opportunity to receive gifts from corporations, foundations, and individuals. A CEO should be involved in nurturing the relationships that philanthropically minded individuals and corporations have with the hospital. It is difficult to solicit funds from individuals or corporations not familiar with the hospital and the most successful philanthropy is built on longstanding relationships.

Fundraising is not the only reason for having solid relationships with individuals and corporations in the community. At a time when hospitals are frequently criticized for the cost of services, it is important to have people who can interpret the hospital's position. It is important that corporate leaders have an understanding of the hospital's programs and services and the relationship between quality and cost. In addition to individual contacts with community leaders, the CEO can tell the hospital story through participation in service organizations such as Rotary and Kiwanis and by serving on the boards and committees of community organizations.

While most hospitals have a personnel director or human resource manger, the CEO is nevertheless the chief manager of human resources. Approximately 60 to 66 percent of every dollar in the budget is expended for wages and fringe benefits. The quality of care provided is, in addition to other factors such as the quality of the medical staff, directly related to the quality and motivation of the hospital's employees. It is the CEO's responsibility to establish the philosophy of human resource management. A successful philosophy is built upon the obligation of the hospital to provide competitive wages and fringe benefits, equal opportunity for all employees, an opportunity to help shape the work environment, effective two-way communications, and opportunities for individual growth and self-actualization. While this philosophy may sound like "motherhood and apple pie" there are hospitals that would not embrace it in deed if not word. Even hospitals that willingly embrace it will not be successful in implementing it without a major commitment of time and effort on the part of the management team.

The governing board, as previously stated, has ultimate responsibility for the quality of care. It is to the CEO, however, that the mandate falls for assuring that the quality of care meets or exceeds appropriate standards. Most hospitals in the United States are eligible for accreditation by the Joint Commission on Accreditation of Healthcare Organizations. In addition, many states have licensing or approval programs. While it is incumbent upon a hospital to meet the minimum standards necessary for accreditation and licensing, the hospital should strive to exceed the standards promulgated by regulatory and quasi-regulatory bodies.

Quality in hospitals can be measured in terms of both process and outcome. As an example, when a patient is admitted to a hospital with an admitting diagnosis of "rule out myocardial infarction" or heart attack, certain baseline diagnostic procedures should be undertaken. If the patient is found to have suffered a myocardial infarction, then the course of treatment should follow generally accepted patterns of practice. The review of quality of patient care on this basis is process evaluation. In contrast if one reviews the number of deaths and complications such as infection, one is looking at outcome measurements of quality. It is the CEO's responsibility to see to it that the hospital has a comprehensive quality assurance program. A good quality assurance program deals with the quality of medical care, the quality of nursing care, and the quality of all the services provided to patients. Process and outcome measurements of quality can be developed for nursing practice, housekeeping, pharmacy, laundry, food service, and most other services. A quality assurance program must embody a well-organized approach to establishing standards, determining how adherence can be measured, data collection and analysis, and taking remedial action through changes in policies and procedures, education and, when necessary, disciplinary action.

Juxtaposed with the quality assurance program is the risk management program, the purpose of which is the reduction of risk to patients, employees, and the public of unintended consequences of receiving care, visiting, or working in the hospital. The primary goal is to prevent harm to patients, visitors, and employees and as a result of so doing, control the cost of insurance. The cost of liability and casualty insurance is a major element of hospital budgets, and one that can be controlled through effective management.

What are the characteristics of a successful chief executive officer? First and foremost, a CEO should have the qualities of an effective leader. A CEO has to motivate others and exercise authority without appearing to use it. The CEO should be able to delegate authority and hold those to whom authority is delegated accountable. The ability to communicate both orally and in writing, easily and well, is very important. The successful CEO should be committed to helping people and should enjoy personal contact with large numbers of individuals. In fact, interpersonal relationships are such an integral part of hospital management that anyone who does not enjoy people and human interaction should not be a health services administrator. A CEO should have highly developed conceptual skills in addition to the ability to become immersed in detail.

A familiarity with economics and financial management are critical in today's environment. The ability to analyze financial statements, and an understanding of basic concepts of internal controls, budgeting, capital financing, reimbursement, and cost benefit analysis are important. While one need not be a computer expert, a knowledge of information systems and the role of computers is essential. A successful hospital administrator should be well grounded in sociology, behavioral and industrial psychology, political science, public administration, and management science. A grounding in public health and medical care concepts is also required. These disciplines can provide a theoretical and conceptual framework for working with people within complex organizations.

Most junior level administrators aspire to assume the role of CEO. Experience largely separates a graduate of a health administration program who is qualified to be a CEO from one who is qualified to assume another administrative role. As one moves up the administrative hierarchy, authority and responsibility increase significantly. The content of the CEO's job is also far more directed at planning, marketing and external relationships than day-to-day operations. The author believes that some individuals have a mix of experience and skills that enable them to function effectively as a vice president or chief operating officer but not do as well as chief executive officer. Some very successful midlevel hospital executives could function well as a CEO, but do not seek the opportunity because it represents a job that they would not like. Management at all levels is critical to the success of the hospital, and it is important that a career decision not to become a CEO be viewed as a reasonable judgment.

Traditionally, hospital executives were trained as administrative generalists. One can define an administrative generalist as someone who knows a little about everything. Today, some programs in health services administration enable students to concentrate in a management discipline such as labor relations, finance, or economics. It is also possible in some programs to concentrate in a content area such as ambulatory care management. The author believes completion of a concentration in either a management discipline or a content area will lead to more opportunities and offers more to potential employers.

Opportunities in management within hospitals are many and varied. Larger hospitals will have a chief operating officer who reports to the CEO and has responsibility for the day-to-day operations. The professional and support service departments will usually be functionally divided up and assigned to one or more administrative generalists with titles such as assistant administrator, vice president or assistant vice president. In addition to their line responsibilities, individuals functioning at this level often have staff responsibilities such as liaison with medical staff or board committees, and responsibility for specially assigned projects.

There are many staff functions that provide opportunities for program graduates. Quality assurance, risk management, and medical staff relations are important functions that also provide an excellent learning experience for a junior executive. It is not unusual for a CEO to have an administrative assistant for special projects and assignments. Administrative assistant positions also provide entry level management opportunities.

Emphasis has been placed on the importance of human resources. The management of human resources encompasses compensation planning and administration, recruitment, training and development, and labor relations. This area provides an excellent opportunity for individuals interested in becoming a management specialist during the initial phase of their career. Traditionally, the primary route to becoming a CEO was through operations. Today, because of the increased importance placed on planning and marketing, senior planning and marketing executives are often being tapped to lead hospitals. The contributions of planning and marketing to a successful hospital have been recognized only recently and there are many opportunities for individuals who have either experience or an interest in becoming involved in these areas.

Some of the large professional departments, such as radiology and pathology, are under the direction of a physician. The medical directors of these departments are often assisted by managers who rose through the ranks as technicians before being appointed as department administrators. However, in radiology and pathology as well as nursing, the operating rooms, and other professional departments, departmental administrator positions are increasingly being filled by graduates of health administration programs. The opportunities for health administration graduates in institutional management are many and varied.

NATIONAL ALLIANCES

A word about national alliances. The opportunities for health administrators in investor-owned and nonprofit multihospital systems are described elsewhere in this book. The development of large investor-owned and non-profit multihospital systems, has led to the development of national alliances of individual nonprofit hospitals. Alliances provide opportunities for the participant hospitals that they could not achieve on their own. The national alliances have concentrated their efforts in purchasing, financial services, and marketing. The purchasing programs generally concentrate on large dollar, high volume items such as IV solutions and pharmaceuticals, and on big ticket items such as major capital equipment. Financial services include bond insurance and cash management programs. Market share programs include investments in health maintenance organizations and preferred provider organizations, professional liability insurance, market research, and programming for geriatric services.

The largest of the national alliances is the Voluntary Hospitals of America with 79 shareholders (that is, principal owner hospitals) and 463 participating hospitals [18]. Other major national alliances include Premier Hospitals Alliance with 40 owner hospitals; American Health Care System with 33 owners and 292 hospitals; and Sunhealth, Inc. with 38 owners and 102 hospitals [19]. In total, alliances had 267 owners and 1,132 participating hospitals in 1986 [20].

Alliances are a relatively new phenomenon in the health care field. Whether they are a passing phenomenon or will have staying power is not yet clear. However, national alliances provide excellent employment opportunities for junior level, midcareer, and senior hospital executives.

REFERENCES

1. Kane, D. A. The Organization of Hospitals in Medieval England. *Hospital Administration* 18 (Winter): 44–52, 1973.
2. Kane, D. A. See 1.
3. Kane, D. A. See 1.
4. *The World Book Encyclopedia*. New York: Field Enterprises Education Corp., 1972, 335.
5. *Webster's Third New International Dictionary*, Springfield, MA: Merriam-Webster Inc., 1971, 733.
6. American Hospital Association. *Hospital Statistics* 1986. Chicago: The Association, 1987, Table 2A.
7. American Hospital Association. See 6.

8. Catholic Health Association of the United States. St. Louis, MO.
9. American Protestant Health Association. Schaumberg, IL.
10. Premier Hospitals Alliance.
11. Kanigel, R. Have Jewish Hospitals Outlived Their Purpose. *The Detroit Jewish News* 90 (February 13, 1987): 22–28.
12. Division of Clinical Services, Association of American Medical Colleges. Washington, D.C. 20036.
13. Greene, J. HMO's Posted Large Gains in Enrollment but Most Saw Profits Decline During 1986. *Modern Healthcare* (June 5) 17: 118–26, 1987.
14. Greene, J. See 13.
15. Oppenheimer & Co. Hospital Management Industry. *Industry Review* (April 21): 12, 1987.
16. Oppenheimer & Co. See 15, 6.
17. Oppenheimer & Co. See 15, 6.
18. Premier Hospitals Alliance. Competitive Analysis of Hospital Management Companies and Hospital Alliances. Westchester, IL, 1986.
19. Premier Hospitals Alliance. See 18.
20. Premier Hospitals Alliance. See 18.

BIBLIOGRAPHY

American College of Healthcare Administrators. *The Evolving Role of the Hospital Chief Executive Officer*. Chicago: The Foundation of the American College of Healthcare Administrators, 1984.

American Hospital Association. *Hospital Statistics 1986*. Chicago: The Association, 1987.

Gantenberg, James B. Who Leads America's Hospitals. *Hospital Health Services Administration* 30 (March-April): 46–53, 1985.

Greene, Jay. HMO's Posted Large Gains in Enrollment but Most Saw Profits Decline During 1986. *Modern Healthcare* (June): 118–26, 1987.

Harvey, James D. Evaluating the Chief Executive Officer. *Hospital and Health Services Administration* 23 (Spring): 5–21, 1978.

Kane, Daniel A. The Organization of Hospitals in Medieval England. *Hospital Administration* 18 (Winter): 44–52, 1973.

Kanigel, Robert. Have Jewish Hospitals Outlived Their Purpose. *The Detroit Jewish News* (February): 22–28, 1987.

Kirk, W. Richard. *Your Future in Hospital Administration*. New York: Richards Rosen Press, Inc., 1963.

Longest, Beaufort B., Jr. The Contemporary Hospital Chief Executive Officer. *Health Care Management Review* 3 (Spring): 43–53, 1978.

McGeorge, R. K. Relationship of the Chief Executive Officer to the Hospital Board. *Hospital Administration in Canada* 18 (June): 48–49, 1976.

Moses, Richard P. *Evaluation of the Hospital Board and the Chief Executive Officer*. American Hospital Publishing, Inc., 1986.

Oppenheimer & Co. Hospital Management Industry. *Industry Review* (April): 12, 1987.

Premier Hospitals Alliance. Competitive Analysis of Hospital Management Companies and Hospital Alliances. 1986.

Reed, David H., and J. Robert Harman, Jr. Selecting a Chief Executive Officer. *Trustee* 28 (August): 14–18, 1975.

Umbdenstock, Richard J., and Winifred M. Hageman. *Hospital Corporate Leadership: The Board and Chief Executive Officer Relationship*. Chicago: American Hospital Publishing, Inc., 1984.

Webster's Third New International Dictionary of English Language Unabridged. Springfield, MA: Merrian-Webster, Inc., 1971, 733.

Weil, Peter A., and Leo Stam. Transitions in the Hierarchy of Authority in Hospitals: Implications for the Role of the Chief Executive Officer. *Journal of Health and Social Behavior*, 27 (June, 1986): 179–192.

World Book Encyclopedia. (New York: Field Enterprises Education Corp., 1972), 335.

3

MULTIHOSPITAL SYSTEMS: APPLYING CORPORATE STRUCTURES AND STRATEGIES TO HEALTH SERVICES

S. DOUGLAS SMITH AND PHYLLIS M. VIRGIL

In the early 1960s, the term multihospital system (multis) was virtually nonexistent. Today, multihospital systems hold a significant place in the health care industry. They are for-profit and not-for-profit organizations that account for approximately 35 percent of the nation's nonfederal hospitals [1].

System activity can be traced back to 1961 with 5 hospital consolidations. During the early 1970s, hospitals were consolidating into systems at a rate of 50 per year. Recognizing that hospitals could be operated in an efficient and effective manner, initial system growth was led by investor-owned firms. These early investors were able to purchase system hospitals by acquiring capital from debt and equity (or stock) markets. That investor-owned firms were able to issue stock as a means to acquire capital funding

S. Douglas Smith is president, HCA Management Company of the Hospital Corporation of America. Mr. Smith holds an M.H.A. degree from Duke University and a B.S. degree in business administration from Abilene Christian University. Phyllis M. Virgil is director of strategic planning, HCA Management Company. Ms. Virgil received an M.H.A. degree from The George Washington University and a B.S. degree in health planning and administration from The Pennsylvania State University.

was a major event; it indicated that investors believed that hospitals could be operated in a businesslike manner. Systems provided many small, more rural hospitals with the ability to make needed capital improvements, gain economies of scale through shared resources, and enhance management expertise. While nonprofit multihospital systems, such as religious chains, have long existed, the consolidation of independent nonprofit hospitals did not become widely practiced until the mid-1970s.

In 1987, there were approximately 250 systems with 2,400 hospitals. According to a 1984 Delphi study by Arthur Andersen and the American College of Healthcare Executives (ACHE), multis are predicted to account for 53 percent of all hospitals by 1995 [2]. Moreover, a 1987 study by Arthur Andersen and the American Hospital Association predicts that the number of hospitals operated by multis will grow from 2,400 today to 2,862 in 1990 and 3,408 in 1995, a 42 percent total increase [3] (see Figure 1).

Edward Stolman enumerates the advantages that a multihospital system has:

1. Multihospital systems have been effective in raising needed capital for expansion, acquisition, remodeling and replacement of physical facilities.

2. They are making possible significant economies of scale and the sharing of scarce human and technological resources.

3. Multihospital systems are developing effective governing structures, capable of responsiveness, decisive corporate action, sensitivity to local needs and variations, as well as growth and adaptability.

4. And they have demonstrated their ability to attract, retain, and develop high-quality management talent [4].

Multis come in all shapes and sizes. They vary on a number of dimensions including ownership, service focus, location, number of facilities, and management style. Their common heritage is that all systems own, lease, or manage two or more facilities.

OWNERSHIP

Multis are commonly categorized by ownership type. In their 1986 survey of multihospital systems, *Modern Healthcare* reported 26 investor-owned systems with 967 hospitals. Not-for-profit systems accounted for 1,064 hospitals under 138 systems [5].

A recent survey of health care leaders predicts that the percentage of investor owned systems will grow from 21 percent today to 29 percent of all

FIGURE 1: System Growth

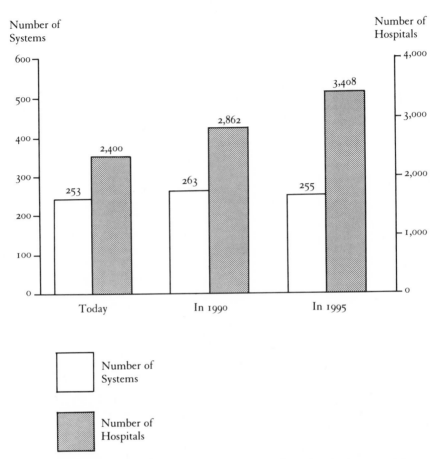

SOURCE: Multi-hospital Systems: Perspectives and Trends, Arthur Andersen, and the American Hospital Association, 1987.

systems in 1995. Not-for-profit systems are predicted to decrease slightly to 71 percent by 1995 [6] (see Figure 2).

Not-for-profit systems are frequently subclassified into the following three ownership categories: secular, religious, and public. In 1986, *Modern Healthcare* reported 67 secular, 57 religious, and 14 public hospital systems operating 442, 516, and 106 hospitals respectively [7].

SERVICES

Looking at service focus, the majority of multihospital systems evolved from a base of general acute care hospitals. Depending on size and location

FIGURE 2: How Will the Percentage of Investor-Owned and Not-For-Profit Systems Change?

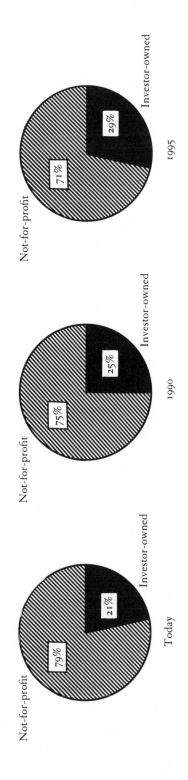

Not-for-profit
79%

Investor-owned
21%

Today

Not-for-profit
75%

Investor-owned
25%

1990

Not-for-profit
71%

Investor-owned
29%

1995

SOURCE: Multihospital Systems: Perspectives and Trends, Arthur Andersen and the American Hospital Association, 1987.

TABLE 1: HCA Hospital Services or Programs

MARKET-ORIENTED PROGRAMS	Number of Hospitals
Adult day care	13
Alzheimer's care unit or center	3
Women's packaged health program	45
Pain rehabilitation	32
Sports medicine	47
Walk-in clinic (hospital-based)	31

TERTIARY SERVICES	Number of Hospitals
Burn care	7
Cardiac catheterization	52
Open-heart surgery	30
Spinal cord and brain injury	9

GENERAL MEDICAL AND SURGICAL BEDS CONVERTED TO ALTERNATIVE USES IN 1985	Total Beds
Alcohol or chemical dependency	94
Hotel	25
Hospice	4
Psychiatric	52
Rehabilitation	42
Stress unit	43
Swing beds	42

Source: HCA, October 1987.

of the hospital, system facilities will range from a primary or secondary focus to a tertiary focus. In addition to their acute-care base, many systems today have other lines of health care business. For example, Hospital Corporation of America (HCA) has a psychiatric company which operates 50 psychiatric hospitals [8]. According to *Modern Healthcare*, multihospital systems operated 293 psychiatric facilities in 1986 [9]. HCA also owns a laboratory company that runs seven regional reference laboratories, and an ambulance company that operates five ambulance units. Humana has a network of urgent care centers and a captive preferred provider organization, and National Medical Enterprises (NME) has a number of nursing homes and rehabilitation facilities [10].

In addition to diversification at the top, many system general acute care hospitals have gone into specialized services and programs. Services and programs that HCA hospitals operate range from Alzheimers care to open-heart surgery to rehabilitation care [11] (see Table 1).

In the recent past, nonprofits have been more active than their for-profit counterparts in diversification at the hospital level. Due to today's demands on market share, the transitioning of the industry from hospital care to health care, and the widespread opinion that health care is a locally driven business, for-profit system hospitals are more actively entering alternative lines of business.

As Table 2 indicates, the mix of services in investor-owned multisystem facilities are comparable to freestanding nonprofit institutions, and for the most part differences between investor-owned and not-for-profit systems are minimal [12].

In addition to systems with an acute care base of hospitals, there are a number of specialty hospital systems. With 2,374 owned or managed facilities, nursing home chains are the largest group of specialty systems. Independent psychiatric hospital systems have also gained a substantial market presence with 35 units containing 3,034 beds [13]. Up and coming specialty systems include rehabilitation chains, urgent care chains, and diabetes center chains. Systems with a specialty focus are predominantly investor-owned concerns.

LOCATION AND SIZE

Systems also differ by geographic location and size. Investor-owned systems have an average of 35 hospitals per system [14]. For the most part, they have a national presence, which is skewed toward the South Atlantic and West South-Central states. There are many small- to medium-sized facilities in the investor-owned segment of the industry averaging 145 beds per hospital. For the most part these hospitals are located in suburban or rural areas.

Not-for-profit systems tend to be more regional in nature. They own, lease, or operate an average of nine hospitals per system and are concentrated in the West North-Central region of the United States. Nonprofit system hospitals are somewhat larger than their for-profit counterparts. The majority of nonprofit system hospitals fall in the 150- to 250-bed size range, with an average of 200 beds per hospital (see Table 2).

ORGANIZATION

The most visible difference between multisystem hospitals and freestanding hospitals is the existence of a system corporate structure.

Multihospital systems are typically organized into a structure that consists of two primary parts; corporate (systemwide executives plus staff experts) and field (facility operating managers). This basic structure will expand or contract based on the size of the system. For example, smaller regional systems may have a lean corporate office which consists of system executives

TABLE 2: Florida Facilities and Services (Percentage of Hospitals With) 1981

	% NONPROFIT	% INVESTOR-OWNED TOTAL	% INVESTOR-OWNED SYSTEMS
Postoperative recovery room	90.2	83.1	88.9
Pharmacy with registered pharmacist (full time)	84.2	83.0	88.9
Pharmacy with registered pharmacist (part time)	7.8	1.7	2.2
Histopathology laboratory	76.5	72.9	77.8
Electroencephalography	86.3	79.7	86.7
Respiratory therapy services	92.5	83.1	88.9
Physical therapy services	90.2	83.0	91.1
Occupational therapy services	23.1	30.5	31.1
Dental services	56.8	33.9	40.0
Podiatric services	45.1	44.1	53.3
Speech pathology services	39.2	40.7	40.0
Volunteer services department	58.8	61.0	64.4
Patient representative services	56.9	44.1	51.1
Social work services	86.3	76.3	82.2
Hospital auxiliary	78.4	37.6	64.4
Premature nursery	29.4	5.1	6.7
Abortion services (inpatient)	31.4	32.2	33.3
Abortion services (outpatient)	11.8	16.9	20.0
Hospice	2.0	3.4	4.4
Emergency department	72.5	71.2	80.0
Organized outpatient department	43.1	32.2	40.0
Rehabilitation outpatient services	17.6	11.9	15.6
Organ bank	0.0	1.7	2.2
Blood bank	60.8	69.4	73.3
Genetic counseling services	0.0	0.0	0.0
Open-heart surgery facilities	13.7	6.8	8.9
Alcoholism chemical dependency outpatient services	7.8	3.4	4.4
Psychiatric services:			
Emergency	21.6	11.9	15.6
Outpatient	9.8	5.1	6.7
Partial hospitalization	9.8	1.7	0.0
Foster and/or home care	0.0	0.0	0.0
Consultation and education	23.5	13.6	15.6
Clinical psychology services	9.8	10.2	13.3
Radiation therapy:			
X-ray	13.7	11.9	15.6
Megavoltage	11.8	5.1	6.7
Radioactive implants	27.5	15.3	17.8
Radioisotope facilities:			
Diagnostic	80.3	76.3	60.0
Therapeutic	19.6	13.6	13.3
Family planning services	2.0	0.0	0.0
Home care department	7.8	3.4	2.2
CT scanners	39.2	27.1	24.4
Cardiac catheterization	15.7	6.8	8.9
Number of hospitals in data base	52	60	45

Source: Sloan, Frank A., Ph.D. and Robert A. Vraciu, Ph.D., "Investor-Owned and Not-For-Profit Hospitals: Addressing Some Issues," *Health Affairs,* Spring 1983, Vol. 2, No. 1.

TABLE 3: Systems' U.S. Acute Care Hospitals

		TOTAL					
		BEDS			UNITS		
TYPE	NUMBER REPORTING	1986	1985	% CHANGE	1986	1985	% CHANGE
Investor-owned not-for-profit	26	140,289	144,380	(2.8)	967	950	1.8
Secular not-for-profit	67	71,790	71,481	0.4	442	445	(0.7)
Catholic	37	85,035	81,124	4.8	358	339	5.6
Other religious	20	35,837	32,974	8.7	158	157	0.6
Public	14	22,908	23,261	(1.5)	106	107	(0.9)
Total	164	355,859	353,220	0.7	2,031	1,998	1.7

Source: *Modern Healthcare*, June 5, 1987.

who are responsible for overall system management, and a small staff of specialists to provide expertise in specific areas (finance, marketing, personnel, and so on).

In larger systems, like HCA, this structure is expanded. Economies of scale are realized in providing more specialized experts within the system. While HCA staff experts primarily work out of the corporate office, some are part of regional field offices. Due to the large number and multiple locations of HCA hospitals, regional field offices exist to bring executives responsible for multiple hospital operations closer to the administrator.

At the hospital level, formal reporting relationships typically differ by system type—investor owned versus not for profit. The most common reporting relationship for the investor-owned hospital chief executive officer (CEO) is to a corporate officer. CEOs in nonprofit system hospitals may report to any of the following three sources of authority:

1. Hospital board of trustees
2. System corporate executive in charge of operations
3. Corporate board of directors

Nonprofit system administrators more frequently report to a group (hospital or corporate board) rather than a single corporate executive.

ADMINISTRATOR ROLE

Stanley Kleiner, in his survey of 42 administrators in 11 multihospital systems found that all administrators, regardless of system type or system affiliation, view their roles as similar. Drawing from these interviews, Kleiner

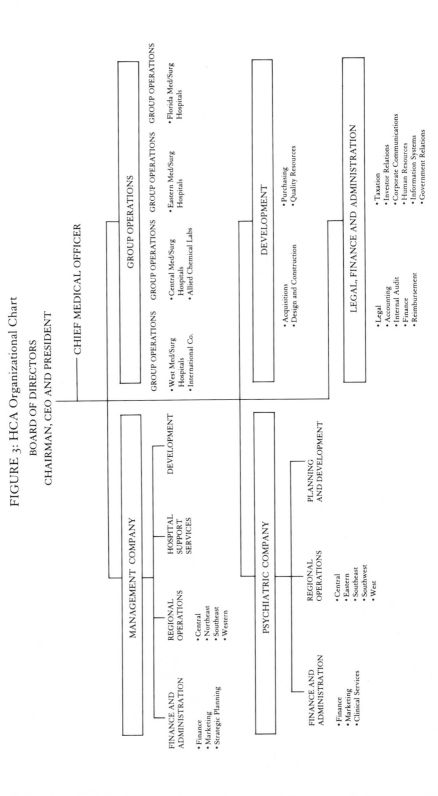

FIGURE 3: HCA Organizational Chart

BOARD OF DIRECTORS

CHAIRMAN, CEO AND PRESIDENT

CHIEF MEDICAL OFFICER

MANAGEMENT COMPANY

FINANCE AND ADMINISTRATION
- Finance
- Marketing
- Strategic Planning

REGIONAL OPERATIONS
- Central
- Northeast
- Southeast
- Western

HOSPITAL SUPPORT SERVICES

DEVELOPMENT

PSYCHIATRIC COMPANY

FINANCE AND ADMINISTRATION
- Finance
- Marketing
- Clinical Services

REGIONAL OPERATIONS
- Central
- Eastern
- Southeast
- Southwest
- West

PLANNING AND DEVELOPMENT

GROUP OPERATIONS

GROUP OPERATIONS
- West Med/Surg Hospitals
- International Co.

GROUP OPERATIONS
- Central Med/Surg Hospitals
- Allied Chemical Labs

GROUP OPERATIONS
- Eastern Med/Surg Hospitals

GROUP OPERATIONS
- Florida Med/Surg Hospitals

DEVELOPMENT
- Acquisitions
- Design and Construction
- Purchasing
- Quality Resources

LEGAL, FINANCE AND ADMINISTRATION
- Legal
- Accounting
- Internal Audit
- Finance
- Reimbursement
- Taxation
- Investor Relations
- Corporate Communications
- Human Resources
- Information Systems
- Government Relations

describes the multihospital system administrator as "The key individual interfacing between the hospital and the corporate structure responsible for a complex organization while also answerable to the corporation, and the local community" [15].

Responsibilities for planning and policymaking, financial management, human resource management, organizational design, and clinical services are common to all types of administrators. In addition, virtually all administrators responding to a survey of both system and nonsystem hospital CEOs view themselves as autonomous [16] (see Figure 3).

Despite real and perceived similarities between system and nonsystem hospitals, some differences in functions and roles do exist.

CORPORATE GUIDANCE, SUPPORT, AND ACTIVITIES

Unlike freestanding institutions, system facilities are both subject to, and the beneficiary of, guidance and support from their corporate parent. The existence of corporatewide policies vary by hospital system. Depending on management style, some systems are managed on a more centralized basis, and others are managed on a more decentralized basis. For example, with the exception of policies which standardize reporting systems (financial, human resource, and information systems), policies governing HCA hospitals are de-emphasized in favor of greater local autonomy.

Kleiner's 1984 survey found that while all multihospital system administrators had some degree of corporate oversight, for-profit system administrators perceived a higher degree of corporate guidance in the area of planning and policymaking, financial management, and human resource management than their nonprofit system peers [17]. Although both groups were actively involved in developing future hospital plans, nonprofit system administrators were more involved in planning with their local boards. Conversely for-profit system administrators worked more closely with corporate staff in developing future plans. Only 5 percent of all surveyed multihospital system administrators (nonprofit and for profit) indicated that their activities were constrained by corporate advisers.

Kleiner also found that for-profit system administrators have the highest overall perception of corporate control, viewing it as very supportive to mildly supportive. Both groups felt a high degree of responsibility for maximizing their use of corporate resources including technical experts, operating systems, and financial resources. Working as intermediaries between the corporate level and the hospital, all multihospital system administrators viewed establishing and maintaining good corporate level relationships as crucial to their facilities. These relationships were seen as based on mutual needs, trust, and personal ties.

CAPITAL MANAGEMENT

System hospitals also vary in the area of CEO financial responsibilities. While all hospitals have capital budgets, the administrator's role in creating and investing capital differs by hospital type. CEOs of investor-owned systems have fewer responsibilities in creating capital. This is largely due to the traditional role of corporate officers in gaining access to capital through debt and equity (stock) markets. In addition, compared to freestanding hospitals, both investor-owned and nonprofit system hospitals must typically receive corporate approval to make expenditures beyond their yearly budgets.

The capital approval process for for-profit hospitals is generally through the corporate structure. Nonprofit system hospitals may have to receive capital approval from both their local governing board and corporate board or officer.

IMMEDIATE ISSUES

While generalizations due to system affiliation are difficult to draw, a 1984 ACHE survey found a slight difference in the immediate focus of hospital CEOs.

— CEOs in investor-owned system hospitals were more concerned and involved in marketing issues.

— Nonprofit system CEOs were disproportionally involved in external relations, joining a political action committee (PAC), and recruiting new board members.

— Freestanding nonprofit system CEOs were involved to a higher degree in corporate reorganization, improving efficiency, staff communication, and issues concerning a satellite facility.

These differences in focus, however, may be due to factors such as local market conditions, organizational mission, hospital size and complexity, quality of medical staff, and administrator personality as much as they are a function of hospital system affiliation [18].

SKILLS OF HIGH PERFORMERS

Today's winning hospitals are led by CEOs who demand sound financial management, who have clear strategic objectives, who are willing to take risks, and who find appropriate ways to integrate the physicians into their operations. While there is no single trait that signals an outstanding leader,

Montague Brown and Barbara McCool, through research and interviews with numerous multihospital system managers, found some of the following behavioral traits and skills to be characteristic of high performers in multihospital systems.

1. The drive and ability to improve continuously is perhaps the most critical trait of successful managers. There has to be a sense of restlessness in striving for systematic, ongoing improvement. A concern for providing the best patient care possible, and determination to measure progress over time make for high-performing managers in all types of hospitals or systems.

2. Personal characteristics include an enjoyment of the job, high ethical standards, sound judgment, and extraordinarily good interpersonal skills.

3. Entrepreneurship and an attitude of "can do" are frequently a part of the multihospital system culture and a necessary behavior trait. This means having a sense of where to take an organization and working diligently to get the job done.

4. Successful executives also have to be able to network, and build relationships to benefit their organizations. There is not much formal authority for hospital administrators when the biggest customer, namely the physician, does not report to the administrator. To work successfully with doctors, administrators must build sound physician relationships. In addition to physician networking, the multihospital system administrator must build and cultivate relationships with other parts of the organization, whether that be with line managers in field offices, or specialized corporate staff.

5. Strong organization skills enable administrators to direct and oversee people within the institution while providing for effective interrelationships with external groups.

6. The ability to analyze and evaluate is critical. Analytical skills must be coupled with the ability to develop a "professional instinct" and know what will work in a given situation.

7. Multihospital system administrators should be energetic and hard working. In many multis there tend to be smaller administrative staffs at the local hospital level. Economies of scale accrue by providing corporate staff to assist the hospital executive.

8. The qualities of creativity and innovation are especially important in today's changing health care environment. These qualities make the essential successes of marketing more likely.

9. It is essential to be able to implement new ideas. This requires

strong people management skills. The bottom line means getting things done through other people.

10. Though energetic, successful multihospital system executives are also patient and keep calm in the midst of a storm [19].

The traits outlined, while true of high performers in multis, can be applied to most any leadership position. Although no one individual will have all of these traits, those who have most are individuals who aspire to continuously improve, and strive for excellence in performance.

EMPLOYMENT OPPORTUNITIES

Along with the growth of multihospital systems, have come a wide range of opportunities for employment in the health industry. As a source of alternative careers, multis can offer unique opportunities in both line and staff employment.

LINE EMPLOYMENT

In multihospital systems a longer term career ladder can be realized through a single employer. As individuals develop their skills and experience level, upward career movements may be afforded. In hospital management, individuals can progress from assistant administrator, to administrator of a small hospital, to CEO of a larger hospital, and then perhaps, to CEO of a tertiary facility. In addition, there are multihospital system management positions where individuals can have responsibility for a group of hospitals.

A career in a system hospital can also provide a reasonably structured learning opportunity for new job entrants. One can start off in a hospital level position that is commensurate with one's experience, and learn rapidly by having a gradient level of stress applied through successive levels of responsibility. Along the way, counseling and coaching can be provided by experienced executives. In addition, specialized corporate consultants can provide staff assistance to hospital administrators. Promotions then can be based on the performance and degree of preparation for the next position in the career ladder.

Some systems have developed structured management trainee programs which provide new graduates with the opportunity to learn in progressively complex hospitals and environments. Other multis proactively use hospital administrative residencies to find and train new graduates. For example, Humana has developed a formal residency program to screen and select new talent. Facing two problems, how to attract and develop prospective management, Lutheran Hospital and Homes Society of America (LHHS), a system based in Fargo, North Dakota, developed a postgraduate fellowship program that spurs interest in the company while grooming potential managers. In conjunction with Concordia College in Moorehead, Minnesota, LHHS developed a fellowship consisting of seven weeks of intensive instruction followed by 12 months of field work in the setting (long-term, rural, or urban hospitals) of the student's choice [20]. In addition, some multis have a variety of inhouse education programs aimed at developing management talent.

In the past, progression with many multis, especially the larger systems, was rapid. Tenure in any one position averaged two to four years. Due to the increasing complexity of running hospitals coupled with a more stable system growth rate, this fast track has slowed down. Today's average tenure is four years with a usual range of three to five years. The average time in any one hospital position, however, will vary by the nature of the hospital and the capabilities of the individual. There is increasing evidence that measurable improvement in hospitalwide quality is compromised by the rapid turnover of CEOs. Therefore, career growth opportunities in terms of tenure must be balanced with institutional quality objectives.

Another advantage of employment in a system hospital relates to CEO turnover. There are frequently political reasons for hospital CEOs' terminations. In freestanding hospitals administrators may be "on the street" through no fault of their own. Some of the high risk relationships with medical staffs and boards of trustees can be assuaged by system management. If relationship problems become unsolvable, one can move to new opportunities within the multihospital system instead of being fired when such an alternative is necessary.

The average turnover rate for all hospital CEOs in 1986–87 was 24.2 percent [21]. In comparison, the turnover rate for administrators leaving HCA hospitals was 10.5 percent [22].

In systems, professionals can enjoy the opportunity to learn the varied market, regulatory, and reimbursement systems that exist in different regions of the country. For example, in larger systems individuals can move from Tennessee to New York and gain firsthand experience in the significant differences that exist. Not only is this possible in the domestic workplace, but through international assignments as well. In an international assignment, one can experience firsthand the health policy and cultural differences between countries. Such an experience can broaden a professional's perspective on both health care delivery and world affairs.

The opportunity for movement can also afford individuals the ability to seek employment in areas of their choice personally. While new careerists typically move to job sites for professional reasons, as opposed to personal preference, more seasoned managers frequently are able to structure moves to accommodate both professional and personal interests. Contrary to many beliefs, movement within systems, when requested and appropriate, can frequently be accommodated. There are benefits to the employer who keeps well trained competent people, and benefits to the employee who is productive and pleased with variation and growth.

When I (Doug Smith) started in health care management, the idea was to find a good administrator with a well run hospital, work there three to five years, get promoted, or find a new opportunity in another hospital. Today, only relevant experience counts. As long as administrators are expanding their horizons, considering a change may be counterproductive both to themselves and the organizations.

I (Doug Smith) started as the administrator for a little county hospital on the eastern slope of the Sierra Nevada mountains in 1962. After graduate school at Duke University, I served in several administrative capacities including assistant to the dean of the medical school and assistant director of the hospital. In 1968 I heard Jack Massey (one of HCA's founding fathers) speak about the concept of an investor-owned hospital organization. Mr. Massey said some exciting things about the growth opportunities for managers in hospital systems and that hospitals should be run like a business. That belief prompted me to join the Greenville Hospital System, where I worked for several years before joining Humana as a regional operations manager. HCA stayed in my mind, however. I was impressed with the maturity of top management, as well as the pride and local autonomy that characterized the HCA administrators in Texas, my home state.

I joined HCA in 1977 as vice president of the HCA Management Company, a unit that manages community hospitals in return for a fee. Then, in September of 1980, when a new, owned division was created in Tennessee, I became division vice president. My next assignment beginning in 1983, was to head up a corporate staff support department in the areas of planning, research, and management development. Then in 1985, I was reappointed to the HCA Management Company as the unit's president. I have found great stimulation and learning in both a line management role and a corporate staff role in the areas of planning, research, and management development.

I believe that today, as never before, there must be dedicated professionals who will provide leadership for the definition and measurement of quality. The difficult health care management field which is under severe pressures for efficiency and downsizing, needs competent, open minded, and enthusiastic leadership for continuous improvement. The bottom line and an organization's mission to meet the needs of its customers without rework and waste are highly correlated. A multihospital system can bring this philosophy, and associated statistical skills to achieve improvement, to a great number of health care organizations. What could be more satisfying than to feel that you can use your own talents in an organization that is committed to raise the standards of care—a commitment that results in continuous improvement in the health care services and products.

STAFF EMPLOYMENT

In addition to line management positions, multis can offer a wide array of specialized staff opportunities in corporate headquarters, regional offices, or hospitals. Among new graduates from master's programs in health services administration, staff positions are more frequently a source of entry level employment. In a recent survey of master's in health administration/ MHA graduates by Korn/Ferry International and AUPHA, the number of students reporting employment in a multihospital system's corporate office increased from 2.7 percent in 1983 to 4.9 percent in 1985 [23]. In addition, more graduates reported employment in a specialty area including planning (13 percent), information systems (8.2 percent), marketing (4.3 percent), personnel management (3.1 percent), and quality assurance (3.1 percent).

Although staff career progression is not as clearly defined as line career progression, entry into a multi through a staff role can provide unique opportunities. First, at the corporate level one can learn the structure and operations of a multi from a systemwide vantage point. Understanding the dynamics and complexity of the overall structure can provide early careerists with a systems perspective which is not obtained as easily at the hospital level.

Second, staff positions, if managed well, can lead to a variety of career paths. One can advance within a specialty, or through appropriate networking move to a new specialty position. In addition, movement to a hospital can be afforded to those who wish to progress to an operating position.

Third, the opportunity to network with a wide variety of both hospital and corporate personnel can be an excellent benefit of a corporate staff position. Developing both formal and informal ties to multihospital system managers is an advantage which can last a lifetime.

In addition to corporate jobs, staff positions can be found in regional and hospital environments. If capitalized upon, such positions can offer similar career opportunities.

Since joining HCA, I (Phyllis Virgil) have been able to realize professional growth and advancement through a corporate staff position in strategic planning. I came to corporate headquarters in 1983 as coordinator of strategic planning. In this entry level job, I had responsibility for managing multiple projects and providing analytical support related to the corporation's strategy development process. Two years later after taking on increasing amounts of responsibility, I was promoted to manager of strategic planning. I was responsible for managing the annual strategic planning process for several of the company's key lines of business. Today, as director of strategic planning for the HCA Management Company, a subsidiary which manages over 200 hospitals, I work with the unit's executives in developing strategies, business plans, and implementation plans for the overall unit, its key lines of business, and products.

To me, working as a corporate staff specialist has provided experience, exposure, and opportunities that will benefit my career for a lifetime. Over the years, I have had the opportunity to work with top management executives, have provided planning support for the majority of the corporation's key strategic moves, and perhaps most important, have always felt that my work was respected, appreciated, and used by the company.

My advice to anyone who is considering a staff position in a multihospital system is:

1. No matter how large or small a project may be, always produce a quality product.

2. Treat those you work with and for as customers, remembering that you are producing a service which others must see as valuable.

3. Network, and get to know the organization inside and out—its people, systems, and culture.

4. Always take on a challenge. Continually push yourself to your limit.

5. Ask your immediate supervisor for support and advice on career planning. It is your responsibility to act, and your supervisor's responsibility to help.

6. Keep an open mind on where you can take your career. If you work hard and excel, the opportunities for advancement, within your chosen staff area or outside of it, can be tremendous.

OPPORTUNITIES FOR WOMEN

In line with national trends, more and more women are entering the field of health services administration. According to the 1987 Korn/Ferry and AUPHA report, over half of the 1985 MHA graduates (55.2 percent) were women compared to only 40 percent in 1979 [24]. While it is still atypical to find women in top management positions, the doors to those positions appear to be opening.

From a personal perspective, I (Phyllis Virgil) have gotten to know a number of extremely talented, successful women, both within and outside HCA. What is very exciting is the fact that I see a number of dynamic women leaders in the field and a wealth of up-and-coming women who have the motivation and talent to become future leaders in health care.

The larger percentage of women managers entering the industry, coupled with increasing numbers of female physicians and board members, will likely lead to increasing opportunities for all types of women health care professionals. As this trend develops, systems can afford qualified female executives greater flexibility for matching opportunities with capabilities.

DEGREES AND EXPERIENCE EXPECTATIONS

Entry into many health care management positions today requires a master's degree. Statistics show that the educational level of American College of Healthcare Executives (ACHE) affiliates has increased over time. In 1973, 30 percent of all ACHE members had less than a master's degree. In 1982, only 17 percent of all affiliates had less than a master's degree [25].

The degree of choice in the health care field has historically been the MHA. In HCA, 69 percent of the assistant administrators hired in 1986 had an MHA. This degree differentiates an individual as a specialist in health care, and has augered well for individuals staying in the field and competing successfully. While the MHA is still predominant today, there are increasing numbers of individuals in the field with a master's degree in business administration (MBA). In 1982, 10 percent of all ACHE affiliates had an MBA compared to 5 percent in 1973 [26].

Regardless of degree, a recurring theme is that a sharp sense of business, combined with a sound understanding of the dynamics of health care services is mandatory in today's environment. Given that MHA programs have greatly enhanced their business curriculum over the past five years, and more of today's students pursue combined MHA and MBA degrees, the differences between pure MHA and MBA degrees will likely lessen.

Although a master's education, and in particular an MHA, remains the predominate degree, entry into multis can be achieved with an undergraduate education. For example, specialty corporate level positions in accounting, information systems, marketing, and human resources are functions that do not necessarily require advanced degrees. At HCA 63 percent of all corporate professional staff have less than a master's degree [27].

In addition, entry into system hospitals as a department manager or assistant manager can provide opportunity for individuals at the bachelor's level. In a number of cases, career advancement for department incumbents can be enhanced by pursuing advanced education on a part-time basis. In the future, we may find that individuals with clinical backgrounds who pursue an advanced education are the most valued job candidates.

SALARIES AND BENEFITS

According to Korn/Ferry International, 1985 MHA graduates were starting at an average salary of $29,773 [28]. At the entry level, multis typically pay market rates to new employees. Actual salaries received in assistant positions, however, will vary by hospital size, experience level of the candidate, and individual multi practices. For example, HCA has been successful in recruiting excellent people, and targets salaries at the median market rate. Other systems may pay at rates slightly below market, and actively reward outstanding job performance after new employees gain experience.

Looking at hospital CEOs, 1983 data show that the more highly remunerated hospital CEOs were those in nonprofit freestanding and system hospitals. Those least well remunerated were in state and local government facilities. Investor-owned hospital CEOs fell in the middle income level [29].

A 1987 survey profiled in *Hospitals*, found that multihospital systems tend to pay their top hospital executives about 15 percent more than single freestanding facilities. For example, the typical multi's vice president of operations is paid $76,000. The comparable position at a single facility receives an average of $59,000 [30].

In addition to salaries and bonus pay, investor-owned multis may provide stock options to eligible employees. Options are granted to select staff at established rates, to be purchased in a future time period. Depending on market conditions, the value of stock options can be considerable.

JOB SEARCH

There is no single, best path to obtain a position in a multihospital system, nor is there any single way in which multis find talented candidates. Companies use a variety of search methods ranging from resumé screening, to onsite campus visits, to residency programs, to word of mouth, and networking. For example, I (Phyllis Virgil) came to HCA from a residency position in one of the company's hospitals. Getting to know HCA staff, and actively communicating my interest in a corporate planning position gave me my entry into the company. According to one Humana officer, due to the high volume of candidates seeking employment, Humana rarely searches for job candidates, relying instead on its hospital residency programs to screen and select new management talent.

In looking for employment in a multihospital system, there are a number of excellent sources of information including

— The American Hospital Association (AHA) Guide to Multi-Hospital Systems

— The Federation of American Health Systems (FAHS) Directory of Investor-Owned Systems

— The SMG Marketing Group, Inc. Guide to Multihospital Systems

— *Modern Healthcare*'s annual Multi-Unit Provider Survey

— Annual stockholders reports of investor-owned systems

These sources provide background for identifying possible employers and are useful in preparing for interviews. In addition, ACHE publishes a directory of postgraduate fellowships. Matching fellowship sites with multihospital affiliation can produce a number of potential job entry options.

Professional associations and societies are also excellent sources of information. Some professional organizations publish job openings. In addition, some have active student chapters. Often, student membership fees are available at reduced rates. Major health care professional associations are

— American College of Healthcare Executives (ACHE)

— American Hospital Association (AHA)

— Federation of American Health Systems (FAHS)

The importance of networking with alumni, members of professional societies and associations, and staff within multihospital systems should not be overlooked. Networking can lead to a wealth of information on career opportunities. Making new professional acquaintances, distributing resumés, interviewing, and seeking out information is a must in any personal placement effort. No matter how talented an individual is, the key to a successful job search lies in self-motivation.

CONCLUSION

The nature and the extent of change in the health care environment from 1983 through 1987 has been extensive. Just as health care consumers have more choice over what, where, and how services will be provided to them, health care professionals have more choices about their professional contributions to the health care industry. Hospitals, ambulatory care centers, consulting companies, and multihospital systems are among a few of the choices to be considered.

The variety of opportunities, the scope of activities, and the fast track growth within multihospital systems has attracted many bright young achievers into these organizations. The experience of most has proved to be rewarding professionally and financially.

Health care is an important social commitment in North America. Innovative solutions in the delivery of quality services will continue to be a priority of the public. Professionals are needed in multis who will respond to this opportunity to provide leadership throughout their careers by bringing quality service to patients, physicians, and the public at a price that represents value to those customers.

We have described the industry, the opportunities, and something about the qualities needed to be successful. In our opinion, there has never been a better time for competent young people to choose a career in health care.

REFERENCES

1. 1987 Multi-Unit Provider Survey. *Modern Healthcare* (June 5) pg. 52, 1987, and Hospital Statistics 1987 Edition, American Hospital Association, Chicago, 1987.
2. Arthur Andersen and Co. and the American College of Hospital Administrators. *Health Care in the 1990s: Trends and Strategies.* Chicago: Arthur Andersen, 1984.
3. Arthur Andersen and Co. and the American Hospital Association. *Multihospital Systems: Perspectives and Trends.* Chicago: Arthur Andersen, 1984.
4. Stolman, E.R. Toward a Health Care Policy for the 1990s. *Issues in Health Care* 1(1): 1980.
5. *Modern Healthcare*. See number 1.
6. Arthur Andersen and Co. and the American Hospital Association. See number 2.
7. *Modern Healthcare*. See number 1.
8. Investor Relations, HCA U.S. Affiliated Hospitals by State, *Hospital Corporation of America*, Nashville, TN, December, 1987.
9. *Modern Healthcare*. See number 1.
10. National Medical Enterprises Annual Depart, 1986, *National Medical Enterprises*, Los Angeles, 1987.
11. The Center for Health Studies, 1987 HCA Annual Hospital Survey, *The Center for Health Studies*, Nashville, TN, 1987.
12. Sloan, F.A. and R.A. Vraciu. Investor-Owned and Not-for-Profit Hospitals: Addressing Some Issues. *Health Affairs* 2(1): 25–37, 1983.
13. *Modern Healthcare*. See number 1.
14. *Modern Healthcare*. See number 1.
15. Kleiner, S.G. The Role of Hospital Administrators in Multihospital Sys-

tems. *Hospital and Health Service Administration* (March/April): 27–44, 1984.

16. Foundation of the American College of Hospital Administrators. *The Evolving Role of the Hospital Chief Executive Officer, A Report of the Ad Hoc Committee on the Evolving Role of the Hospital Chief Executive Officer*. Chicago: The Foundation, 1984.

17. Kleiner, S.G. See number 14.

18. Foundation of the American College of Hospital Administrators. See 15.

19. Brown, M. and B.P. McCool. High-Performing Managers: Leadership Attributes for the 1990s. *Health Care Management Review* 12(2): 69–75, 1987.

20. Multis Send Executives Back to School. *Hospitals* (January 20): 44–46, 1986.

21. Draft study, CEO Turnover, AHA, ACHE. Heidrick and Struggles, December 1988.

22. Human Resources Department. Administrator Turnover. Nashville, TN: Hospital Corporation of America, 1987.

23. Korn/Ferry International and AUPHA. Health Administration Employment: A Survey of Early Career Opportunities. New York: Korn/Ferry, 1987.

24. Korn/Ferry International and AUPHA. See number 23.

25. Weil, P.A. and J.O. Lanier. The Changing Profile: Affiliates of the American College of Hospital Administrators, 1973 and 1982. *Hospital and Health Services Administration* (March/April): 6–25, 1984.

26. Weil, P.A. and J.O. Lanier. See number 25.

27. Human Resources Department. Education level. Nashville, TN: Hospital Corporation of America, 1987.

28. Korn/Ferry International and AUPHA. See number 23.

29. Foundation of the American College of Hospital Administrators. See number 16.

30. Multis: Executive Salaries: Multis Still Top "Singles." *Hospitals* (June 5): 68 (A/10), 1987.

4

RURAL HOSPITALS: BIG IMPACT IN SMALL COMMUNITIES

DAVID J. ROBERTSON

Administering a rural hospital offers tremendous challenges and rewards for today's health services administrator. While logic might dictate that the challenge of hospital administration increases in direct proportion to an institution's bed size, this is an erroneous assumption. The unique environment in which rural hospitals operate, the high visibility of the rural hospital administrator, the vital role of the hospital in maintaining the economic stability of the community, the frequent absence of many of the traditional administrative support functions available in urban institutions, and the ever-tightening fiscal constraints on the hospital are but a sampling of those factors which make rural hospitals extremely complex and challenging to administer.

It takes a special type of individual, equipped with a unique set of skills, to function effectively as a rural hospital administrator. Although programs in health services administration significantly differentiate their training programs for various segments of the health administration field (for example, ambulatory care administration, mental health administration, and long-term care administration) there is little, if any, differentiation among hospital administration programs with regard to the rural and urban hospital environments. It is frequently assumed that the only significant difference between urban and rural health care institutions is their size; however, nothing could be further from the truth. Certainly, an institution's size is a

David J. Robertson holds an M.S.P.H. and an M.B.A. from the University of Missouri-Columbia, and also earned a B.S. in health care administration from Wichita State University.

major determining factor in the scope of services which are offered and the resulting personnel requirements, but more important are the vast differences in the functional roles and relationships of the administrator, the public and intra-institutional visibility, available support resources, and unique issues such as rural reimbursement inequities and health manpower shortages.

Administrators frequently enter the field of rural hospital administration without a good base of knowledge as to the challenges, pressures, and frustrations which they will encounter. While the challenges can be overwhelming, the rewards can be equally uplifting. In no other sector of health administration can an individual have as dramatic an impact on the health care of a community. Likewise, there may be no area in the field of health administration where the critical need for highly skilled professional administrators is as great.

CHARACTERISTICS AND IMPORTANCE OF THE RURAL HOSPITAL

Rural hospitals serve as the primary point of access to health care services for millions of people, and as such provide a significant portion of the hospital care delivered in this country. A rural hospital is defined as being any hospital which falls outside one of the 281 U.S. metropolitan statistical areas [1]. Using this definition, figures released by the American Hospital Association indicate that in 1986 rural hospitals comprised 46 percent of the total number of U.S. hospitals and represented 2,638 individual institutions [2]. These hospitals serve an area encompassing approximately 42 percent of the population, or an estimated 95 million people [3].

A total of 345 rural hospitals serve as their communities' sole source of health care due to factors such as the isolated location of the community and restrictive geography [4]. Although only a small minority of rural hospitals serve as the only available source of health care for their community, it is important to recognize that the lack of public transportation in rural areas effectively isolates a significant proportion of the rural elderly and indigent populations. Consequently, a much higher number of rural hospitals functionally serve as the sole available source of health care for the elderly and indigent within their service area since transportation to other facilities is not readily available.

Despite the fact that rural hospitals account for a significant proportion of the total of U.S. hospitals and hospital utilization, the future of the rural hospital is in question. In a 1986 survey of hospital executives conducted by Touche Ross & Co., the most frequently cited institutions at risk of failure

TABLE 1: Number of U.S. Rural Hospitals by Bed Size
(1984)

SIZE	NUMBER	%
6–24 Beds	175	7
25–49 Beds	809	31
50–99 Beds	908	34
100–199 Beds	576	22
200+ Beds	170	6
Total	2,638	100

SOURCE: *Profile of Small or Rural Hospitals*, 1980–86, copyright 1988
by the American Hospital Association.

TABLE 2: Percentage of U.S. Rural Staffed Beds by
Hospital Bed Size (1986)

SIZE	%
6–24 Beds	1
25–49 Beds	14
50–99 Beds	29
100–199 Beds	35
200+ Beds	21
Total	100

SOURCE: *Profile of Small or Rural Hospitals*, 1980–86, copyright 1988
by the American Hospital Association.

were rural hospitals under 100 beds in size. Furthermore, 59 percent of the administrators of hospitals under 100 beds indicated that they believed that their institutions were at risk of failure [5]. If this analysis is accurate, it certainly portends that difficult times are ahead for the majority of rural hospitals. As can be seen in Table 1, 72 percent of U.S. rural hospitals are less than 100 beds in size, with 44 percent of all staffed rural hospital beds being in institutions with fewer than 100 beds (Table 2).

The lack of certainty of hospital executives as to the future of their institutions is understandable as one examines the financial distress facing many rural hospitals. By some estimates, as many as 600 rural institutions are projected to close by 1990 [6]. While closure for some may indeed be appropriate, most rural hospitals are vital to the communities which they serve. These institutions frequently serve patients in dangerous occupations where access to emergency medical care is critical. In addition, a rural hospital is often the largest employer in the community and closure often begins or

TABLE 3: U.S. Small and Rural Hospital Ownership (1986)

OWNERSHIP	% HOSPITALS
Voluntary	49
Government	35
Investor-owned	16

SOURCE: *Profile of Small or Rural Hospitals*, 1980–86, copyright 1988 by the American Hospital Association.

accelerates the economic demise of a community. While only time will answer the question as to the number of closures which will occur, in the period from 1980 to 1985 the level of rural hospital mergers and closures was consistent with the hospital industry as a whole. However, in 1986, for the first time this decade, the number of rural hospital closures (37) exceeded the number of urban closures (31) [7]. The greatest risk exists in communities which have two or more hospitals where declining utilization and the need for cost efficiency will dictate that a consolidation occur. Certainly, closures will occur, but strong and creative administrative leadership can play a significant role in assuring the continued viability of the majority of rural hospitals by guiding them through the turbulent times which lie ahead for the entire hospital industry.

As Table 3 illustrates, rural hospitals are primarily voluntary, nonprofit organizations or government institutions. These categories of institutions are typically governed by a board of trustees and have tax-exempt status. This designation means that they are exempt from federal tax, and use their net revenues (profits) to offset future operating costs as well as costs associated with modernization. Investor-owned proprietary institutions are required to pay federal tax on any profits that they generate. It is a frequent misconception that a nonprofit hospital does not, and should not, make a profit. It is essential that all hospitals, whether profit or nonprofit, generate an excess of revenues over expenses if they are to continue to meet the health care needs of the populace which they serve. The distinction between a nonprofit and for-profit institution lies not in whether a profit is made but, rather, in how those profits are used. In the nonprofit institution profits are re-invested in the institution, where in the proprietary institution the profits are distributed among the shareholders.

Multihospital systems are continually increasing their involvement with rural hospitals, with a total of 30 percent of rural institutions being either owned, leased, or managed by a multihospital system. In addition, 47 percent of the hospitals comprising multihospital systems have fewer than 100 beds [8]. Rural institutions have linked with both proprietary hospital systems (for example, Hospital Corporation of America) and not-for-profit systems (for example, Voluntary Hospitals of America), but regardless of the structure of the system the end result is to link rural institutions to secondary and tertiary providers. This linkage is intended to promote the commitment of these multi-institutional systems in working to assure the continued survival of these rural hospitals. Through these linkages, strong administrative talent is frequently provided along with support functions such as physician recruitment expertise, marketing and public relations expertise, personnel expertise, and strong financial analysis capabilities.

It is difficult to describe the typical rural hospital in terms of the services which it provides for there is a broad diversity of service mixes. On one end of the spectrum are those institutions providing basic primary care, offering only the minimum level of services necessary to be recognized as a hospital. In contrast, there are many rural institutions that provide secondary and tertiary services and function as regional referral centers. These institutions provide a full spectrum of medical and surgical services. Thus, rural hospital administrators need not fear functioning in an antiquated medical environment, for through administrative creativity and motivation, modern technology can be made available to the vast majority of rural institutions. Shared service arrangements, joint venture financing, philanthropic support, advanced communications technology, and solid marketing efforts are but a few examples of techniques that have made modern medical technology a realizable dream for many rural hospitals.

MAJOR ENVIRONMENTAL FACTORS AFFECTING RURAL LIFE

Any social institution, whether it be a school, church, or hospital, must monitor the environment in which it operates in order to respond effectively to changes which are continually occurring. Rural life is undergoing dramatic change, and as a result rural hospitals are being forced to re-evaluate the roles which they play within the community. Among the environmental factors that affect rural hospitals are

1. The depressed rural economy
2. Population trends
3. An increasing elderly population
4. The increasing competition in the hospital industry
5. Declining hospital utilization
6. Deteriorating hospital financial conditions

DEPRESSED RURAL ECONOMY. The rural economy is largely dependent on the agriculture, forestry, mining, petroleum, and natural gas industries. Each of these industries has been negatively affected in the last few years by high interest rates and declining prices. This depressed state has resulted in a decline in rural hospital payments for services rendered, philanthropy, and tax subsidies. This decline in receipts is largely attributable to the inability of individuals to pay for the services which they receive. One in every seven rural Americans has an income below the poverty level compared with one in ten nationally [9]. Compounding this problem is the fact that approximately 50 percent of all rural hospitals receive subsidies through local taxation, and as the economy has deteriorated the level of tax collections has also diminished [10].

POPULATION TRENDS. From 1970 to 1980, rural America experienced a 14 percent growth rate which significantly exceeded the 10 percent urban rate of growth. However, the 1980s have seen a reversal in this trend with urban growth (5 percent) exceeding rural growth (3 percent) [11]. This significant decline in rural population growth has had a dramatic downward impact on the utilization of rural hospitals, tremendously affecting their financial condition. In addition, this decline is a significant factor in the planning of future services, a critical task of the health administrator.

INCREASING ELDERLY POPULATION. Nationally, between 1980 and 1986, the elderly population grew as follows:

— age 65–74   11%
— age 75–84   16%
— age 85 +   25% [12]

With a large segment of the elderly population residing in rural areas, this growth has had a major impact on rural hospitals. In addition, as the economy has deteriorated, there has been an outmigration of young people to urban areas. Outmigration has had a dual impact on the rural hospital resulting in both an overall decline in the number of people served as well as increasing the average age of the remaining population.

Since rural hospitals provide services to a significantly more elderly and low-income populace than urban institutions, they are more dependent on Medicare and Medicaid as a source of reimbursement. The percentage of Medicare patients served in rural institutions is very high, but only 15 percent of total national Medicare payments goes to small or rural hospitals [13]. Thus, small changes in reimbursement to rural institutions may have only a minor impact on the overall Medicare program, but a dramatic impact on the viability of rural institutions. Table 4 illustrates the significant dependence of the rural hospital on Medicare and Medicaid reimbursement.

TABLE 4: Distribution of Hospitals by Percentage of Medicare and Medicaid Net Patient Revenue, Registered Community Hospitals, 1986

	NUMBER OF HOSPITALS	PERCENTAGE OF MEDICARE NET REVENUE			TOTAL %
		0–42% (AT OR BELOW AVERAGE)	43–52% (ABOVE AVERAGE)	53+% (WELL ABOVE AVERAGE)	
Total U.S. Hospitals	5,676	53	38	9	100
Rural Hospitals (Bed size)					
6–24	175	75	12	13	100
25–49	809	23	61	16	100
50–99	908	26	64	10	100
100–199	576	74	21	6	100
200+	170	67	31	3	100
Total	2,638	41	48	11	100

	NUMBER OF HOSPITALS	PERCENTAGE OF MEDICAID NET REVENUE			TOTAL %
		0–8% (AT OR BELOW AVERAGE)	9–14% (ABOVE AVERAGE)	15+% (WELL ABOVE AVERAGE)	
Total U.S. Hospitals	5,676	47	43	10	100
Rural Hospitals (Bed size)					
6–24	175	48	46	6	100
25–49	809	29	66	5	100
50–99	908	39	50	11	100
100–199	576	45	44	11	100
200+	170	48	38	15	100
Total	2,638	38	52	9	100

Percentages do not add to exactly 100% due to rounding.

SOURCE: *Profile of Small or Rural Hospitals*, 1980–86, copyright 1988 by the American Hospital Association.

TABLE 5: U.S. Hospital Admission Trends

	% 1980–1984	% 1984–1985	% 1985–1986
All U.S. Hospitals	−3	−5	−3
Rural Hospitals			
6–24 Beds	−25	−13	−7
25–49 Beds	−9	−8	−5
50–99 Beds	−18	−10	−6
100–199 Beds	−13	−7	−10
200+ Beds	−27	−10	−5
Total Rural	−18	−8	−7

SOURCE: *Profile of Small or Rural Hospitals*, 1980–86, copyright 1988 by the American Hospital Association.

INCREASE IN COMPETITION. Rural hospitals are facing increasing competition from neighboring institutions, urban hospitals, multi-institutional systems, freestanding diagnostic centers and ambulatory surgical centers, to name but a few. These competitors frequently target younger populations, thus compounding the problem of losing the opportunity to serve these individuals. Developing plans to compete effectively in the marketplace and monitoring the impact of competition are the administrator's responsibility.

DECLINING UTILIZATION. Hospitals throughout the country are faced with declining utilization rates. However, nowhere is this trend more dramatic than in the rural setting. In spite of the increasing health care needs of the elderly, hospital inpatient utilization continues to decline. Utilization of health care services is affected by a myriad of industrywide factors that include, but are not limited to, federal cost-containment efforts, the Medicare prospective payment system, increased competition, negotiated payment rates with the government and other third-party payers, the trend toward wellness, holistic health care, preventive medicine, and outpatient care coupled with increasing levels of consumer awareness of health issues and involvement in health care decisions.

The declines in utilization are primarily the result of decreasing rates of admission and average length of stay. Table 5 illustrates that during the period from 1980 through 1984, rural admissions declined at a rate greater than six times the national average, while the rate of decline for rural hospitals between 1984 and 1986, following the advent of the Medicare prospective pricing system, was twice the national rate.

The combination of this declining admission trend and the fact that the average length of stay in rural hospitals under 100 beds is less than the national average for all hospitals (see Table 6), has resulted in average daily

TABLE 6: Average Length of Stay in U.S. Hospitals (1986)

	DAYS
All U.S. Hospitals	7.1
Rural Hospitals:	
6–24 Beds	5.0
25–49 Beds	5.5
50–99 Beds	7.0
100–199 Beds	7.4
200+ Beds	7.5
Total Rural	7.1

SOURCE: *Profile of Small or Rural Hospitals*, 1980–86, copyright 1988 by the American Hospital Association.

TABLE 7: Trends in Average Daily Census in U.S. Hospitals (1980–86)

	% 1980–1984	% 1984–1985	% 1985–1986
All U.S. Hospitals	−4.7	−7.4	−1.8
Rural Hospitals:			
6–24 Beds	−22.2	0.0	−14.3
25–49 Beds	−15.8	−6.3	−6.7
50–99 Beds	−10.9	−9.8	0.0
100–199 Beds	−9.2	−6.7	−2.4
200+ Beds	−8.8	−7.1	−1.6
Total Rural	−13.3	−7.7	−2.1

SOURCE: *Profile of Small or Rural Hospitals*, 1980–86, copyright 1988 by the American Hospital Association.

census declines in rural hospitals which continue to outpace the hospital industry as a whole (Table 7).

The rural health administrator is challenged to find alternative uses for facilities which may no longer be necessary to meet the declining acute care needs of the community due to these changing patterns of utilization. Certainly, abolishment of all acute care services is generally not desirable, but frequently more cost effective and needed health care service delivery options exist.

Among the options being considered are

— Long-term care

— Skilled nursing care

— Mental health services

— Substance abuse centers

— Hospices

— Ambulatory surgery facilities

— Day care services

— Professional offices

— Birthing centers

— Wellness centers

— Congregate housing

— Home health care

— Community education

— Catering services

DETERIORATING HOSPITAL FINANCIAL CONDITIONS. The combined impact of the major environmental factors described thus far is amplified by changing hospital reimbursement formulas which frequently penalize the rural institution, resulting in a significant deterioration in the financial condition of these institutions. As shown in Table 8, in 1986 38 percent of rural hospitals had a deficit of 6 percent or more, while only 22 percent of urban institutions saw this level of deficit. Table 9 illustrates that average net margins are particularly poor in the smallest of rural hospitals. With deteriorating financial conditions come increased difficulties in physician recruitment, retention of key staff members, and maintenance and upgrading of the physical plant. The role of the health administrator in providing financial planning and financial guidance can be instrumental in assuring the institution's ability to deal effectively with these challenges.

MAJOR CHALLENGES FOR THE RURAL ADMINISTRATOR

To fully understand the role and nature of the rural hospital administrator, it is important to understand some of the key management challenges faced in the rural hospital environment. While many issues affect all hospitals regardless of location or size, there are many which provide a disparately greater challenge to administrators in the rural setting.

RETENTION AND RECRUITMENT OF A WELL-STRUCTURED GOVERNING BOARD. One of the paramount prerequisites for institutional success is strong leadership at both the administrative and governing board levels. There is a critical need for strong administrative leadership and similarly there is a critical need for strong governing board leadership. As Bruce Amundson, director of the Kellogg Foundation's rural hospital project, has stated, "Board leadership is particularly poor in many commu-

TABLE 8: U.S. Hospital Operating Margins (1984)

	% DEFICIT OF 6%+	% DEFICIT OF 3.0-5.9%	% DEFICIT OF .1-2.9%	% PROFIT OF 0-2.9%	% PROFIT OF 3.0-5.9%	% PROFIT OF 6%+
All U.S. Hospitals	29	12	12	19	14	14
Rural Hospitals:						
Under 50 Beds	57	9	7	9	12	10
50-99 Beds	36	15	15	17	10	8
100+ Beds	18	15	14	23	10	8
Total Rural	38	13	12	16	12	10

SOURCE: *Profile of Small or Rural Hospitals*, 1980–86, copyright 1988 by the American Hospital Association.

TABLE 9: U.S. Hospital Average Net Margins (1986)

	%
All U.S. Hospitals	−2.0
Rural Hospitals:	
6–24 Beds	−20.7
25–49 Beds	−8.6
50–99 Beds	−2.9
100–199 Beds	.3
200+ Beds	.9
Total Rural	−1.5

SOURCE: *Profile of Small or Rural Hospitals*, 1980–86, copyright 1988 by the American Hospital Association.

nity hospitals" [14]. Rural hospital boards frequently do not consist of individuals with strong backgrounds in strategic planning, financial planning, or policy setting. Consequently, there is a tendency for rural governing boards to become operationally oriented rather than serving in a planning and policymaking role. One of the critical challenges facing the administrator is to help educate governing board members on the role of the governing board, the pressures and challenges which are affecting the institution, and to focus their decision making on appropriate issues and planning horizons. In the rural community, there is no shortage of dedicated individuals willing and committed to serving the best interests of the hospital; the challenge is helping them grow into sound hospital leaders.

It is very common that the rural hospital administrator has a higher level of education, responsibility, and income than do the individual members of the governing board. This can create awkward situations at times, and require the rural administrator to respond with diplomacy and tact. As more and more highly skilled and well-trained administrators choose to serve rural areas, the frequency of this problem is bound to increase.

RECRUITMENT AND RETENTION OF QUALIFIED MEDICAL STAFF. Recruitment of physicians to rural communities has traditionally been a problem, and while the supply of physicians continues to increase, there does not seem to be any significant resolution to the shortage of physicians in rural areas. Physicians tend to be extremely reluctant to locate their practices in rural areas due to the lack of an adequate population base to support selected specialty practices, inaccurate perceptions of income potential, a lack of peer support and practice coverage, a lack of specialized technology, a lack of cultural and educational opportunities, and fear of professional obsolescence. The administrator must recognize these negative components, both real and perceived, of a rural medical practice and aggressively work to counteract and eliminate them where possible, and to assure a positive presentation of the community in the recruitment process.

RECRUITMENT AND RETENTION OF QUALIFIED EMPLOYEE STAFF. A common frustration experienced by rural hospital administrators is the inability to recruit and retain qualified departmental management and professional staff. Administrators are faced with the dilemma that, while the services provided by an individual may not be optimal, it may be difficult if not impossible to recruit a suitable or more appropriate replacement. Other problems develop from the demands on managerial staff to play significant roles in direct patient care in addition to their administrative functions. Typically, good technicians are promoted to administrative roles with very little administrative training or experience. However, success as a technician in no way assures managerial success. Unfortunately, those individuals who do prove to be excellent managers frequently move on to other institutions due to the limited potential for upward advancement within a rural hospital. It is therefore essential that the rural administrator serve as both an educator and motivator in developing and retaining a sound management staff.

In addition to the challenges associated with recruiting qualified managers and professional staff, providing adequate staffing levels is at times difficult. Rural hospitals typically function with significantly fewer employees per occupied bed than the national average for all hospitals. Rural hospitals frequently have cross-training programs in order to use individuals in multiple areas of an institution to help alleviate the problem. Typical examples of this include cross training in admissions and business office, x-ray and laboratory, and surgery and sterile supply.

CREDENTIALING AND PEER REVIEW PROBLEMS. The small size and diversity of the rural medical staff frequently makes effective peer review and credentialing quite difficult to achieve. In a community where there is only one general surgeon, who is capable of reviewing the care rendered by that individual? When a community has a need for ten physicians but actually has only four, is it reasonable to expect that the time spent on peer review activities will diminish a physician's ability to practice medicine, thereby exacerbating the shortage? In rural environments, every member of the medical community is vital, and consequently there frequently exist both institutional and community pressure to bypass or minimize quality problems. The administrator and governing board must function as the community's advocate and work with the medical staff to find ways to maximize their effectiveness and enhance the peer review process to assure the provision of high-quality medical services.

LACK OF ADMINISTRATIVE SUPPORT RESOURCES. In most urban institutions, as well as in larger rural institutions, administrative resources and support functions in the areas of finance, planning, marketing, data processing, as well as day-to-day administration exist; however, in many small rural institutions administrators are on their own. Thus, they must be "jacks-of-all-trades" with a broad level of knowledge sufficient to support decision making across a wide spectrum of issues. Rural administrators must possess the ability to identify those areas in which their expertise is not sufficient, and know when to call in outside assistance. Outside assistance might come from members of the governing board, the business community, health administration colleagues, hospital association resources, or consultants.

Figure 1 is the organization chart of Duncan Regional Hospital, a rural hospital consisting of 152 licensed beds for which I serve as administrator. This hospital is larger than the average rural facility, but despite this fact it is readily apparent that the number of administrative personnel is much less than what you would typically see in a metropolitan hospital of similar size. No formal assistant administrator or administrative assistant positions exist and all professional service departments report directly to the administrator. This "flat" organizational structure is fairly typical in rural institutions and illustrates the point made earlier of the need for the administrator to deal with a broad variety of issues and personalities.

Prior to my association with Duncan Regional Hospital in Duncan, Oklahoma, I served as the administrator of the 85-bed Shelby County Myrtue Memorial Hospital located in Harlan, Iowa. This institution likewise had a "flat" organizational structure; however, the hospital was somewhat less specialized, and therefore had fewer total departments. While the challenges of administration are similar in both institutions, without question the levels of management expertise are greater in the larger institution. As mentioned earlier, rural health care department managers typically have risen to their position due to the fact that they are excellent technicians, but as institutions become larger, the ability to attract department managers with strong managerial skills increases. Without question, this lifts some of the burden from the administrator as it is easier to delegate tasks and responsibilities to individuals with stronger management skills.

INCREASING REGULATION. More and more frequently, rural hospitals are finding themselves with insufficient resources to respond to the continual increase in regulations being placed on hospitals. It is easy to feel as if this deluge of regulations is never ending and is intended specifically to close rural institutions. The administrator must be an advocate of the insti-

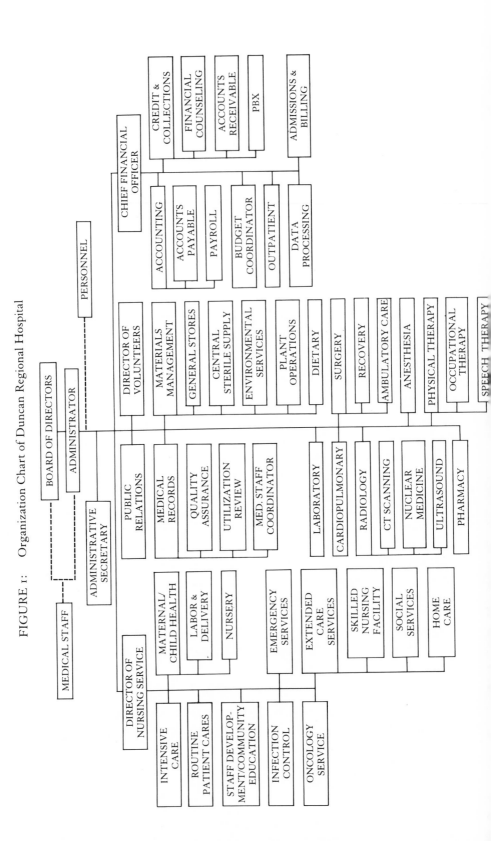

FIGURE 1: Organization Chart of Duncan Regional Hospital

tution and attempt to shape legislation through informing state and national legislators of the impact of proposed legislation. Frequently, rural hospitals find it easier to discontinue services rather than to meet the additional requirements imposed by legislation. The fallacy of this course of action is that as services are discontinued the fixed costs of the institution must be spread over a smaller volume of services, thus decreasing the overall profitability of the remaining services and moving the institution one step closer to financial ruin.

LACK OF ADEQUATE INFORMATION SYSTEMS. The administrator must obtain the best information reasonably possible, and use sound management and decision-making skills in charting the course for the future. Rural hospitals do not generally enjoy the luxury of sophisticated management information systems or data analysis support and consequently sound information on which to base managerial decisions is frequently not available. Large quantities of information can neither be developed nor analyzed by a small staff, so the focus must be on identifying critical information needed for sound decision making and assuring that it is provided on a timely basis.

INDIGENT CARE. The funding of indigent care is an issue that is receiving broad attention and it affects virtually every hospital. However, in rural settings the issue of indigent care has some unique elements not typically present in urban settings. The lack of resources with which to fund indigent care is a problem that exists in most institutions; however, with the small budget size of the average rural institution and low or nonexistent profit margins, a few indigent care cases can push an institution perilously close to financial disaster. These strong financial implications, coupled with the fact that most communities have no other viable source of care for the indigent, present a true dilemma. Due to the close relationship which rural institutions typically have with their patients and the high visibility of the hospital, decisions to do anything but treat indigent patients can create significant public relations problems. This issue is very complex and it is one of the greatest long-term challenges to be faced by rural hospital administrators.

FUNDING OF SERVICES. With utilization declining, dramatic shifts in profitability, declining levels of Medicare and other third-party reimbursements, increased competition, and declining percentages of the community's populace who are insured, the future sources of funding for rural hospital services are of great concern. Certainly, third-party reimbursement will continue to be the most significant funding source; however, as payments decline it is critical that administrators identify new sources of revenue to assure that hospitals will continue to have the ability to provide services meeting the broad needs of the community. Corporate restructuring, development of charitable foundations, new service development, provision of nontraditional services, and even development of alternative delivery systems are being pursued in an attempt to help alleviate funding shortfalls and assure a steady patient base. These developments present exciting opportunities for creative managers.

CORPORATE CITIZEN. Rural communities look to the hospital as a major corporate citizen of the community. The rural hospital plays a much more integral role in all aspects of community life than does the metropolitan institution, and with this leadership role comes a high level of visibility. The institution, as well as individuals associated with it, is expected to provide civic leadership and the expectations of the administrator in this regard are high. Rural administrators can be deluged with demands on their time and a balance must be maintained between the commitment of time devoted to the institution, community, and family. Despite the demands, the experience of community involvement, leadership, and the feeling that as an individual you truly *can* make a difference can be infinitely rewarding.

KEY RELATIONSHIPS OF THE RURAL ADMINISTRATOR

Hospital administrators, whether urban or rural, hold the same key relationships, among the most important of which are those relationships with the following groups: (1) governing board, (2) medical staff, (3) employees, (4) patients, (5) business community, (6) community-at-large, (7) the health care industry. Despite the fact that the urban and rural hospital administrator must interact with the same groups, significant differences exist with regard to the nature of these relationships. Rural administrators typically have a much closer working relationship with their governing board, employees, medical staff, patients, business community, and community-at-large. These relationships are high among the tremendous rewards of rural health services administration because they provide opportunities to be an integral part of a truly personalized health care delivery system. However, administrators are also highly visible and consequently subject to intense scrutiny by each of these key groups since there is great awareness of administrators and their daily activities. Rural administrators are constant representatives of their institutions throughout the community, and at times may feel that their personal lives are somewhat compromised as a result of the ever-present institutional shadow.

Governing boards frequently play a much greater role than do their urban counterparts in the day-to-day operations of the institution, and they generally desire high levels of knowledge and awareness of daily activities in order to function in their capacity as informed trustees. While this desire for knowledge and involvement is understandable, the successful rural administrator must maintain a delicate balance between appropriate interest and improper involvement. Due to the small size of the medical community, the administrator will also typically function in a much closer relationship with the medical staff, providing the opportunity to build much stronger interdependent relationships with this important group than is typical in an urban setting.

The rural administrator has an opportunity to work very closely with employees, patients, and members of the business community through both hospital and civic activities. As a result, relationships with these groups have the potential to be more personal and rewarding than is possible in the metropolitan institution. However, while most of the key relationships which develop tend to be much closer than those of urban administrators, the rural administrator often finds it difficult to have a strong tie with the health care industry and other hospital administration colleagues. Interactions with other administrators is limited. This can create feelings of isolation, and if efforts are not made to stay in touch with changes in the industry, administrative obsolescence may result.

CHARACTERISTICS OF THE SUCCESSFUL HOSPITAL ADMINISTRATOR

While it is impossible to predict the success which a single individual will enjoy in any profession, there are a number of characteristics which many successful rural hospital administrators have in common. Among these are the following:

1. Technical Competence
Administrators must have a broad knowledge of the internal workings of the hospital, the role which the hospital plays within the community, and must strive to stay abreast of changes occurring within the environment in which the hospital operates.

2. Self-Confidence
In the rural setting, there is a lack of internal administrative support and, therefore, administrators must have the confidence necessary to make decisions across a broad spectrum of functional areas and provide the leadership to which others look for guidance. Administrators must

be willing to stand by principles and decisions in which they believe but yet remain open to the viewpoints of others.

3. Strong Communication Skills

Administrators must be able to communicate with individuals at all levels of the organization and community. As the most visible representative of the institution, these skills are a major factor in developing the overall image which the community holds of the hospital.

4. Strong Board and Medical Staff Relations

This skill is critical to the success of any administrator, and in rural hospitals is even more vital because of the closer working relationships between administrators and individual members of these two groups.

5. Motivation

Successful administrators must be self-starters, be able to recognize areas requiring attention, and be able to conceptualize ways to resolve problems. In addition, administrators must be able to motivate others in striving toward the common goals of the institution.

6. Innovation

Future success of rural hospitals is dependent upon the ability to see creative new solutions to both old and new problems.

7. Integration

Administrators must be able to integrate the various functions of the institution into an efficient operating whole.

8. Educator

Administrators must play a vital role in educating the governing board and administrative personnel as to the roles which they play.

9. Visibility

Rural administrators must take an active role within the community, and be perceived as an integral, constructive part of the community. If viewed as disinterested outsiders, the effectiveness of administrators will diminish and the institution will ultimately suffer.

10. Planning

Administrators must be able to see the big picture and continually work to move their institutions toward their ultimate objectives.

11. Resiliency

The pressures of rural administration are great, and administrators must be able to rebound from the frustrations of today and recognize that tomorrow is another day with its own challenges and rewards.

12. A Sense of Humor

Without a sense of humor and the ability to leave the office behind, rural health administration provides an environment which can rapidly create administrative burnout.

EDUCATION AND CAREER OPPORTUNITIES

In the past, it was quite common for rural health administrators to lack any formal training or education in administration, and in fact, many administrators of the past did not have any formal management training of any type. Those days are over, and today a master's degree in hospital or business administration, or both, is a virtual prerequisite for any top rural administrative positions. Individuals with a BA in health administration might expect to find a middle management position but the obtainment of a master's degree will be important to future career advancement. In addition to formal training, most institutions seek individuals who have a minimum of five years' administrative experience when filling top administrative positions. This administrative experience may reasonably be obtained in either rural or urban settings. Those obtaining their experience in urban settings frequently have exposure to health services and medical specialties unavailable in many rural institutions, thus bringing a broad technical background to the institution. However, these individuals frequently lack the understanding of the role and environment of the rural hospital which those receiving experience in the rural setting possess. Either experiential track provides a strong background and will be favorably considered in the evaluation process.

Rural health service administration salaries are becoming competitive with their urban counterparts, and as the qualifications of rural administrators increase, parity in salaries will occur. Graduates of master's degree health administration programs obtaining positions as administrative assistants or assistant administrators in rural hospitals can reasonably anticipate starting salaries in the range of $24,000 to $30,000.

REWARDS OF RURAL HOSPITAL ADMINISTRATION

It is important to recognize the tremendous rewards which exist with a career in rural hospital administration. Nowhere is there an opportunity for an individual to have a greater impact on the overall health care of a community. It is an environment where the impact of management decisions and managerial effort can be seen very rapidly. For example, the addition of a single physician in a community with 10 physicians certainly has much greater impact than the addition of that same physician in a community with 200 physicians. Thus, personal satisfaction in rural hospital administration is often much more tangible and immediate than in other settings.

It has been stated that rural administrators must be "jacks-of-all-trades," and this broad exposure to health service administration and the total institution can be extremely rewarding. Rather than becoming isolated in a single department or function, the rural administrator has the opportunity to become involved in every aspect of the institution. Rural institutions tend to be smaller and more personal with a greater tendency to take on the personality of a family rather than an impersonal corporate personality and philosophy. Communication is generally easier and certainly less formal.

Just as the rural administrator has the tremendous opportunity to affect the community through the hospital, I do not feel that any environment offers an individual a greater opportunity to affect a community outside of the hospital. The administrator has the ability to become involved in the total community, and in fact, the community will expect it. The Chamber of Commerce, service and civic organizations, school, and church are some of the many areas of potential community involvement. This involvement is very gratifying and has always made me feel that "I do indeed make a difference!"

As rural hospitals restructure themselves to respond to the changing rural environment, changes in the scope and configuration of hospital services can be anticipated. The following are some of the many options which rural hospitals will be forced to consider:

1. Closure of inpatient services and development of emergency medical systems

2. Limitation of inpatient hospital services

3. Development of a comprehensive community health center approach

4. Development of regional health care networks through partnerships with neighboring institutions

5. Development of alternative delivery systems such as health maintenance organizations and preferred provider organizations

6. Expansion of the continuum of care to include services such as skilled nursing facilities, intensive care, retirement housing, and psychiatric services

7. Networking of services through development of satellite clinics, or alliances with secondary and tertiary providers of care

8. Diversification into nontraditional services such as adult day care, hospice, health promotion and wellness programs

Regardless of the direction which individual rural hospitals take, it is certain that the status quo is not an option. The public will always need rural hospital services, and it is imperative that institutions respond to the changing environment in order to position themselves best to meet these needs. The rural hospital administrator is the leader of this process and a career in rural administration provides great challenges and rewards for those willing to commit themselves to the effort.

REFERENCES

1. Lutz, S. Rural Hospitals Offer New Services, Seek Affiliations in Effort to Survive. *Modern Healthcare* 17 (13): 30, 1987.
2. American Hospital Association. *Profile of Small or Rural Hospitals 1980–1986.* Chicago: The Association, 1988, p. 4.
3. Robert Wood Johnson Foundation. *A Call for Proposals ... Hospital-Based Rural Health Care Program.* Princeton: The Foundation, February, 1987, p. 3.
4. Robert Wood Johnson Foundation. See 3.
5. Touche Ross. The Future of U.S. Hospitals. New York: Touche Ross, April, 1987, p. 7.
6. Robert Wood Johnson Foundation. See 3, p. 3.
7. Oklahoma Hospital Association and Price Waterhouse. Rural Hospital Survival Test. 1987, p. 1.
8. Schmitt, G. H. Multis and Small/Rural Hospitals: A Ripe Opportunity for Innovation. AHA News 23 (6): 4, 1987.
9. Kelley, E. Rural Health Care Worsening, Studies Say. The Daily Oklahoman (June 15): 1, 1987.
10. Robert Wood Johnson Foundation. See 3, p. 3.
11. American Hospital Association. *Profile of Small or Rural Hospitals 1980–1984,* Chicago: The Association, 1986, p. 2.
12. Kelley, E. See 9, p. 1.
13. American Hospital Association. See 2, p. 21.
14. American Hospital Association. Letter from Bruce Amundson to Jim Schuman. In Draft Report of the Management Strategies Subcommittee of the Special Committee on Rural Hospital Care. Chicago: The Association, March 16, 1987.

BIBLIOGRAPHY

American Hospital Association. Letter from Bruce Amundson to Jim Schuman. In Draft Report of the Management Strategies Subcommittee of the Special Committee on Rural Hospital Care. Chicago: The Association, March 16, 1987.

American Hospital Association. *Meeting the Rural Health Care Challenge.* Chicago: The Association, 1987.

American Hospital Association. Profile of Small or Rural Hospitals 1980–1984. Chicago: The Association, 1986.

American Hospital Association. Profile of Small or Rural Hospitals 1980–1984. Chicago: The Association, 1988.

Bailey, R. S. The Plight of Rural Hospitals: There's No Single Cure. *Health Management Quarterly* IX (2): 16–18, 1987.

Johnson, E. A., and R. L. Johnson. *Hospitals in Transition.* Rockville, MD: Aspen Publications, 1982.

Robert Wood Johnson Foundation. A Call for Proposals . . . Hospital-Based Rural Health Care Program. Princeton: The Foundation, 1987.

Kelley, E. Rural Health Care Worsening, Studies Say. *The Daily Oklahoman* (June 15): 1, 1987.

Kovner, A. R. *Really Trying: A Career Guide for the Health Services Manager.* Ann Arbor, MI: AUPHA Press, 1984.

Lutz, S. Rural Hospitals Offer New Services, Seek Affiliations in Effort to Survive. *Modern Healthcare* 17 (13): 30–43, 1987.

Oklahoma Hospital Association and Price Waterhouse. *Rural Hospital Survival Test.* 1987.

Schmitt, G. H. Multis and Small/Rural Hospitals: A Ripe Opportunity for Innovation. *AHA News* 23 (6): 4, 1987.

Touche Ross. The Future of U.S. Hospitals. New York: Touche Ross, April 1987.

Touche Ross. U.S. Hospitals: The Next Five Years. New York: Touche Ross, August 1986.

5

THE NURSING HOME: WHERE MANAGEMENT SHAPES THE QUALITY OF LIFE

MINER L. BROWN

AND

JOHN R. KRESS

The graying of the United States and Canada is a complicated, serious problem. It also presents an enormous challenge and opportunity for the health services administrator to apply talent and creativity to the evolution of the long-term care system including policy development, service provision, integration, financing, and quality assurance. The goal of these activities is to maintain the quality of life and optimal functioning of elderly and impaired citizens. While the terms long-term care and long-term care administration are commonly associated with the elderly and nursing homes, they encompass multiple levels of care for all age groups. They focus on chronic conditions and services which are required over an extended or continuing time period. Thus the physically handicapped, mentally impaired, physically ill, and those of all ages unable to negotiate activities of daily

Miner L. Brown is the executive director of the Jewish Center for the Aged in Chesterfield, MO. Mr. Brown holds an M.H.A. from Washington University in St. Louis, and has also received an A.B. in sociology from St. Laurence University. *John R. Kress* is director of long-term care and aging for the Association of University Programs in Health Administration in Arlington, VA. Mr. Kress holds an M.H.A. from Columbia University and a bachelor's degree in sociology from the City University of New York.

living fit into the definition of long-term care. The long-term care executive must, regardless of the service setting, be an excellent manager with special knowledge of and sensitivities to the broader life needs of the client, resident, or patient, rather than focusing solely on more narrowly defined health care needs.

LONG-TERM HEALTH CARE—AN EXPANDING HORIZON

The U.S. population, as the world population, is aging. People are living longer and the elderly represent a growing percentage of the population. The U.S. Census Bureau projects the over-65 population in the year 2020 at an estimated 51 million persons or 17 percent of the population, an increase from the current 12 percent level. The 85 and over age cohort is the fastest growing segment of the U.S. population representing 1 percent of the population in 1980 and projected to grow to 2.8 percent or 8.6 million people in 2030 [1].

Currently, life expectancy beyond age 65 for males and females is 14.4 and 18.8 years respectively [2]. Assuming continued growth in life expectancy, we will be faced with an even larger impaired population. According to the 1982 National Plan for Research on Aging, "There is no substantial evidence that the elderly of today have better or worse health than the elderly of yesterday" [3].

Over 20 percent of the U.S. population will live in nursing homes before they die. In 1980, 5.2 percent of the U.S. population resided in nursing homes (1,300,000 people). There were 19,000 nursing homes with in excess of 1,624,000 beds [4]. Growth projections for the year 2000 are estimated by some to be 1.2 million, an increase of 73 percent [4]. Nursing homes are broadening their service base beyond skilled or intermediate nursing services to include a wider array of long-term care activities. Home health services, adult day care, respite care, meals programs, assisted living, housing for the elderly, and special units or facilities for AIDS (acquired immune deficiency syndrome) patients, Alzheimer's victims, or brain-injured, and related ventures are expanding rapidly.

While nursing homes are at the center of the provision of institutionally based long-term care services, other service providers are experiencing similar growth prospects. Hospitals, whose censuses reflect a rising number of elderly patients, are looking to the aging services field for vertical integration and growth opportunities [5]. The American Hospital Association's fastest growing section is long-term care. Swing beds (as designated in a federal demonstration program permitting small rural hospitals to provide long-term care in underutilized acute care beds), nursing home services operated as separate facilities or as units of the hospital, home health services, and numerous ventures in community-based long-term care are examples of hospital-sponsored services.

Continuing care retirement communities are growing with an estimated 1,700 operating currently and 2,500 projected for the turn of the century [6]. These organized communities provide elderly citizens a full spectrum of services from independent unassisted living to skilled nursing facilities, assuring a secure environment with most needed services available for the resident, often for the duration of their lives.

Home health services, as skilled nursing facilities, have expanded dramatically since the enactment of Medicare and more recently, the institution of prospective hospital payment through the diagnosis-related group (DRG) mechanism. Some analysts estimate that there are two persons in the community who are equally impaired for every occupant of a nursing home bed. Currently, there are some 5,900 Medicare certified home care agencies and an estimated 3,700 non-certified agencies. Certification assures that a minimum predefined set of federal standards have been met by the agency before it can provide services to Medicare beneficiaries. Some researchers estimate that services by these agencies represent only 30 percent of all such care rendered, the balance provided by friends and relatives of service recipients [7].

The number of agencies and organizations providing community-based long-term care services that assist the elderly and impaired to function optimally in the home or community setting is enormous and growing. They include adult day health care centers, adult day and respite care programs, hospice services, home delivered and congregate meals, chore services, case management, housing for the elderly and assistance for living independently. All offer opportunities for the health services administrator, particularly as government and private insurers and corporate purchasers of long-term care services seek managed care opportunities through fringe benefit packages that support movement to the most appropriate level of care.

Health maintenance organizations (HMOs), long absent from the elder care market, are now moving aggressively into this area. Their penetration of the field will grow considerably along with related mechanisms of managed care. Further, the development of expanded HMO-like programs which combine long-term care with acute care, such as social HMOs and community-based life care programs, are examples of creative attempts to provide the client with a broader range of coordinated service.

Nursing home administration is a relatively new profession stimulated by the enactment of Medicare and Medicaid, requirements for state licensure, and minimum standards for management practice in skilled and intermediate care facilities. Of the 19,100 nursing homes recorded in the 1985 National Nursing Home Survey, 75 percent were proprietary. Not-for-profit and government ownership accounted for 20 and 5 percent respectively. Some 41 percent of the homes, representing 49 percent of the beds, were chain owned and operated. Chains increased nursing home ownership from 28 to 41 percent of all homes between the 1977 and 1985 National Nursing Home Surveys. Nursing home occupancy rates between the two surveys rose from 85 to 92 percent. The age of nursing home residents is increasing with the median age currently at 79 years [8].

Facilities offer a wide range of services with increasing complexity, intensity, and variety. Nursing home occupants represent differing populations. Service needs range from short-term stays of under two months for those recovering from an acute illness or other conditions requiring nursing and rehabilitation attention to those residing in the facility for the balance of their life. Some facilities specialize in treating certain conditions, for example, stroke rehabilitation, Alzheimer's-related disorders, and others. Regardless of the nature of the resident population, nursing home administrators are responsible for the quality of care in those facilities. The role of the geriatric long-term care facility administrator is unlike that of any other in the health care field and it is particularly different from a hospital administrator. Granted, significant similarities do exist and management principles and skills are transferable. However, the role is different because the needs of those being served in the two institutional settings are quite different. The acute care hospital environment is one of patient dependence, high technology, and short-term stay. The nursing home or geriatric center is occupied by residents, not patients, who fall across a broad spectrum of psychosocial, economic, and service dependency. It is a last refuge—even a home—for most residents.

Given resident stays ranging from months to years (the average length of stay is 401 days), the nursing home administrator must deal with the total life needs of residents over extended time periods [9]. The average hospital patient is discharged within a week of admission with nutritional, social, emotional, and broader needs of secondary importance in the priority of concerns for the hospital administrator. In addition to quality of care, the nursing home administrator is responsible for the resident's quality of life. The "home" in nursing home is no misnomer. The nursing home resident lives at the home, having left house and community behind. The administrator and staff must provide the qualities of family and home for persons who have nursing care needs but whose social, emotional, recreational, spiritual, nutritional, legal, financial, and related needs frequently take on equal if not greater importance. The administrator and staff must work toward maintaining the resident at the highest possible level of functioning.

The commonly held belief that quality of care equals quality of management is particularly true in the nursing home. Nursing homes are generally small (fewer than 100 beds) with limited levels of management at the facility level. The administrator, director of nursing service, and supervisors of dietary, housekeeping, and activities departments are the principal managers. Unlike their hospital counterparts, who often have associate administrative staff in addition to a wide array of expertise in numerous department heads, nursing home administrators are much closer to decisions directly affecting patient services. The nursing home administrator is less insulated from the impact of those decisions, and has greater contact with residents and their families. This contact is critical for the emotional support of both resident and family as well as for marketing and facility image building. The size of the average nursing home fosters closer ties with staff at all levels which further influences patient care.

Another major difference between the nursing home and the hospital is availability of medical support. Medical supervision of all residents is required by law, with most services provided by the nursing staff. Medical presence is considerably less evident in the nursing home than in an acute care facility. This is changing. Licensure laws, federal regulations governing nursing home operations, increased attention to geriatrics in medical school curricula, growing interest by physicians in working with nursing home residents, and an increase in the severity of illness will increase medical attention to the long-term patient. Nevertheless, nursing home administrators spend less time with physicians and with medical concerns than their acute care counterparts.

NURSING HOME MANAGEMENT TASKS

The job descriptions for nursing home chief executive officers vary considerably with facility sponsorship (private, church related, for profit), size, single versus facilities that are part of a larger system, corporation, site, or location. There are, however, several features universal to the position:

1. Accountability for defining the organization's objectives in concert with the institution's corporate leadership

2. Responsibility for assisting the board of directors in making policy decisions, participating in board committee activities, and involving board members in the institution's activities

3. Responsibility for developing, implementing, coordinating, evaluating, and modifying programs

4. Selection of senior staff and overseeing the overall human services (personnel) program

5. Accountability for fund-raising and financial management

6. Representation of the facility

7. Participation in professional long-term care organizations and civic, community, and charitable affairs

Nursing home administrators are required by federal law to be licensed by the state, the only such requirement in the health administration field. In 1985, the National Association of Boards of Examiners for Nursing Home Administrators (NAB), and the Foundation of the American College of Health Care Administrators (FACHCA), had the Professional Examination Service (PES), conduct a role delineation study of nursing home administrators. The purpose was to define the knowledge, skills, and abilities required for entry-level practice. PES isolated six "domains of practice" with attendant standards within each domain to ensure adequate practice and quality of care. The domains include: patient care; laws, regulatory codes, and governing boards; financial management; personnel management; physical resource management; and marketing and public relations. The average administrator's work day (in terms of percentage of time) was spent as follows: patient care (26 percent); personnel management (22 percent); financial management (18 percent); laws, regulatory codes, and governing boards (13 percent); marketing and public relations (10 percent); and physical resource management (10 percent). Task definitions within each domain delineated the role as follows:

1. Patient care
   a. Plan, implement, and evaluate nursing services provided to residents and patients to maintain their maximum health potential.
   b. Plan, implement, and evaluate a social services program for residents and patients that will meet their psychological and social needs and rights.
   c. Plan, implement, and evaluate a food service program designed to meet the dietary needs of residents and patients.
   d. Plan, implement, and evaluate with the medical director, a program to ensure that residents and patients receive the appropriate medical care.
   e. Plan, implement, and evaluate social and therapeutic recrea-

tional activities programs to meet the needs of residents and patients.

   f. Plan, implement, and evaluate an appropriate medical records program for resident and patient care, with consultation.

   g. Plan, implement, and evaluate a rehabilitation program that will maximize the potential of residents and patients.

2. Personnel management

   a. Create a positive atmosphere for communication between management and the work force through receptive management and the use of various media.

   b. Plan, implement, and evaluate a program that will provide an opportunity for the personal growth and development of employees through a performance evaluation process.

   c. Recruit individuals through appropriate referral sources to care for residents and patients directly or to assist in the care of residents and patients.

   d. Interview individuals to determine their suitability for employment in a nursing home.

   e. Fill vacancies by selecting prospective staff members from a pool of applicants based upon interview results.

   f. Plan, implement, and evaluate a training program to facilitate adjustment of employees to the organization and the job through appropriate educational methodology.

   g. Plan, implement, and evaluate an employee health and safety program that minimizes the nursing home's exposure to liability through an employee health and safety education program.

   h. Create personnel policies applicable to all employees to provide a basis for employee conduct and performance.

3. Financial management

   a. Develop an integrated budget for the facility to allocate fiscal resources properly, meet regulatory requirements, and provide services at a reasonable cost, using a data collection accounting system and budget format.

   b. Plan, implement, and evaluate an integrated financial plan to meet the facility's goals.

   c. Develop a cash management system, or audit the existing one, to ensure financial viability.

   d. Use generally accepted accounting principles and procedures to ensure accurate financial records.

4. Marketing and public relations

    a. Plan, implement, and evaluate a public relations program to inform and educate the public about the positive attributes of the facility.

    b. Plan, implement, and evaluate a marketing program to advertise and sell the services of the facility.

5. Physical-resource management

    a. Plan, implement, and evaluate a program for maintenance of building, grounds, and equipment.

    b. Plan, implement, and evaluate a program of environmental services that will provide a clean and attractive home for residents and patients.

    c. Plan, implement, and evaluate a safety program that will ensure the health, welfare, and safety of residents, patients, staff, and visitors.

    d. Plan, implement, and evaluate a fire and disaster policy to protect the safety and welfare of residents, patients, staff, and property.

6. Laws, regulatory codes, and governing boards

    a. Plan, implement, and evaluate policies and procedures that are in compliance with federal laws and regulations.

    b. Plan, implement, and evaluate policies and procedures that are in compliance with directives of the governing boards [10].

Clearly, the role delineation study and standards support the contention of nursing home administrators that their relationship to patients, staff, residents, and direct care is closer than their acute care hospital counterparts and that the corresponding impact of their decisions has more direct implications for patient care.

NURSING HOME ADMINISTRATION— AN EXPANDING HORIZON

The maturing profession of nursing home administration is evolving in two directions; it is becoming more specific and complex at the facility level while encompassing a broader range of services as nursing homes enter the world of housing, social health maintenance organizations, respite programs, hospice care, home health care, long-term health care insurance, and planned community development, among others. The field offers a tremendous diversity of size, corporate complexity, and specialization. These practice areas are expanding in an era of major demographic upheaval and heightened realization of service need.

A great deal of mythology surrounds the environment called a nursing home. Many popular conceptions are archaic and outmoded. The nursing home is defined in numerous governmental regulations, zoning ordinances, licensing rules, and reimbursement documents which attempt to express what long-term care facilities are, definitions projecting both positive and negative images. The most important issue, however, is what takes place in and through the institution, its staff, and programs. Herein lie the challenges that make the nursing home administrator's job so exciting. Herbert Shore, the executive director of Golden Acres, the Dallas Home for Jewish Aged and a professor at North Texas State University, expressed it well when he wrote "The major challenge is to provide for a continuity of life experience—but meaningful life—with freedom of choice, when and if to participate—a program of social health, personal identity, independence, privacy, stability, self direction, re-engagement, rediscovery, reinstitution of normal elements of daily social living" [11].

The process by which a person selects and pursues a vocation or profession is a very personal one. The pattern varies as widely as the personalities involved. Historically, many long-term care administrators entered this field by some twist of fate or chance. Their backgrounds varied from minister and social worker to nurse and businessman. That is no longer the case. Now most nursing home administrators have at least a bachelor's degree with some exposure to gerontology. The trend is toward a master's degree in health care administration with an emphasis in long-term care and gerontology. In looking back over my (Brown) career pathway, the decision-making process was a combination of both planning and fate.

I originally entered the hospital administration field because I was committed to being part of a Gemeinschaft—a community of shared beliefs, values, ideals. Over the years, I observed a shift to a Gesellschaft environment—an impersonal setting requiring a strict codification of rules where trust could not be assumed. Numerous careers encompass a community of shared beliefs, values, and ideas; why long-term care management? There was a time when I saw no challenge and little future in managing the care of institutionally bound old people. Raised in a small village in upstate New York where our father served as the only physician covering a large geographic area, the importance of community service was instilled in us, through parental example at an early age. I can recall assisting my father as he placed casts on broken legs and holding a child so that an open wound could be sutured. The need to pursue a helping profession grew.

Entering a small liberal arts college, I explored various interests as a sociology major with minors in business and history. My varied interests in business, community organization, and health converged and I began to give thought to a career called hospital administration, having worked summers as a recreational therapist and as stores clerk at a local hospital. As a senior, I took courses in physiology and accounting expecting they would be helpful in defining a career direction. I applied to graduate schools with little guidance, and in retrospect, less than a full understanding of their requirements. My applications were rejected. In one rejection letter, the program director suggested that I look into a specially designed hospital personnel internship which was then offered at Aultman Hospital, a teaching institution, located in Canton, Ohio. My application was accepted for a one-year internship and it was during this experience that I came under the mentorship of the hospital's director. This exposure prompted my re-application and subsequent acceptance by several graduate schools; I chose to attend Washington University in St. Louis, entering as the second youngest graduate student, but with a well-developed appreciation of the hospital environment.

Following graduate studies, I served as an administrative resident at Cedars of Lebanon Hospital in Miami, Florida, where I remained as administrative assistant for an additional year. I moved on to serve as administrative assistant at the 300-bed State University Hospital of the Upstate Medical Center in Syracuse, New York, where I remained for three years. Then I joined an exciting program at Marlborough Hospital in the Greater Boston Area, starting as assistant, and later becoming the associate director. While relatively small in size, 153 beds, the hospital had a complete management engineering program, the first hospitalwide education department in the New England area, was on its third generation of computers, and had a unique planning and building program which featured a team representing four consulting firms, architects, and hospital management. However, as a direct result of a significant decrease in hospital utilization, the expansion program was ended after the schematic design phase was completed, and I began to plan to relocate. Each of the preceding positions were carefully selected to provide different management responsibilities in different settings under different sponsorships.

I now felt well equipped to assume a hospital administrator position, but it was unlikely that I could land one in the New England area at the age of 31 and I was hesitant to uproot my family. So, I accepted a lateral move to a hospital in an adjoining community. Just three weeks later, I was approached by the director of a large teaching geriatric center (475 beds) in Boston. The result was an offer to join that facility as assistant director. After much soul searching, I joined the Hebrew Rehabilitation Center for the Aged. I did so for four reasons: an opportunity to learn about a new field, an invitation to join a nationally acclaimed facility, a chance to serve an ethnically compatible population, and a growing feeling that the higher I moved in the hospital hierarchy, the more impersonal the environment became.

I have never for one moment regretted making that professional career move. Long-term care administration has changed significantly in the 15 years since, and the career potential offered is more promising today than it was then. The number and variety of positions, along with the prestige afforded is higher. Nursing home administrators enjoy the respect of their hospital peers and the general public because of the great strides and positive achievements made in long-term care institutions. With increased recognition has come commensurate salary and benefits packages, which are always important factors in career decisions.

FUTURE PROSPECTS

Employment possibilities in long-term care will continue to grow. At the facility level, job titles include assistant, associate, and chief executive positions. As nursing homes expand in size and complexity, the number of associate and assistant administrator positions will also expand. Within multifacility nursing home or chain organizations, whether not-for-profit or proprietary in sponsorship, employment opportunities include positions at the facility, regional, and corporate levels. The regional level positions generally include responsibility for supervising multiple nursing homes within a given geographic area and require a knowledge of facility operations as well as broader management skills. Corporate headquarters positions are also available for those with the requisite skills and expertise.

Executives with nursing home administrator training and experience are sought increasingly by other organizations. As hospitals, continuing care retirement communities, residential care, and related programs expand to offer skilled or intermediate nursing facility services, they often must place a licensed nursing home administrator in charge of their long-term care services to obtain certification for Medicare or Medicaid reimbursement. As marketing directors and strategic planners search for new venture opportunities, they are turning to nursing home administrators for consultation and assistance. Rather than staying in a "dead-end job," those with this dimension to their health services administration preparation can capitalize on the growing advantages in the broader market. Wage and fringe benefit packages, which traditionally have lagged behind their hospital counterparts, have improved dramatically over the past few years. According to a recent survey conducted by the ACHCA, the average nursing home administrator compensation package is $45,000 ranging from $25,000 to $70,000 and is related directly to education, previous experience, and the size, type, and location of the long-term care facility [12]. Significantly higher salary ranges can be found in the larger multilevel teaching nursing homes.

Students interested in long-term care should seek field experience through a residency or postgraduate fellowship in a nursing home setting to provide exposure to the special qualities of management practice found therein. The field work should be coupled with the administrator-in-training (AIT) requirements for licensure in many states. State licensure requirements often dictate the minimum preparation required of entry level administrators. Since state requirements differ dramatically, aspirants should discuss regulations early in their academic career and as part of their choice of academic programs.

The NAB has recommended that the baccalaureate degree be the minimum entry level academic preparation for nursing home administrators. Those who plan to work in this field should choose a program with a focus on applications of management disciplines to long-term care. Special grounding in gerontological issues, interpreted as the social, psychological, physical, and related needs of the elderly or chronically impaired person, is highly recommended.

In summary, you will find successful nursing home administrators who are quiet, somber, and reserved and others who are exuberant and determined. Occasionally, you will see a charismatic personality. But you will find them all enthusiastic. They love their work, they care for the residents they serve, and they respect their employees. Further, successful administrators possess the critical elements of a clear sense of purpose and direction, a good sense of priorities and balance, and a sense of humor.

The field of nursing home administration is changing rapidly, demanding leaders who possess both managerial excellence and sensitivity to the multifaceted needs of the elderly resident. As the population ages, you have the opportunity to join in the design of the programs which enhance the quality of life and provide the quality of service which our elderly citizens need and deserve.

REFERENCES

1. U.S. Senate Special Committee on Aging/American Association of Retired Persons. Aging America: Trends and Projections. Washington, DC, Undated, 3-18.
2. U.S. Senate Special Committee on Aging/American Association of Retired Persons. Aging America: Trends and Projections. Washington, DC, Undated, 11.

3. National Research on Aging Planning Panel. *Toward an Independent Old Age: A National Plan for Research on Aging*. U.S. DHHS Pub. No. (NIH) 82–2453, Washington, DC: U.S. Government Printing Office, 1982.

4. Strahan, Genevieve. Nursing Home Characteristics: Preliminary Data From The 1985 National Nursing Home Survey U.S. Department of Health and Human Service. NCHS Advanced Data 131 (March 27): 1987.

5. Valiente, John D., The Capital Requirements for Long-Term Care Services. In Long Term Care: Challenges and Opportunities. A 16-Article Compilation from Healthcare Financial Management. Healthcare Financial Management Association. Oak Brook, IL, 1985, 38-42.

6. Valiente, John D. See number 5.

7. Doty, Pamela, Korbin Liu and Joshua Wiener. An Overview of Long-Term Care. *Health Care Financing Review* (Spring): 70, 1985.

8. National Center for Health Statistics. U.S. Department of Health & Human Services. *1985 National Nursing Home Survey*. Unpublished data.

9. See number 8.

10. Schoon, C.G. and S.K. Hayez. The Entry-Level Role of Nursing Home Administrators. *The Journal of Long-Term Care Administration* (Fall): 16, 1987.

11. Shore, Herbert, Ed.D. "Improving the Quality of Life for the Aged, The Changes of the Seventies," in *Adventures in Group Living* by Herbert Shore, Ed.D. and the Staff of Golden Acres, The Dallas Home for Jewish Aged. Dallas, Golden Acres, 1972.

12. American College of Health Care Administrators. Are You Considering A Career In Long-Term Health Care Administration? Bethesda, MD: The College, no date.

6

MENTAL HEALTH SERVICES: THE SYSTEM AND ITS MANAGEMENT MOVE TO THE MAINSTREAM

AARON LIBERMAN, Ph.D.

The expanding managerial specialty of mental health administration offers unlimited potential for professional involvement and personal growth. It affords the conscientious executive opportunities for steady advancement, job satisfaction, and contact with intelligent and dedicated professionals. The consequent psychic income represents an incentive for an enduring commitment to service.

At the same time, it is important to note that contemporary mental health administration has evolved considerably from the once held perception of the manager as an order giver in the most traditional of senses. Today, the successful mental health administrator employs a multiplicity of skills which encompass entrepreneurship, risk and insurance management, marketing theory, financial and strategic planning, and human resources administration. Together and in concert with one another, these skills form the nucleus for dealing with a watchword of 1980s style leadership—management competition [1].

Aaron Liberman is an associate professor of public administration and director of the Bureau of Business Research and Services at California State University, Dominguez Hills. Dr. Liberman is also the president of Health System Reviews, Inc., an insurance and risk management consulting firm located in Mission Viejo, CA and holds an M.A. and Ph.D. in health administration from the University of Iowa. He also holds an A.B. in psychology from Baylor University and an M.S. in psychology from Indiana University.

This chapter will review the characteristics of mental health administration as a specialty of health services administration. Analysis of the relationship between mental health itself and the administration of services to mentally ill patients will show how the competent administrator can facilitate the clinical process. Comments on academic and experiential preparation for mental health administration and remarks on applying human relations skills are included in this initial section. Succeeding sections will speak of the social value of mental health administration to the patient and to society. Other later sections will discuss ethical practices, the politics of administration, and job mobility.

As a beginning, it is essential to acquaint the prospective administrator with the evolution of mental health administration as a component of health administration. Therefore, a brief historical perspective of the mental health movement follows.

AN ORGANIZED MOVEMENT

The beginnings of an organized mental health movement in the United States have been traced to Clifford Beers, who in 1908 founded the first state mental health association, the Connecticut Society for Mental Hygiene [2]. Through his personal experience as a patient, Beers had become acutely aware of the wretched conditions existing in the institutions of the day, detailed in this book, *A Mind That Found Itself*.

One of the earliest federal activities in mental health was medical inspection of immigrants arriving at our nation's eastern seaports during the period of highest influx, 1900 to 1920. Brand has cited the high rate of immigrant admissions to mental hospitals as evidence of the seriousness of mental illness as a national health problem [3].

The first noninstitutional (outpatient) psychiatric clinic was established in 1909 at the Institute of Juvenile Research in Chicago. Within a relatively short period of time a philosophy embracing the psychiatric clinic as a social institution began to take hold. The appearance of demonstration clinics in 1922 and the founding of the American Psychiatric Association in 1927 added impetus to this philosophical orientation [4].

Mental health was relegated to a position of lesser importance in the midst of the nation's preoccupation with economic survival during the Great Depression years and later in relation to the problems of social and cultural survival during the Second World War. Nevertheless, the seeds for an organized community mental health movement had been sown.

Daniels suggested that much of the communitywide approach to mental health began in the practice of psychiatric medicine during the war. Physicians not only provided clinical services to the individual soldier but also advised the general command about such matters as the organization of psychiatric and social services, education for soldiers, policy formulation, and problems of morale. Daniels had intimated that herein was the forerunner of the therapeutic communities, milieu therapy, the open hospital system, and tranquilizing drugs [5].

At the end of World War II, the National Committee for Mental Hygiene convened in Hershey, Pennsylvania, to discuss the question of postwar psychiatric rehabilitation. In attendance were distinguished health leaders who had been summoned from throughout the nation. The committee was faced with numerous problems. Some 500,000 servicemen had been discharged from active duty during the war and subsequently classified as psychiatric casualties. An additional 1,750,000 men had been rejected by the respective military service branches for failing to meet the minimum personality or mental health standards for admission. Only 4,000 psychiatrists existed at this time in the entire United States.

An additional 10,000 clinicians would have been needed just to meet the immediate postwar needs of the country. Institutions began seriously to consider using nonmedical administrators to free physicians for more direct patient care.

Moreover, facilities were inadequate owing to the geographic isolation of mental hospitals with advanced scientific standards, the social stigma attached to mental deficiencies and emotional disturbances, and the lack of adequate financial support. In addition, the capacity for research and training was severely limited [6].

A published report of the National Committee for Mental Hygiene directed public awareness to the need for increased research, training, and services in all phases of mental health. Subsequent demands for action led to the eventual passage of the National Mental Health Act of 1946. "Under this legislation, the federal government launched a major program of support for specific projects and assistance to states and privately supported institutions" [7].

As a result of this legislation, the National Institute of Mental Health (NIMH), founded in 1949, was assigned responsibility for the following: (1) assisting in the development of state and community mental health services; (2) supporting research into the causes, prevention, and treatment of mental illness; and (3) supporting the training of psychiatrists, psychologists, psychiatric social workers, and psychiatric nurses [8].

NIMH assisted the states in upgrading local mental health activities and planning programs by allocating federal funds according to population and financial need.

A COMMUNITY-BASED APPROACH TO MENTAL HEALTH SERVICES

The founding of NIMH marked the official entry of the term "community" as a conceptual framework for treatment and prevention. Previously, a traditional institutional approach had been employed. Clinicians and administrators alike began to recognize the importance of fostering a comprehensive approach to providing mental health services. The change in focus added complexities to the delivery of services and directed attention to the need for competent administration and well-trained mental health administrators.

President Dwight D. Eisenhower established a Joint Commission on Mental Illness and Health in 1955. This working group assessed the nation's mental health needs and recommended a series of new approaches to bring about an improved system of health care. So extensive was the approach taken that six years were required to collect and collate the full text of the report. When published in 1961, *Action for Mental Health* "shocked the nation into a new awareness of the need to improve mental health services" [9].

The Kennedy Administration expressed deep concern about the Commission's findings. In his 1963 message to Congress the President called for "a new type of health facility, one which will return mental health care to the mainstream of American medicine and at the same time upgrade mental health services" [10]. Congress responded to the President's plea by passing Public Law 88–164, which authorized $150 million for fiscal years 1965 through 1967 to assist in the construction of community mental health centers which were intended to form the nucleus of the new federal program [11].

The development of community-based programs did provide an alternative resource to an overburdened and complacent state hospital system but the establishment of community-based resources did not include an infrastructure through which persons discharged from state hospitals could readily be admitted to a community program. This in turn resulted in a hailstorm of controversy as well as a concerted call for more stringent controls on the development of and decision making in community mental health programs.

In 1972, Morgan Martin, Superintendent of Norwich Hospital in Norwich, Connecticut, cited several of what he called "big ideas" that community mental health programs had developed. They were identified as accessibility, availability, and equity of care without regard for ability to pay; provision of adequate living conditions within each program; total population coverage and an ample opportunity for community involvement in treatment and evaluation programs; primary programs for prevention; continuity of responsibility for care; and better use of state mental hospitals.

Essentially, Martin seemed to be most concerned about the overlap in responsibilities between state institutions and community programs in the absence of adequate cooperation and coordination. He also criticized the existence of state hospitals and community mental health centers as separate functioning systems. Truly coming to grips with the issues as they affected both community- and state-operated programs, he felt, would mandate cooperation between the community-based endeavors and the state hospital systems [12].

Further complicating the matter of program development is the controversy surrounding the funding and marketing of mental health programs. The reality of the 1980s is that there are fewer financing alternatives outside of an increased census of patients. Additionally, the competition for patient dollars is demanding that providers establish more flexible admissions criteria and more attractive program alternatives. This in turn has led to creative marketing practices and an increased emphasis on program accessibility. This traditional approach to marketing attaches significant importance to project development, services management, and sales development [13].

Much of the emphasis on marketing practices in mental health has been exemplified by a renewed goal of achieving a true continuity of care along with developing the internal mechanics to guide program development [14]. One of the stark realities being played out is the fact that as few as 5 percent of those persons with serious mental and emotional problems receive any community support or rehabilitation [15].

SIGNIFICANCE OF LEGAL ACTIONS

Much of the current concern about the cost and accessibility of care has resulted from several individual state and court decisions regarding the care and treatment of patients on a long-term basis in state hospitals and in other mental health facilities. In Massachusetts, for example, a 1971 law provides that an involuntary commitment in a state facility is limited to those cases in which there is a substantial likelihood of serious harm to the individual or to others. The law further ensures early discharge and follow-up services in the community.

Possibly the most significant actions, with ramifications affecting virtually all facets of cost and quality of mental health care today, was the landmark decision handed down by Alabama Federal District Judge Frank Johnson in a case styled *Wyatt* v. *Stickney* [16]. Foremost in the jurist's decision was a finding that there exists a constitutional right to adequate treatment for those who are involuntarily institutionalized. In addition, Judge Johnson set forth the following guidelines involving patient rights: a humane psychological and physical environment; a qualified staff in sufficient numbers to provide treatment; and a requirement of individual treatment plans for each patient [17].

Implicit in this historical perspective is an appeal for continuity and access to patient care throughout the domain of mental health services.

RELATIONSHIP OF ADMINISTRATION TO THE PROVISION OF MENTAL HEALTH SERVICES

There is a consensus that more effective working relationships need to be established among the disparate programs that provide complementary and competing services to the mentally and emotionally disturbed. This is consistent with the need to eliminate costly duplication of health services. The mental health administrator needs to expand working relationships with related agencies. Thoughtful referrals, admissions, and transfer agreements between long-term care programs, such as state hospitals, and community-based programs can exert a positive effect on quality of care and on control of costs.

IMPLICATIONS OF HEALTH SERVICES ADMINISTRATOR'S INVOLVEMENT

It was once not uncommon for physicians to serve both as primary therapists and as administrators of mental health programs. At times they established a rigid pecking order. With the maturation of the community mental health movement, the power position of the psychiatrist began to shift, and other clinical professionals have emerged as clinical and administrative partners. The role of social workers, psychologists, and nurses has become more prominent. The shift has helped create a breach between those clinicians who favor the traditional medical model of treatment and management and those who endorse a social process model [18].

Strain inevitably has developed in many state institutions. Some who found themselves on the defensive correctly interpreted community mental health as an instrument that would close state hospitals and return mentally impaired people to the community where they could live and function while receiving ongoing care. Indeed, this philosophy eventually became one important outcome measure of effectiveness of the community program in various locales.

It is essential that the mental health administrator work closely with the clinical practitioner to enhance the quality of care. At best, the two should be able to give and take advice and criticism, although conflicts sometimes arise when the practitioner and administrator view their areas of responsibility as overlapping.

The clinician may develop a protective relationship with the patient and be simultaneously protective of professional prerogatives. The administrator may try to modify the behavior of the clinician on behalf of the patient. The clinician may judge such an attempt on the part of the administrator to be illegitimate and incursive. It is incumbent upon both the clinician and the administrator, each acting in good faith, to be sensitive to one another's professional needs. Taking precedence over all of these needs, of course, are the needs of the patient whom both claim to serve. The challenge to the mental health administrator becomes one of assisting the clinician to work through clinical difficulties and circumvent organizational blocks in order to achieve the objective of the organization—the best possible care for the mentally ill.

Achieving common objectives requires a thoughtful process of planning and goal development with the active participation of clinical and administrative personnel at all levels of the organization. This places clinicians and administrators in like positions of contributing to their future as members of an agency's professional team. It further establishes a contractual form of obligation in which the planning and goal attainment process becomes an end result toward which all members of the staff have committed themselves. The services which thus emerge have a higher probability of representing a quality product for the benefit of the community.

PREPARATION OF THE MENTAL HEALTH ADMINISTRATOR

Future mental health administrators would be well advised to take formal courses relating to clinical practice, general psychology, and human resources administration. Moreover, the importance of certain strictly managerial areas of knowledge deserves reiteration here: included are personnel administration, policy analysis, health economics, data processing, statistics, marketing, and financial management [19].

A frequently observed fault of the young mental health administrator is the lack of fundamental writing and verbal skills. In a field notorious for its jargon, clarity of expression is particularly essential. Excellent writing and verbal skills will complement one's ability to plan, organize, and direct a staff. This point was emphasized some years ago when several scholars representing the fields of psychiatry, psychology, and social work were victims of an instructive hoax. The speaker, a dynamic man who professed to be an expert, was an impostor with a gift for verbal fluff. The responses to his presentation were overwhelmingly favorable, and the resulting paper describing this folly became known as the Dr. Fox Paradigm [20].

Other academic preparation one might undertake to secure a position in mental health administration depends upon individual circumstances and needs. Premedical students, aspiring psychologists, business administration candidates, and others who have reconsidered their academic and career goals may be found among the ranks of those destined to become future leaders in mental health administration.

The professional administrator with a master's degree will understandably doubt the abilities of anyone who has not received graduate training in health services administration. On the other hand, formal education in mental health administration is no substitute for instructive experience under professional supervision in the real world of work.

SOCIAL VALUE OF MENTAL HEALTH ADMINISTRATION

The mental health administrator should ponder how contributions to the organization reflect the stress put upon maintaining human dignity in our political system. It needs to be remembered from time to time that serving the patient is the overt, professional raison d'être of the mental health administrator.

The social value of managerial performance is closely related to the administrator's attentiveness to detail—a most important consideration as the complexities of the mental health agency increase. For example, the seemingly mundane accomplishment of reducing the patient's waiting time by improving scheduling will contribute to more responsive and more efficiently delivered care. Improved administrative practices can motivate employees to deal more humanely with patients and can do a great deal to improve the public's current perception of today's health services as being largely inaccessible and impersonal.

Mental illness not only affects the person suffering from the problems but also a large number of people who are either influenced by or are directly related to that person. Mental and emotional problems, if unchecked, can debilitate an entire family. The family can lose potential income, and their contacts with others can be severely disrupted. Transferring the disturbed person from that environment to a long-term care institution can alleviate some of the more immediate short-range problems affecting the family unit.

On the other hand, the long-term effects of losing an integral family member can harm other members of the family unit, particularly children. An agency's ability to keep a mentally ill person functioning in the community can lessen the probability of a complete breakdown within that family unit and the consequent problems with other family members which then may adversely affect still other people in that community. The dedicated mental health administrator contributes to the larger social universe by establishing workable, efficient, and effective therapeutic and preventive systems in mental health.

STRENGTHS REQUIRED OF THE MENTAL HEALTH ADMINISTRATOR

In mental health administration, as in all areas of health administration, the executive needs to develop those skills that strengthen human relations within an organization. Successful mental health administration depends on the proper management of human resources—perhaps the most challenging requirement placed upon a manager. In the course of managing an organization that furnishes mental health services to its clientele, as much as 75 percent of a typical work day may be devoted to decision making directly involving employees and their interrelationships.

Invariably some employees become rankled when particular decisions affect their professional lives and their livelihood. It is prudent to anticipate people's predictable reactions to a particular issue and to take action preventing breakdown in communication. Such a management philosophy requires that the administrator solicit and include staff opinions when developing plans for a major policy shift or a program recommendation. Few other areas of health administration can be more perilous to an administrator's ability to function than the failure to deal with the human needs of the organization. No academic sequence exists that will guarantee success in dealing with employees. Most human relations skills require on-the-job learning. *Remember always: Good judgment comes from experience; experience comes from bad judgment.*

Every successful executive has learned to live within budgetary considerations. Herzlinger has suggested that "perhaps the most important step administrators can take is in educating doctors and other providers of care in economics and aspects of management" [21]. If providers remain ignorant about their impact on costs, they may remain convinced that only administrators affect cost of care. The potential administrator needs both to learn financial management at an academic level and to translate these academic skills into the ability to draw from colleagues the desire to serve the organization's objectives.

The administrator must also assess employee performance. Rensis Likert has stated: "Clearly there is a need to help supervisors and managers to appreciate deficiencies which can and should be corrected" [22]. This may be approached by developing evaluation procedures which objectify as much as possible the process of assessing employee performance. An evaluation can be used to develop a consistent system of wage and salary administration. This in turn assists the staff to view realistically their relative positions and their future with the organization.

The mental health administrator who is able to develop and implement complementary systems such as fiscal controls and employee management procedures can largely chart a pattern of success for the mental health agency. This is particularly true when the financial impact of the employee's salary upon the budget of the organization is to be considered. The less subjective the management practices of an organization, the greater will be its credibility with employees.

Another professional strength required of managers is related to ethical practices. Ethics refer both to the business and management practices of the organization. Sound ethical practices carry implications which reverberate throughout the mental health agency and the health industry as a whole. Medicare and Medicaid abuses by hospital and by clinicians have been notorious. Understandably, the regulatory bodies governing the practices of the nation's health organizations have tightened their powers of oversight and evaluation. In mental health administration, strong ethical practices are synonymous with good management.

THE POLITICS OF MENTAL HEALTH ADMINISTRATION

The political process is nothing foreign to the world of health administration. With the advent of federal involvement in our nation's financing and delivery systems, principally in Medicare and Medicaid programs, the intensity and scope of political practices have escalated. Today, health care providers engage in intensive lobbying efforts which rival those of almost any member of our nation's military and industrial complex.

The organized efforts of mental health supporters to influence governmental actions at the federal, state, and local levels extend back many years. But the politics of mental health go well beyond the efforts of organized interest groups to influence favorably the actions of federal and state legislative bodies. Political activities include board and staff relations, community affairs, and interorganizational relationships.

At the board level, politics are a pervasive and integral part of managing a mental health program. In community programs where board members are selected from among citizen representatives, the administrator must respond to a diversity of views. Often individual board members represent special interest groups which in turn have several concerns in need of conscientious expression. How well managers relate to the board of directors may inevitably determine their professional survival.

Sometimes training or interests may cloud the judgment of board members. In one situation involving the author, a board member who was of an ethnic minority was interested in protecting the rights of all minority staff members. This board member was asked to serve on the personnel committee, where he could oversee on a first-hand basis all activities affecting the employee relations program. This assignment purposefully channeled the energies of the board member in a constructive direction, and in turn encouraged a responsible approach to the adjudication of most employee matters. In short, an administrator must understand motivations and work closely with board members in policymaking to achieve the organization's aims.

Intermeshed with governing board politics are those activities which influence staff relations both directly and indirectly. In mental health, as in other facets of the health field, staff members often have their own political constituencies both within and outside the agency structure. Consequently, the rapport existing between the executive and the staff is most important in ensuring continuing forward movement for the mental health agency.

Committees are not the most efficient way to administer a mental health program, nor do they facilitate decision making. However, they do maintain a flow of communication. Staff members who are intimately involved in helping to formulate decisions affecting an organization are much more supportive of their administration and leader.

Staff members and board members will communicate on an informal level no matter how rigid the formal communication network of the organization may be. It is prudent for the mental health administrator to recognize those relationships and to use them to further the agency's best interests. Such an effort not only maintains harmony between the board and the executive, but also produces timely and informal feedback about cogent matters.

One potentially major problem area can, if ignored, hobble the administrator and the agency: the antipathy that can arise between the executive and the board. Sometimes when individual board members become disenchanted with the performance of their executive, rather than facing the problem on a formal level with all board members in attendance, they may choose to leak the news to the community. Such public displays can only be a detriment to the management and operation of the agency.

The board's politics and community relations are closely related, since most board members belong to the community and represent at least a portion of that community. Such relationships in mental health have been further enhanced by the formation of mandated advisory committees to provide boards of trustees with citizens' views on the development and implementation of mental health services. While this phenomenon may seem to constitute a threat to the executive's authority, if properly used, it can ensure a flow of information between the board and the community.

Another facet of community relations to be weighed by the administrator is the role played by groups such as mental health associations and associations for retarded citizens. These associations represent the interests of afflicted persons both before the mental health organization and its board of trustees and among legislators at the federal and state levels.

Frequently, inadequate relationships between complementary and otherwise competing mental health organizations can cause tension. State hospitals, under political and financial pressures to reduce patient census, may discharge patients before they are ready to be returned to the community. Without formal referral, admission, and discharge agreements between state hospital systems and community agencies, these patients can easily be lost. This lack of integration not only creates a source of friction but also exacerbates competition for federal and state dollars. In recent years efforts to achieve better interagency coordination are slowly resulting in a more rational deployment of services—but there is a long way to go.

The new mental health administrator, then, has a chance to practice diverse management techniques which actualize the political process on behalf of patients. Included in the commitment to make the system of health care work for the people are the following elements: the positive use of board members, the mobilization of staff members to provide quality information and services, the maximization of community resources to ensure that the message of community need is present in the minds of lawmakers, and, finally, the use of interagency relationships to further the provisions of health.

MOBILITY AND CAREER ADVANCEMENT

In recent years mental health administrators' salaries have risen significantly, in part due to a recognition of the importance of the administrator in making the patient services process work for patients and their families. Occasionally administrators may have to change jobs in order to increase their income. Some administrators have done well financially by remaining in place and qualifying for seniority and merit salary increases. At present, opportunities in the field are numerous, with chances for advancement depending on the personal aspirations and conscientiousness of the individual candidate.

The modern mental health administrator must become accustomed to working and surviving in a professional care-giving world marked by advancing technology, an omnipotent political process, and sometimes abrasive interpersonal relationships within a community services structure. Armed with patience, understanding, perseverance, and optimism, the mental health administrator will successfully manage the systems of care for the mentally ill and help alleviate their psychosocial disabilities.

REFERENCES

1. Shalowitz, D. Competition Can Control Costs: Professor. *Business Insurance*, July 13, 1987, 63.
2. Ridenour, N. *Mental Health in the United States: A Fifty Year History*. Cambridge, MA: Harvard University Press, 1961, 1.
3. Brand, J. L. The United States: A Historical Perspective. In *Community Mental Health: An International Perspective*, eds. R. H. Williams and L. D. Ozarin, 18–44. San Francisco: Jossey-Bass, Inc., 1968.
4. N.Y. State Department of Mental Hygiene. *A Guide to Communities in the Establishment and Operation of Psychiatric Clinics*. New York: The Department, 1959, 1.
5. Daniels, R. S. Community Psychiatry—A New Profession, A Developing Subspecialty or Effective Clinical Psychiatry? *Community Mental Health Journal* 2 (Spring): 51, 1966.
6. Annual Report. National Committee for Mental Hygiene, Inc. Finding a Way in Mental Hygiene. New York: The Committee, 1945, 2.
7. U.S. Department of Health, Education and Welfare. *The National Mental Health Program and the States*. Washington, D.C.: The Department, 1965, 11.
8. U.S. Department of Health, Education and Welfare. *Mental Illness and Its Treatment: Past and Present*. Washington, D.C.: The Department, 1965, 11.
9. U.S. Department of Health, Education and Welfare. See 8.
10. Ansberry, C. Community Facilities for the Mentally Ill Are Few and Overburdened. *The Wall Street Journal* 117 (September 25): 1, 1987.
11. U.S. Department of Health, Education and Welfare. *Community Mental Health Advances*. Bethesda, MD: The Department, 1964, 1.
12. Martin, M. Community Mental Health Centers: Coming to Grips with Big Ideas. *American Journal of Psychiatry* 129 (August): 126, 1972.
13. Super, K. and R. Mazzoni. Marketing, Take Two. *Modern Healthcare* 17 (April 10): 46, 1987.
14. Landsberg, G., R. Fletcher, and T. Maxwell. Developing a Comprehen-

sive Care System for the Mentally Ill, Retarded. *Community Mental Health Journal* 23 (September): 132, 1987.

15. Ansberry, C. See 10.

16. Wyatt v. Stickney, 325 F. Supp. 781 (D.C. Ala. 1971).

17. Johnson, R. and M. Fraser. Right to Treatment. *Mental Hygiene* 56 (Summer): 13–16, 1972.

18. William Nathan, Chairman of the Board, Vista Health Corporation, Los Angeles, California, 1987. Personal Communication, January 20, 1988.

19. Super, K. and R. Mazzoni. See 13.

20. Naftulin, D. H., J. E. Ware, Jr., and F. A. Donelly. The Dr. Fox Lecture: A Paradigm of Educational Seduction. *Journal of Medical Education* 68 (July): 630–35, 1973.

21. Herzlinger, R. Can We Control Health Care Costs? *Harvard Business Review* 56 (March-April): 108, 1978.

22. Likert, R. Motivational Approach to Management Development. *Guideposts to Executive Growth*. Cambridge, MA: Harvard University Press, 1965, 25.

PART III

NONINSTITUTIONAL SERVICES

7

MANAGED CARE: ADMINISTERING EMERGING COMPREHENSIVE CARE SYSTEMS

GAIL L. WARDEN

While the clinical practice of medicine has experienced unprecedented change in recent times, so too has there been revolutionary change in both the organization and financing of health services. Many of these remarkable and fortuitous changes have occurred in the field of managed health care. Significant victories in the cost containment war and the ongoing effort to lead the population into healthier lifestyles are being won by managed health care organizations. Today, the managed care sector of health administration offers a broad assortment of employment opportunities on the forefront of a rapidly evolving industry. This chapter discusses managed care systems from three perspectives: first, their historical development, growth, and key characteristics; second, their unique attributes as compared with common forms of health services organization, including descriptions of key jobs within them; and third, an evaluation of career opportunities within them.

THE MANAGED CARE MOVEMENT AND ITS HISTORY

Managed, or prepaid health care, today accounts for a substantial and rapidly growing segment of the health care establishment. But this was not always so. As a method of organizing the financing and delivery of health

Gail L. Warden is president and chief executive officer of Henry Ford Health Care Corporation in Detroit, MI. He received an M.H.A. from the University of Michigan and also holds a B.A. degree from Dartmouth College.

services, the managed care movement began as an alternative and routinely embattled exile from the traditional world of fee-for-service medicine.

The idea of delivering a slate of health care services as needed, over time, and for a fee set in advance first became a reality in the United States during the 18th century. In fact, the Colonial army was served by physicians who worked under contract. Dr. Benjamin Rush, a signer of the Declaration of Independence, organized this provider group and also served as a participating physician [1].

Despite recurring protests from vocal and well-organized segments of the fee-for-service medical establishment, the prepaid movement grew. By 1929, the first of what came to be called HMOs (health maintenance organizations) was organized by Dr. Michael Shadid in Elk City, Oklahoma. But it was not until 1933 that Dr. Sidney Garfield put together the first HMO that resembles contemporary descendants. Dr. Garfield combined medical group practice with an insurance component to provide a wide slate of prepaid health services. This organizational form is considered to be the true ancestor of managed care systems because Dr. Garfield's creation was both insurer and provider of those medical services. Dr. Garfield later became a cofounder of what is today the largest managed care organization in the country—the Kaiser Foundation Health Plan of California with nearly four million subscribers.

By 1987, approximately 660 health systems were operating in the United States on the basis of prepayment [2]. Although these systems have traditionally been called HMOs, or health maintenance organizations, this term no longer reflects the breadth and scope of prepaid practices. Many feel it is more accurate to use the term "managed care organization" (MCO) to define the group. Canada and the United Kingdom sponsor managed care systems covering the health care needs of all citizens.

CHARACTERISTICS OF MANAGED CARE SYSTEMS

A managed care system may be broadly defined as a single legal entity that has assumed responsibility for both financing and providing a defined slate of health care and related services to its enrollees. Instead of paying for services as they are rendered, as in the fee-for-service world, members of managed care systems prepay for services in the form of dues. Dues are usually collected monthly. Enrollment within the system entitles members to receive all health services covered by the plan as need arises, and at no extra charge aside from small co-payments or deductibles. Thus, the managed care organization is at financial risk for a package of covered services, it is rewarded for controlling both cost and utilization, and it is responsible to its members for the quality within and access to a defined system of care.

While traditional fee-for-service medicine attracts those seeking immediate help in becoming well, managed care attracts those seeking long-term help in staying well.

By virtue of the prepayment model, managed health organizations eliminate the fee-for-service system's natural incentive for providing an excess of health services. In most cases, managed care organizations give the primary care physician lead responsibility for the care of their patients as it is delivered throughout the system. Hospital-based care is normally de-emphasized for most treatment programs, while less costly alternatives are promoted, such as outpatient and home-based care.

A managed care system directly provides health services through its own staff and facilities, contracts for health services from outside hospitals, clinics, physician groups, labs, and so forth, or does a combination of both.

In addition to the provider network, an insurance function is maintained. This means that the organization designs health care policies and sets the level of dues, co-payments, and possibly deductibles. Further, managed care systems today are deeply involved with marketing their services. This entails sales, advertising, and public relations.

Aside from the how, what, and where of managed care, there is the why. Why promote a managed care system? Most managed care systems are philosophical descendants of the HMO movement in that a common philosophy runs through a great many—to give quality health care at the lowest appropriate cost and to take an active role in improving the health status of their communities. The ideal of maintaining and potentially improving the health status of the membership is a primary tenet of the managed care system.

Managed care administrators are dedicated to the outcomes and basic principles which guided the pioneers of the HMO movement as they sought an alternative to fee-for-service medicine.

VARIOUS MODELS OF MANAGED CARE SYSTEMS

Four models of organization dominate the field of managed care: the staff model, the group model, the network model, and the independent practice association. These models are so named by virtue of the legal and contractual relationship between the organization that finances and markets the care and the organization or organizations which provide the care.

Staff and group models deliver the majority of care within facilities they either own or lease. Their physicians see only patients who are members of the plan. The difference between the staff and group model is that while the physicians of staff model plans work directly for the organization that insures the care and enrolls the subscribers, under the group model the physicians form a separate corporation which in turn contracts with the insurance plan to provide health services exclusively to plan members. (See Figure 1.)

According to InterStudy, the Minnesota-based health research group, of the 30 largest managed care plans (ranked by enrollment), 10 are group or staff model plans. In general, these plans are the oldest and largest of managed care systems. Of the group model organizations, Kaiser Health Plan of Northern California is by far the largest with just over 2 million members. By contrast, the largest staff model plans are CIGNA Healthplans of California, and Group Health Cooperative of Puget Sound, with 398,000 and 381,500 members, respectively [3].

Network and independent practice association (IPA) model plans are the two other varieties of managed care systems. The network model operates like the group model except that instead of contracting with one physician group to provide health services to its members, it contracts with several. As with the group model, contracting medical providers see only patients of the managed care plan.

IPAs, the fastest growing segment of the managed care industry, contract with individual physicians under a capitation (per person) agreement. IPA physicians typically are already in practice and usually continue to see patients not covered by the IPA plan. IPAs select provider physicians according to many factors including location, quality of care, practice style, and commitment to cost-effective health care. To receive care, IPA enrollees use these physicians exclusively, who may in turn refer patients to such diagnostic clinics, hospitals, and other facilities as are covered under the plan.

GROWTH TRENDS IN MANAGED CARE

For many years, great potential was the only claim to fame for the managed care industry. Government agencies and many consumer groups liked the concept, but it did not receive much attention in the marketplace until the cost explosion of the 1970s and 1980s sent the government and private employers searching for options. Today, managed care is the fastest growing forest on the health care continent.

The reasons for this growth spurt in the managed care sector are many: the doctor glut, the need to control federal health care expenditures, the inability of employers to support unlimited expansion of the acute care system, and the growing sophistication and cost consciousness of the health care consumer. Because of these and other factors, enrollment in managed care systems has increased at an average annual rate of 21.4 percent from 10.5 million members to nearly 30 million in the five years between 1982

FIGURE 1: Staff Model Managed Care Organization

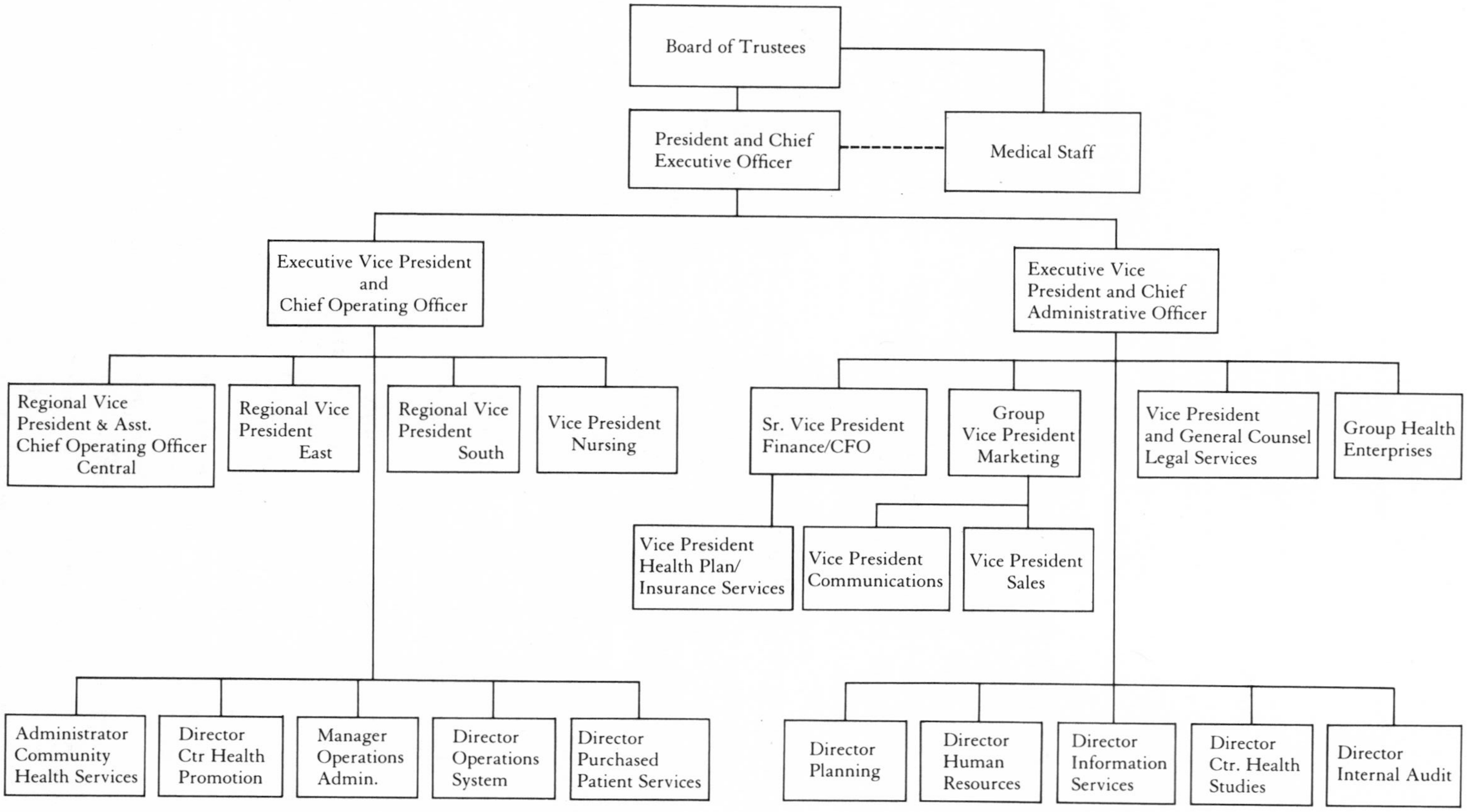

and 1987. During this same period, the number of managed care organizations has increased from 260 to 660 [4].

Today, enrollment growth is slowing from the record pace of 25 percent per year recorded in 1986, but it is still vigorous. However, after five years of proliferation, 1987 saw the number of managed care start-ups slow to a near standstill as demand for managed health services was met by existing plans.

IPAs and for-profit managed care systems have dominated the start-up list since 1984. Since that time, of approximately 350 managed care systems to open their doors, nearly 80 percent have been IPAs. Further, close to 80 percent of the total number of start-ups during this period were organized for profit, many financed by public stock offerings. Competition and rising costs have recently slowed the performance of for-profit managed care systems [5].

Industry observers tend to agree that the trend toward for-profit IPAs will continue. Because the IPAs usually start with health care professionals and facilities already in operation (but often underutilized), their start-up costs are much less than those of other models. And because many urban areas are still oversupplied with physicians, an increasing number are taking advantage of the marketing clout promised by IPAs. However, the IPA route is not a guaranteed road to security. Any managed care organization can experience financial duress if it cannot control utilization and costs. For these reasons, it is recommended that those seeking employment in an MCO consider organizations having a proven track record of success, a strong financial position, and a large and stable enrollment base.

THE CHANGING MARKETPLACE

Like every organization offering either health care services or health care financing to the consumer, the managed care organization operates in a turbulent environment. Consumer demands are increasing and the financial resources to respond to those needs are limited. The largest purchaser of health care—the employer—has become increasingly influential in the design and management of health plans. Employer groups pay over 54 percent of the total spent on health services in the United States. They are demanding accountability and efficiency from the health plans they approve for their employees—not to mention their retirees. For example, one Washington state business organization president recently said that in 1974 the average manufacturing company in the industry had 12 workers supporting the retiree benefits of 1 former worker. Today, that ratio is down to 3 active workers to 1 retiree [6]. Because employers, who already pay the lion's share of the nation's health care tab, are facing even larger outlays in the future, they are currently working to shift a significant portion of this financial burden to their employees and health care providers. The new clout of the employer is changing the way health organizations deliver services, set rates, and market their plans. We can expect this trend to continue.

Meanwhile, individual consumers have become more knowledgeable of medical practices in recent years, and have also become more sensitive to price (due to cost sharing), convenience, and service. This has required health care providers to be more conscious of patient attitudes and expectations than they have been in the past.

Additionally, consumer health care needs are increasing and changing as the population ages. New medical technologies and procedures have increased the cost of acute care across the board. Further, the spread of acquired immune deficiency syndrome (AIDS) is having and will continue to have a significant impact on every health services organization. And the number of uninsured and underinsured continues to grow, presenting a serious challenge to health care systems.

On the supply side of health care services, the physician glut is expected to continue. This will fuel further competition as more physicians seek shelter within MCOs. Competition among hospitals is heated and will remain so for some time. According to one investment banking firm specializing in the health care industry, hospital occupancy stood at 63 percent in 1986, compared to 74.6 percent ten years earlier [7].

In aggregate, cost and service pressures on the demand side, and competitive pressures on the supply side will continue to rock the health care services industry for some time to come. Fortunately, the managed care organization is on the right side of the future to respond effectively to these pressures. Studies by such prestigious organizations as the Rand Corporation have shown managed care organizations to charge 28 percent less for the same slate of services offered in the outside, fee-for-service community [8]. Because they can operate more efficiently and because their emphasis on preventive medicine holds the greatest promise for answering the long-term health needs of the nation, the marketplace will continue to be friendly to the well-managed MCO.

SOME SPECIAL ASPECTS OF MANAGED CARE ADMINISTRATION

THE EPIDEMIOLOGIC PERSPECTIVE

The central features of the managed care system include a defined and relatively stable population of enrollees and the financial investment the organization has in the health status of those enrollees. Accordingly, it is in the best interests of both the MCO and its members that the MCO not only track the health status of its population, but be committed to improving it through the practice of preventive medicine.

Some preventive medicine is simply medicine well practiced. Early detection and treatment of life-threatening diseases is something every capable physician will seek to accomplish during routine physical examinations. But preventive medicine can be more than advising patients to lose weight and handing out brochures on breast cancer and heart disease.

MCOs can make preventive health care more systematic by modifying their primary care practices to make use of epidemiological research. For example, if we know that women who are most likely to develop breast cancer are likely to first show signs of it between the ages of 35 and 45, it makes good economic and medical sense to initiate a cost-effective screening program aimed at early detection of breast cancer in women enrollees of this age group. And from the MCO's standpoint, it makes even better sense to do so if those women would likely be enrolled in the MCO at the time when they would otherwise require radical breast cancer surgery.

MCOs (staff, group, and network models) can take the epidemiological imperative one step further. These organizations, unlike fee-for-service systems, have the ability to collect and analyze complete medical histories of thousands of member individuals over a broad span of time. By virtue of this, the MCO can determine how effective whatever preventive programs it may choose to run have been—effective both in terms of economic and health outcomes.

For example, suppose an MCO knows that a significant percentage of its members are middle-aged men with a high cholesterol count who smoke an average of one and a half packs of cigarettes a day. From this information, the MCO can predict that if these behaviors continue, a certain percentage of these men are likely to develop cardiopulmonary problems of serious magnitude. The insurance specialists within the organization can estimate the costs of treating these future problems. Now the MCOs health promotion specialists may believe that they can change not only the eating habits, but also the smoking habits of these individuals by offering certain health promotion programs, and perhaps giving enrollees a financial incentive to participate actively. Five, 10 and 20 years after running these programs, the MCO can review not only the medical effectiveness of the programs it designed, but also their cost. Armed with both medical and financial information, the MCO can decide whether the preventive programs were cost-effective ways to improve the health status of its members.

The main point is that the MCO administrator's job is fundamentally different from that of the hospital administrator, or the fee-for-service clinic manager. In these latter settings, the organization is not at financial risk for the future health problems of the people who come in for treatment. To the contrary, the MCO administrator knows that improving the health of its members over time will pay off in the form of lower costs, lower dues for the members, and thus an enhanced competitive position for the MCO.

THE INSURANCE SIDE OF THE JOB

The administration of a managed care organization is as much the administration of health insurance plans as it is the management of health care providers and facilities. Unlike the fee-for-service environment where financial success hinges on the timely collection of amounts owing for actual services performed in the past, the survival of managed care organizations depends on their ability to forecast the costs of services which will likely be performed in the future. Thus, the managed care organization is also in the insurance business.

Accordingly, many managed care administrators spend their days in the highly competitive world of health insurance. Should we charge every member the same amount, regardless of age and health status? Should we age rate our plans, offering lower cost policies to younger, healthier members? Should we offer lower priced plans to those willing to pay a deductible? Should we require a mandatory co-payment for each clinic visit? Should covered services include heart transplantation, or will that price us out of the market? What about buying a separate insurance policy to cover our costs in caring for those needing bone marrow transplants? Or should we plan to finance such care from operating reserves built up through a possible increase in regular dues? And what about dental coverage, midwifery, chiropractic, and naturopathic medicine?

These are just a sampling of the kinds of insurance questions that must be answered in the normal course of managed care administration. But when it comes to deciding them, the managed care administrator has another dimension to consider besides the normal run of issues relating to risk, level of subscriber interest, and competition with other insurers. That is the system of medical care itself because, unlike the indemnity insurer, managed care administration has direct control over many cost factors involved in providing the services covered by the plan. For example, if the question on the table is whether or not to add midwifery services to the coverage, it is reasonable to consider how smoothly and cost effectively such a program can be phased into the existing obstetrics and gynecology function. This is a matter over which the MCO administrator has a certain degree of control—particularly in a staff model organization where most facilities and personnel are an integral part of the MCO. In deciding whether to add a service to a normal indemnity plan, insurance executives can only shop around the existing market; they cannot directly influence the product itself.

Your Friend the Actuary

How does the MCO administrator decide the cost of the premiums which entitle subscribers to care within the system? Will deductibles coupled with lower premiums attract or repel potential subscribers? Should all members pay the same premium or should younger members pay less because they use fewer health services? If so, how much less?

In the past, a good many of the insurance-related questions arising within MCOs were decided more by educated guesswork than by analysis, but this is changing. Fierce competition among health care providers and insurers, the advent of new expensive health care providers and insurers, the advent of new expensive medical procedures and technologies, and the changing health needs of the population are among factors which have required managed care organizations to seek extensive guidance from professional actuaries in deciding questions involving rate setting and policy design.

Actuaries bring to MCOs specialized skills and information necessary to evaluate the financial risk of offering new policies, redesigning old ones, and making any number of changes to their program of health services. These actuarial skills include expertise in data collection and analysis, and in computer modeling of different demand scenarios. The information actuaries can bring to an MCO is extensive data on the health care needs of various populations. Thus, actuarial expertise can be vitally important to an MCO hoping to extend its coverage to new user subscriber groups (such as Medicare patients), design special competitive policies for distinct occupational or employee groups (for example, state government workers), make additions to covered services (for example, heart transplantation), expand to a new geographic territory (Boomtown), or construct a unique package of services to answer a pressing social need (for example, long-term care).

Actuaries are rarely employed on a full time basis by MCOs, but are often hired on a project basis and are most often employed as consultants to management. One nationwide firm of independent consulting actuaries lists the following among their services in consulting for MCOs: medical cost and premium development, benefit design, claim liability estimation, management information systems analysis, and small group contract design [9].

ROLES PLAYED BY MANAGED CARE ADMINISTRATORS

While there are scores of distinct jobs available in MCO administration, only a few can be discussed here. The five described below cover a representative cross section of positions available.

Policy and Planning Manager

Policy and planning managers work to set the direction and values of their organizations. Sometimes this work is decidedly tangible, sometimes it is highly theoretical.

On the tangible side, planning managers may be involved in such projects as deciding the best way to handle overcrowding at an outpatient clinic. Should the old one be expanded? Should a new one be built in an adjacent community? Or should a capitation agreement be sought with an existing group practice nearby? Other tangible problems commonly referred to planning managers concern how best to judge the success of new service offerings (such as a new slate of health promotion activities) or the efficiency of current operations (for example, the decision to lease time on a nuclear magnetic resonance scanner rather than purchase one). These sorts of issues concern resource utilization and all are the province of policy and planning managers and their staff.

Some problems presented to policy and planning managers within MCOs do not easily yield to quantitative solutions. Should it be the policy of the MCO to perform legal abortions on request? What about providing naturopathic or chiropractic services? To decide these kinds of "Should we?" questions, MCO administrators must evaluate the merits of ethical, financial, and medical arguments.

Finally, the strategic planning function of the MCO is normally assigned to policy and planning managers. Strategic planning requires gaining consensus on the organization's desired future and then mapping out a path which takes into account the organization's environment and resources. Needless to say, this is difficult and important work. No health organization can take its current political, financial, medical, social, or competitive environment for granted. It is better to choose a future and try to bring it about than merely to accept the consequences of inaction. Policy and planning managers strive to bring about the former.

Perhaps it goes without saying that policy and planning managers do not work in isolation, bringing their results to the board as a *fait accompli*. Policy and planning managers are facilitators of organizationwide decision making. They work to establish processes of problem solving that bring together the affected parties and translate their concerns, interests, and hopes into efficient work plans which yield conclusions all can wholeheartedly support. It is not easy.

The Insurance Services Manager

All the various, component responsibilities involved with managing an insurance function fall to the insurance services manager: publishing membership information on covered services, administering the health contracts themselves (billing for dues and collecting co-payments, collecting overdue accounts, and resolving coverage disputes), maintaining an actuarial data base for use in establishing underwriting criteria and rate setting for new benefits, managing the activities of consulting actuaries, maintaining liaison with the state insurance department concerning state regulation of health plan contracts and rates, and managing the purchasing of health services from nonstaff providers.

The insurance services manager is a key player on the senior management team. In any large managed care organization, the financial relationships holding among the MCO and its enrollees, its provider organizations, government payers, and regulatory agencies can be extremely complex. Typically, the insurance services manager will oversee a large staff of analysts, computer specialists, regulatory experts, billing clerks, accounts payable and receivable personnel, and a wide range of consulting organizations.

Clinic Manager

For plans which own or manage medical facilities, the outpatient clinic is typically the MCO's first line of service. For most MCO subscribers enrolled in such plans, the clinic is the entry point into the vast system of health services available through their plan. A typical clinic will house a group of primary care physicians, a cadre of specialists, a sizeable contingent of nurses, a small diagnostic laboratory capable of performing routine tests, perhaps a pharmacy, and all of the office functions and personnel required to keep the place running smoothly and in harmony with the rest of the MCO system.

The main job of the clinic manager is to oversee daily clinic operations, develop clinic budgets, act as a communication link between MCO administration and on-site staff, supervise clinic administrative personnel, and assure a proper level of maintenance and care for the physical plant and equipment. The role of clinic administrator is pivotal to the middle-management system in the typical HMO. Not only do clinic administrators oversee the most highly used facilities in the MCO system, but they also are the front line in the war against health care cost creep.

Not surprisingly, clinic administrators are highly organized, committed, and detail-oriented people. Success in this job is measured on a daily basis by smooth patient flow, efficient medical staff working in close collaboration with other providers and administrators, and high patient satisfaction with both service and quality of care.

Product Line Manager

In the health care industry it is somewhat heretical to speak of managing products, but products are managed in the MCO. These are normally "bundles" of health and related services which are grouped according to the needs of a select population. The next step is to determine a financing method for the delivery of those services that is not only feasible for the MCO but affordable and attractive to prospective subscribers. One example from Group Health Cooperative is the new product line of long-term care insurance. This is planned as a joint venture between Group Health Cooperative and large insurance underwriters. The insurance package would cover a broad range of long-term health care needs of aging enrollees that are not covered by Medicare—either wholly or in part. Group Health provides the health care and performs the necessary administrative functions involved with dues collection, marketing, and the coordination with Medicare programs. Like their counterparts in the world of consumer and industrial goods, the product-line managers within are intimately concerned with product design, promotion, pricing, timing of market entry, distribution or availability, and of course, profitability.

Product line managers must bring to their work a high degree of skill in health services planning as well as a working knowledge of insurance principles.

Director of Sales

The old adage, "Nothing happens until somebody sells something," is as true within the MCO as it is for the Dow industrials. Without enrollees paying dues and employers purchasing group contracts, clinic managers could close their doors, planners would have nothing to plan, product-line management would deteriorate into an intellectual exercise, and insurance managers would have no policies to manage. In short, a successful sales function is critical to the life of the MCO. And as the competition among providers and insurers has heated up, the sales director's job has become even more vital.

Sales directors are charged with generating new accounts and keeping current ones. Generating new accounts means prospecting for interested purchasers—usually benefit managers for private or public employers—and insurance brokers; working with the marketing managers to design special group contracts for particular employers; pitching the capabilities of the organization to groups of prospective enrollees; and following up on sales calls to determine the causes of consumers selecting or not selecting your plan. Maintaining current accounts means answering questions about price, access, or coverage; keeping purchasers informed of the range and cost effectiveness of the MCO's services; and brainstorming ways to structure or restructure current contracts to bring about cost savings and service efficiencies.

Sales directors achieve sales objectives through a team of sales or account representatives. Typically, sales territories are divided first by geographic region, and then by type of account, such as school districts, unions, private employers with 50 or more employees, and individual enrollees. Government accounts such as Medicare are usually consolidated across geographic boundaries.

Sales directors work in close collaboration with marketing managers to plot sales tactics, analyze the competition, and coordinate sales efforts with promotional activities.

Sales directors for MCOs, like sales managers everywhere, must be disciplined and creative thinkers who can also inspire a sales force to achieve meaningful and difficult goals.

CAREER OPPORTUNITIES IN MANAGED CARE

ADVANTAGES OF MANAGED CARE EMPLOYMENT

Most who enter health services administration as a career want to make a significant contribution toward improving the health status of a community. However, once on the job it becomes painfully apparent that delivering health services is one thing, improving the health status of individuals over time is another. In the hospital or fee-for-service clinic setting, patients generally come and go as their acute care needs arise and subside with care. Little emphasis is put on the systematic practice of preventive medicine because these organizations simply do not have a large stable population to care for—in sickness and in health—over time. There may be a short-term revenue gain for such organizations which choose, for example, to sell time on fitness equipment or market weight-loss clinics. But this is not the same as having a long-term financial investment in wellness.

On the other hand, the managed care organization can and does invest in preventive medicine because it is at financial risk for the future health of its enrollees. This style of operation in turn attracts health professionals with the skills and desire to practice preventive medicine in addition to responding to the immediate needs of their patients. Consequently, managed care administration is about as close as one can get to having genuine responsibility for improving the health status of a community over time—the community being that of the MCOs enrollees.

Inside the managed care organization one has the opportunity to witness the ways in which health care finance and delivery affect each other at the intersection of cost, access, and quality. Accordingly, a career in managed care gives one the opportunity to be schooled on both sides of health care. After several years in a large MCO, senior managers will have gained experience qualifying them for top positions with either insurers of health care or providers of health services.

Managed care settings offer the administrator greater flexibility and control than the typical hospital-based environment. What care to offer, how much to charge for it, how to promote it, and where to deliver it can all be open questions for the managed care administrator. This is normally not so for the hospital administrator, who may have little control over such matters.

Salaries for managed care administrators are typically higher than those of hospital-based administrators. Pay at the middle-management level is typically higher than within the insurance industry.

Only in a managed care setting will one come to understand the unique long-term perspective on health care that comes from running an institution grounded in the principles and practice of preventive medicine and health promotion.

DISADVANTAGES OF MANAGED CARE EMPLOYMENT

Managed care is a growing segment of the world of health care delivery and finance, but it is still a small segment. Of some 200 million people who receive some form of health care within the United States, approximately 28 million are enrolled in managed care organizations. There are only 660 managed care plans functioning at this writing. Consequently, the number of job opportunities in MCOs is considerably smaller than those awaiting elsewhere [10].

Many managed care organizations have suffered through decades of opposition from the medical establishment. It is therefore not uncommon for older MCOs to have developed a "bunker mentality" that has estranged them from other medical care organizations in the community. This can be frustrating for the new employee who seeks collegial relationships in the outside health care community. Similarly, many older MCOs have developed a strong, self-sustaining culture which can take some getting used to.

Because the managed care organization is partly an insurance company and partly a provider organization, it is sometimes regarded by the rest of the health care community as truly neither one. While this conclusion does not follow in the least, the "neither fish nor fowl" attitude does persist and will only be erased by time. One consequence for the managed care administrator can be a lack of acceptance.

Getting a good education in the principles of managed care outside the workplace is difficult because few universities give it much attention in their curricula. This means that prospective managed care administrators must supplement their educations with a higher than normal amount of on-

TABLE 1: Relative Value of Managed Care Positions

The following table compares the relationship between job content, base salary and total cash compensation levels for 23 out of the 32 positions for which there was comparable data year to year. Each factor is compared to the value of the CEO and expressed as a percentage. The display shows the internal value of the job expressed without actual dollars or units of job content.

| | Average as a Percentage of CEO | | | |
| | UNITS OF JOB CONTENT | | BASE SALARY | |
	1987 %	1986 %	1987 %	1986 %
Chief executive officer	100	100	100	100
Chief operating officer	71	72	73	72
Chief financial officer	50	51	59	59
Development executive	44	46	51	52
Regional director of operations	42	42	43	42
Legal executive	39	39	47	41
Marketing executive	39	39	44	41
Planning executive	35	37	39	43
Human resources executive	33	35	37	36
EDP executive	31	31	37	34
Corporate controller	31	30	35	33
Head of construction engineering	29	29	37	33
Treasurer	27	29	31	30
Head of foundation	25	33	35	37
Public relations executive	25	26	29	29
Head of purchasing materials management	25	25	28	29
Head of home health	25	25	26	30
Head of quality assurance	23	22	30	28
Reimbursement executive	22	22	28	25
Head of internal audit	22	23	24	23
Head of management engineering	21	23	30	28
Risk management	20	22	26	25
Regional controller	20	22	24	21

For example, if a company pays the CEO a base salary of $200,000 and the CFO $150,000, the CFO's pay is 75% of the CEO.

SOURCE: The Hay Company, 1987. Reprinted with permission.

the-job training and self-directed study. This translates into longer hours for the working administrator.

COMPENSATION FOR MANAGED CARE ADMINISTRATORS

In general, managed care administrators are well paid in comparison to administrators of other health care organizations. Salary depends on a variety of factors including experience, size and complexity of the organization, true job responsibility, and the financial position of the organization itself.

More specific information on the compensation levels of managed care administrators can be gleaned from the 1987 Health Care Management Company total compensation survey of Hay Management Consultants, the nation's largest human resources consulting organization. The following facts emerge from their survey:

— Managed care administrators are generally paid less than executives in financial and industrial corporations.

— Salaries paid to managed care administrators are generally higher than those paid to hospital administrators and indemnity insurance workers with comparable responsibilities.

— Within the managed care sector, chief administrators of for-profit plans receive greater total remuneration than their counterparts in not-for-profit plans, but this gap is narrowing.

— Taking the health care management industry as a whole, senior executives can expect to receive 66 percent of their total remuneration in base salary, 22 percent in benefits, and 12 percent in annual incentive bonuses [11].

To illustrate the comparative value of various posts in managed care organizations, Table 1 has been extracted from the 1987 Hay Survey. To translate these percentages into base salary approximations, one must know the salary of the chief executive officers. The Hay report indicates that CEO salaries in managed care organizations cover a wide range depending on the complexity of the job, the size of the organization, for-profit or nonprofit status and, of course, the financial performance of the organization.

CONCLUSION

If anything, this report on managed health care portrays an industry which is, as they would say in the old newsreels, "on the move." Keeping up with it is not easy, but it can be done. The following are organizations that are good sources of additional and current information on managed health care:

Group Health Association of America
1129 20th St. N.W. Suite 600
Washington, D.C. 20036

Interstudy
P.O. Box 458
5715 Christmas Lake Road
Excelsior, MN 55331

American Hospital Association
840 N. Lake Shore Drive
Chicago, IL 60611

REFERENCES

1. Berman, H. and D. Berhenne. *The Complete Health Care Advisor*, 2nd Edition. Unpublished manuscript.
2. InterStudy. The InterStudy Edge. Quarterly Report of HMO Growth and Enrollment, Summer 1987, p. 1.
3. InterStudy. See 2, 4–9.
4. InterStudy. See 2, 1.
5. InterStudy. See 2, 10.
6. Kramon, G. Insurance Rates for Health Care Increase Sharply. *New York Times* (January 12) 76: 29, 1988.
7. Hoover, J. B. et al. Managed Health Care in the United States. Robertson, Colman & Stephans–Investment Bankers, November 23, 1987, p. 5.
8. Rand Corporation, Santa Monica, CA.
9. Milliman & Robertson, Inc., Seattle, WA.
10. InterStudy. See 2, 1.
11. 1987 Health Care Management Company Total Compensation Survey. Hay Management Consultants, CA 1987.

SUGGESTED READING LIST

1. Anderson, O. W., et al. *HMO Development, Patterns and Prospects A Comparative Analysis of HMOs*. Chicago: Pluribus Press Inc. 1985.
2. Fuchs, V. *The Health Economy*. MA: Cambridge, Harvard University Press, 1986.
3. Goldfield, N. and S. B. Goldsmith. *Alternative Delivery Systems*. Rockville, MD: Aspen Press, 1987.
4. Luft, H. S. *Health Maintenance Organizations: Dimensions of Performance*. New York: John Wiley and Sons, 1981.
5. Machie, D. L. and D. K. Decker. *Group and IPA HMOs*. Rockville, MD: Aspen Press, 1981.
6. Group Health Foundation. *1987 Proceedings—New Health Care Systems: HMOs & Beyond*. Seattle, WA: Group Health Foundation.
7. Starr, P. *The Social Transformation of American Medicine*. NY: Basic Books, 1982.

8

HOME HEALTH SERVICES: NEW TECHNOLOGIES, NEW ORGANIZATIONS, NEW GROWTH

LOUIS KATZ

Home health care is the delivery of skilled and unskilled medical, rehabilitation, and personal care services to patients in their own homes. While it is the oldest form of health care delivery, home health care is undergoing dramatic changes in the methods and variety of services being offered. It shares with the other segments of health care delivery the goals of promoting, maintaining, and restoring health or minimizing the effects of illness and disability. Home health care delivery, however, is unique in that the providers of care, services, and products come to the patient. While still a relatively small component of the health care industry, when compared with hospital, physician, and nursing home services, home health care is the fastest growing segment in the field.

Home health care is a major part of the dramatic change now occurring in health services delivery. It has introduced new services and products as well as more sophisticated management techniques and control. Most im-

Louis Katz is president of National Health Management Systems, Inc., Cherry Hill, NJ, and was formerly executive vice president of the Home Health Corporation of America. Mr. Katz received an M.B.A. in health administration from Temple University, an M.A. in psychology from Memorial University in Newfoundland, and a B.A. in psychology from Sir George Williams University.

portant, home health services providers are reevaluating not only what their missions are, but who are now their primary market.

Home health care has always been considered an ancillary or add-on service. The challenge for the next decade is for home health services to become part of the mainstream of health care delivery. Home health services have contributed to and shared in the recent dramatic, if not revolutionary, changes in the health care field. In fact, the growth in demand for home health services suggests that these changes may ultimately have a greater impact on home health care than on other health care delivery components. In 1985, 20 to 30 million visits were made to two to three million patients in their homes. It is estimated that by the year 2000, 50 to 60 million visits will have been made to four to five million patients.

The overwhelming majority of the patients (80 percent) receiving care at home currently are elderly with chronic conditions. The mix, however, is rapidly changing as a result of new attitudes, practice patterns, reimbursement mechanisms, and other regulations. The new medical technologies which have allowed complex treatments hitherto provided only in acute care settings to become available at home are also having a profound effect.

This chapter describes the forces of change and some appropriate responses—responses that have required home health service providers to show flexibility and adaptability to change and innovation. The failure to modify traditional home health delivery mechanisms, values, and philosophies by implementing programs and systems that were once considered inappropriate and beyond the scope of home care will lead inevitably to the collapse of some conservative providers. The responses described are not the only ones available, of course, but they have been implemented successfully in my organization.

Several factors have contributed to the increased demand for home care services. Some are related to changes in health care delivery; other influences are related to the economics of the health care delivery system that is simply getting out of control; still other factors relate to consumers' demands for more convenient service. The current trend is to keep the patient out of the acute care setting. This is evidenced by the rapid proliferation of alternative health care delivery systems and ancillary services.

In 1985 there were 350 health maintenance organization (HMO) plans serving 20 million members. With current trends continuing it is estimated that there will be over 500 plans with 50 to 75 million members by the year 2000. Preferred provider organizations (PPOs) are experiencing similar growth. The 350 plans with 3 million members in 1985 are expected to grow to 500 plans with 20 million members by 2000. Other indicators of these trends are the growth of ambulatory care facilities and home health services agencies. In 1985 there were 25 to 30,000 ambulatory care centers. This is expected to climb to 40 to 50,000 by the year 2000. Similarly, home care companies made 20 to 25 million visits to two million patients in 1985. These numbers will more than double by the year 2000.

The elderly have become increasingly independent. They are more active and healthy than generally thought by the public and often have some financial independence by way of social security, home equity, or both. Nursing homes are perceived negatively by these relatively well elderly and generally offer significantly more expensive and intensive care than needed. There has been growth recently in less restrictive environments for this group including life care centers, continuing care facilities, adult congregate living arrangements, and personal care facilities. Home care is the least restrictive and is increasingly being perceived as important in aiding the elderly to maintain their active, self-reliant, independent life styles.

Moving chronically ill and subacute patients out of institutions often has the effect of changing patient expectations toward the future. Fulfilling these expectations can lead to improvement in the quality of life. Patients at home will attempt to surround themselves with as many products and services as are available, convenient, and affordable so that life at home will be as nearly normal as it was prior to the onset of the debilitating condition(s).

Increased demand for home health care also reflects the aging of the population with its associated increase in the prevalence of chronic diseases and disability. It is estimated that by the year 2000, 35 million people or 13.5 percent of the U.S. population will be over 65 years of age, up from 28 million or approximately 11 percent in 1985. Of this group 50 percent will be over 75 years of age. This has produced patients with needs for more intense and frequent postdischarge subacute care.

Currently, Medicare patients account for approximately 50 percent of home health care expenditures. It is projected that by the year 2000 they will account for approximately 55 percent. The over-75 age cohort, which accounts for an even higher percentage of health care expenditures, is increasing at several times the rate of the elderly group as a whole. There are also millions of people under 65 years of age who will be alive having survived acute conditions such as heart attacks and strokes. Millions of others will survive with chronic conditions such as Alzheimer's disease, arthritis, incontinence, and other impairments.

The diagnosis-related group (DRG) hospital reimbursement system has caused an influx of generally sicker patients into the home health system. As a result, home health agencies, already faced with increasing numbers of patients, have found themselves with a population demanding services of an intensity not previously required.

Opportunities exist in home care and related services for providers to have a considerable impact on the life and well-being of patients. The potential also exists to generate a considerable amount of revenue (though not necessarily profit). As those needing home care increase, so do the numbers of new entrants in the field. Whereas the visiting nurse associations (VNAs) were the primary providers of home care a few years ago, the field has become wide open due to continuing efforts to reduce or eliminate hospitalization as well as the perceived lack of resources to fill the growing need.

Hospitals are major new entrants into this field. As patients were being discharged more quickly, hospitals saw occupancy rates drop and sought new sources of patient referrals. Many developed home health agencies for this reason. At the very least, it was felt that the patients could be kept within the system to ensure readmissions when appropriate; moreover, since the DRGs fixed the hospitals' reimbursement, excess revenue could be reduced or "shifted" to cost-reimbursed programs such as home health care. In this period many hospitals were involved in corporate restructuring to allow them to benefit from excess revenues.

Advances in technology have made techniques and treatment modalities possible in the home which were formerly restricted to acute care settings. They include enteral and parenteral nutrition, dialysis, bone growth stimulation, intravenous antibiotic therapy, cancer chemotherapy, drug infusion for congestive heart failure, respiratory therapies, high risk infant monitoring, and phototherapy.

These and other new services have brought millions of new patients into the system and with them many new providers specializing in these services. Existing providers have had to develop such services or face the loss of new patients. Even more serious to these providers is the potential loss of their traditional patients since it is more convenient for referral sources to use agencies that can provide all services to all patients.

While technology, social forces, and some regulations such as the DRGs stimulate the field to expand, certain reimbursement attitudes and regulations are limiting growth. According to data collected by the Health Care Financing Administration (HCFA) the rate of home health visit denials has tripled since the DRGs were instituted.

Nowhere in the home health field have changing regulations affected the system more than with respect to durable medical equipment (DME). Durable medical equipment includes those products ranging from canes, walkers, and commodes to wheelchairs and beds which are supplied to homebound patients. Seeking to increase their excess revenues, hospitals exploited the potential of being in the home health arena and developed relationships with DME and home health companies. At this time DME was a reasonable venture for hospitals to participate in. Not only was it a service for which the hospital patients had need, but Medicare reimbursement, the major payment source, was in most cases reasonable and often even generous. In February of 1984, however, Medicare implemented a new strict lease or purchase policy and ended the age of the "Golden Commode." The change dramatically affected existing companies as well as hospitals that had just entered the field with what has suddenly become unrealizable revenue projections.

In spite of these events, the current marketplace is one filled with opportunity. Private industry, moreover, is just now beginning to recognize fully the total potential of home health care. Commercial insurance companies, realizing the savings potential of replacing hospitalization with home health care, are increasingly offering these services as health benefits. Consumers are also becoming more aware of this service and are demanding these benefits. As a result, millions of people (the under-65 population) are being introduced to a system of care in which they have not recently participated.

To meet the ever-increasing demand and expectations of the consumer, home health agencies have had to increase dramatically the scope of their services. This has led to the implementation of new programs, changing home health care from an ordinary nursing field into a high-tech, or more appropriately, a high-touch service. This has also led to the development of sophisticated systems for patient tracking, management, scheduling, and control. It has forced the traditional voluntary and "mom and pop" providers to become sophisticated business people. However, it is still the availability, scope, and sophistication of services that drives the system. While some additional services were offered a few years ago by a few providers, most must now be offered by any provider wishing to be competitive in the community.

THE SCOPE OF HOME HEALTH SERVICES

CARDIOPULMONARY THERAPY

Pulmonary and cardiac rehabilitation programs are usually offered together but may be run separately. The goals and treatments often coincide, with a major focus of both being to prepare the patient for a more intensive cardiac rehabilitation program in an outpatient facility.

A well-managed program offers a wide variety of nursing and rehabilitation services as well as continuous ventilation to patients who meet predetermined criteria. Once admitted to the program the agency should be able to take care of all the patients' needs including regular arterial blood gases.

Primary objectives of this program include educating and motivating the patient to make the necessary changes in life style to become a functioning member of the family and society. This includes assisting the patient in reducing anxiety and depression and developing emotional stability. The patient is helped to recognize early warning signs to prevent recurrence of potentially acute conditions.

The cardiopulmonary nurse (a registered nurse with specialized training) performs the initial predischarge assessment and provides skilled nursing services in the home, coordinating the other required ancillary services.

INTRAVENOUS THERAPY

Patients are admitted to an intravenous therapy program for the purpose of correcting fluid or electrolyte imbalances, providing nourishment when the patients are unable to eat normally or adequately, administering continuous or intermittent medication, or for the administration of anticoagulants.

Intravenous therapy is provided by registered nurses certified to administer intravenous solutions. The nurse arranges for all equipment, supplies, solutions, and medications. Intravenous solutions are sometimes prepared by the discharging hospital's pharmacy.

Enteral and Parenteral Nutrition

Enteral and parenteral nutrition are provided to patients unable to swallow or digest food normally and who depend on infusion of nutrients for sustenance. Again the patient is managed by a specially trained and certified registered nurse.

A prime objective is to foster independence by teaching the patient and family procedures for safe administration of nutrients.

Oncology

Care and support of the cancer patient is provided through a multidisciplinary team using individualized programs prescribed by the oncologist, hematologist, and surgeon.

The program focuses on helping patients and families understand medications, dosages, disease process, pain control, relaxation techniques, signs and symptoms of side effects of chemotherapy, the purposes of treatments, and other aspects of care. The goals focus on improving the quality of life and increasing independence in activities of daily living.

Chemotherapy

The goals of home chemotherapy include education, cure, control, and palliation.

If properly organized, all supplies and equipment related to the delivery of nutritional support, intravenous and chemotherapy are provided by the home health agency. Chemotherapy agents are administered only by specially trained and certified RNs.

PEDIATRICS

New technology and heightened awareness of home services have increased demands for treatment of neonates and older children at home. Pediatric diagnoses and conditions that may warrant home care include, but are not limited to, bronchiopulmonary dysplasia, ventilator dependence, soft tissue injury requiring intravenous antibiotics, burn injuries, juvenile diabetes, asthma, cystic fibrosis, and other conditions. The goals of these programs include the education of the family and patient in order to allow them independence and participation in some aspects of their care.

While the hospital maintains an undisputed role during the acute phases of illness, the home environment has long been recognized as more therapeutic during recovery. Caring for children in their homes, surrounded by familiar objects and people, has been shown to reduce fear greatly and allow children to continue normal emotional development despite illness. Pediatric programs should allow parents to become actively involved as integral members of the care-giving team.

POSTPARTUM PROGRAMS

Postpartum programs have been developed (often in conjunction with pediatric programs) to promote early discharge from the hospital for those who have experienced uncomplicated vaginal deliveries.

Home visits are provided by pediatric nurse practitioners or RNs knowledgeable in all aspects of postpartum care and assessment of newborns. These nurses perform a thorough assessment of mother and neonate and participate in education in such areas as breast-feeding, maternal nutrition, exercise, infant care and parenting skills for both parents, and response of siblings to the new family member.

Comprehensive pediatric programs also offer specialized services such as phototherapy. One of the most common reasons for lengthened neonatal hospitalization is heightened bilirubin levels prior to discharge. While the treatment is very simple (exposure to ultraviolet radiation) it tends to get expensive as mothers often insist on remaining in the institution until their newborn is discharged. Home phototherapy is a very simple and inexpensive program to implement and its availability can have a tremendous impact on the operation (and occupancy) of any maternity ward.

CARE OF THE TERMINALLY ILL—HOSPICE

While hospice care is only a small part of the total home care picture, it has been receiving a great deal of public attention. Hospice care is a rather vague term used to describe a variety of programs which include inpatient care, hospice care at home as part of a home care program that offers other home health services, and hospice care at home provided by an agency that serves only the terminally ill and their families. Terminally ill patients, defined as those with life expectancies of less than six months, have a unique set of health care needs that often does not fall within the definition of skilled health care. At the same time, these patients require medical management of those aspects of care related to safety, comfort, and pain control as well as emotional support for the patient and family alike. While traditional hospital and home care services do not attempt to meet all these needs, hospice programs do.

Inpatient hospice care is provided in an institutional setting. It can be a designated wing or section of an acute care hospital or an entire freestanding facility. In either case, the services are identical and are provided to the patient who resides in the facility. In this setting the emphasis is on palliation rather than cure, comfort rather than progress. The clergy and social service departments as well as other counseling services help both the patient and family deal with such issues as death and dying and grieving. Issues such as addiction to pain medication and rehabilitation are not important in hospice programs since death is assumed to be imminent and the goal of achieving a normal life is not possible. Patients are not subject to the rigors of hospitalization such as dietary restrictions, testing procedures, and uncomfortable treatments.

A major difference between inpatient and home-hospice care is the extent of family involvement. In the latter setting, the family along with the hospice team assumes responsibility for care 24 hours a day. Because of the amount of direct patient care and contact, intense emotional support for the family and patient is a major feature of this kind of program. In addition to clerical, social service, and counseling support, home-hospice programs rely on volunteer services by the community to allow rest breaks to family members charged with providing care to the patient. Professional staff is available on-call 24 hours a day to meet the unique needs of these patients.

ORGANIZATIONAL CHANGES

Home health care, as was pointed out earlier, is the oldest method of health care delivery. It was not until the early part of this century that this kind of care was delivered in a formal, organized fashion. The early home health agencies were voluntary in nature and organized as not-for-profit organizations. Their primary mission was to provide medical and skilled care to their patients (mostly indigents who could not receive medical attention elsewhere). As home care came into its own and began to be recognized as a valuable service, payers for this service appeared.

Although Medicare and Medicaid have always provided reimbursement of one kind or another for home health services, they limited the recipients of payment to nonprofit organizations. Entrepreneurs who wanted to participate in the programs had to form nonprofit companies to deliver these services. While cynics could argue that their motives were less than purely service oriented, the so-called private nonprofit agencies did provide useful services of high quality and were able to fill what was becoming a growing need.

In fact, because the need was growing faster than it could be filled, legislation was passed allowing for-profit agencies to become eligible to receive federal reimbursement. This had the desired effect, and within a relatively short time, hundreds of new agencies appeared. While these agencies sought to carve a profitable niche for themselves in what had traditionally been a nonprofit field, the existing nonprofit agencies found themselves with aggressive competition.

Very few of the nation's more than 6000 home health care providers were involved in anything but the provision of home health services, leaving the sale, rental, and distribution of equipment and supplies to others. As nonprofit organizations, the existing home health agencies felt that business enterprises per se were not within their organizations' missions.

Two forces acted in concert to change this philosophy: one was the realization that significant opportunities existed to allow the agencies to make a considerable impact on their patients' lives and health, the other was simply the basic will to continue to survive in a competitive environment. So dramatic was the change that many nonprofit agencies reorganized their corporate structures and formed for-profit subsidiaries or holding companies. With for-profit structures in place, these agencies had a potential previously denied them—the ability to finance a whole host of new services.

The addition of new services, moreover, expanded the opportunities for greater revenues and profits as these high-touch services often required equipment that could not only be supplied by the agency but for which there was more than adequate reimbursement. By providing products as well as services, the agencies played an even greater part in their patients' lives offering a central source for all facets of care. This also made the referral process more streamlined and convenient for the physicians and other referral sources who would be more inclined to use an agency where most of the discharged patients' needs could be handled with one phone call.

Until recently the few home health agencies supplying anything beyond services were involved with durable medical equipment. The salient question for these and the rest became how to take advantage of the potential market without losing sight of our jeopardizing their primary mission. The quick and easy answer for many was to participate in joint ventures with other organizations already involved in the desired market. These relationships, where properly structured and organized, have proven to be beneficial to all parties involved.

Home care has grown from a voluntary service to indigent patients to a comprehensive and often technical delivery of sophisticated care to patients of all ages and socioeconomic levels. Until recently those in charge were generally nurses who had come up through the system. Few career-minded individuals chose home care administration deliberately as a career option. Even today, many are not familiar with, or know, until they have need for the services provided, that such organizations exist. Nonetheless, home care is receiving more attention as a career option for those considering health care administration. This is in part due to the fact that while hospitals, the largest single employer of health care professionals, have peaked in terms of growth and growth potential, home care is in an expansionary mode.

Home health care operates in a very service-intensive environment. The majority of services are provided by technical and professional people, with little demand for supportive services that require much administrative time. In addition, most of the services are provided during normal working hours and do not require around-the-clock personnel. As a result, most administrators and all middle managers are required to have expertise—degrees and/or experience or both in the function they are supervising. The small size of many agencies dictates that the administrator function as the director of nursing and, therefore, a master's degree–prepared nurse becomes the only eligible candidate for the position. The level of experience for the position and the type of degree required varies from state to state. Individuals with degrees in health administration are able to fill or create job opportunities in multimillion-dollar multifaceted agencies. Large agencies that are committed to expanding into some of the areas described in this chapter are in need of such individuals. Most middle-management (supervisory) positions in home health services call for at least a baccalaureate degree in nursing. Advanced degrees would be helpful but any incumbent in this job category must be prepared to provide hands-on services to patients.

Because home health agencies have become diversified, they have found more need for individuals who are able to implement and manage new programs. These individuals must possess those skills required to operate what are potentially multimillion-dollar businesses. In addition, as the field grows, opportunities become available with large national as well as multinational companies. In the last few years home health care has entered the business world. Any individual possessing skills related to organizing new ventures, including everything from the development of business plans to arranging for and overseeing new contractual relations, would be an asset to a large home health services company. On the other hand, degreed individuals with no previous home health care experience would have difficulty finding employment with an agency that provides only traditional home health services.

Career opportunities and prerequisites for employment in hospice care are similar to home care. Although there are no specific degrees in hospice care, there is a variety of backgrounds that will help prepare one for this type of work. Graduate degrees in nursing with specialties in areas such as oncology are helpful. Master's-degree-level social workers with specialization in areas of hospice, death and dying, or health care are viable candidates for a variety of positions in the hospice field. Those with master's degrees in health administration must have some type of experience in health care, preferably in a hospital or community health setting to be eligible candidates. Individuals with backgrounds working with volunteer community organizations such as the Red Cross or the American Cancer Society also prove to be viable candidates for hospice positions. Experience in grant proposal writing, planning, outreach programs, or fund-raising is an important background for those wanting to work for hospice programs. Health professionals experienced in working with the terminally ill are in great demand for hospice work. Some of the complex care required demands individuals with master's degrees in particular specialties in staff positions to provide direct care as well as supervise, train, and evaluate other care-givers.

While experience is a vital and necessary aspect for employment in both home care and hospice care, an advanced degree in health administration allows one not only to advance further and more rapidly but also to have more input and provide direction to the organization. On the other hand, an individual with an advanced degree along with technical or professional skills will be most in demand. In other words, a nurse with an advanced degree in health administration will be in an excellent position to achieve a top administrative position.

An area that cannot be overlooked in home health care for those possessing an advanced degree and an independent entrepreneurial spirit is, of course, ownership. Home health care is one area of health care that offers easy entry to the new entrepreneur (as opposed to a hospital or nursing home). The organization is not too complex and financing requirements are minimal as there are no major capital outlays. Ownership, however, is recommended only for those with previous hands-on experience, as even the most educated cannot anticipate all the nuances of operating such a business.

While not complete, the following lists the kind of organizations associated with and participating in the delivery of health care services at home: Medicare home health agencies (for-profit and not-for-profit); private-pay home care companies offering nonfederally reimbursed services such as private duty nursing, home health aides, homemakers, and companions; durable medical equipment companies including soft goods suppliers; sports medicine; respiratory services; nutritional support services; pharmacy services; transportation, ambulance, or paramedic services; rehabilitation services; geriatric consultation services; pediatric services; and other supportive services such as meals-on-wheels, house cleaning, and home repair services. This list of services available in the home is less than complete. It does, however, provide a basis for an understanding of the opportunities in this exciting and rapidly changing field.

BIBLIOGRAPHY

Auerbach, Marly. Changes in Home Health Care Delivery. *Nursing Outlook* (November–December): 290–291, 1985.

Evashwick, Connie. Home Health Care: Current Trends and Future Opportunities. *Journal of Ambulatory Care Management* 8(4): 4–17, 1985.

Home Care Agencies Up 25 Percent Since '84. *Hospitals* (Special Section). May 16, 1985, 64.

Rosenberg, Hilary. Prognosis for Home Health Care. *Financial World*. May 15, 1983, 29–32.

Sharma, Rabinder K. Forecasting Need and Demand for Home Health Care: A Selective Review. *Public Health Reports* 95 (November–December): 572–579, 1980.

Shaw, Stephen. A Home Care Technology: Futuristic Home Health Services. *Caring* (October): 20–22, 1985.

Taylor, Marietta B. The Effect of DRGs on Home Health Care. *Nursing Outlook* (November–December): 288–289, 1985.

Trubo, Richard. Home Health Care Encounters Growing Pains. *Medical World News*. February 10, 1986, 76–88.

United States Senate Special Committee on Aging. The Crises in Home Health Care: Greater Need. Less Care. July 28, 1986.

9

MEDICAL GROUP PRACTICE: WORKING WITH PHYSICIANS

F. KENNETH ACKERMAN, Jr.

The dramatic improvements in American health statistics during the twentieth century stand as landmarks of the progress medicine has achieved. In the last quarter of this century a confluence of social, economic, and political developments and new market forces forever altered the health care environment. Health care economists point to dramatic changes in the national economy and in federal entitlement programs such as Medicare and Medicaid, the strengthened role of regulatory authority and the business sector's power over health care, the oversupply of physicians in some specialties, the skyrocketing cost of malpractice insurance, and the emergence of competition as forces in this new environment.

Exponential increases in the cost of employee health insurance in the 1970s and 1980s transformed employers—and governments—from passive payers to active choosers and monitors of employee insurance plans. The business sector was no longer willing to preserve patients' complete freedom of choice, pay carte blanche charges to hospitals and physicians, or pay "usual, customary, and reasonable" rates [1]. Employers who are willing to intervene in the doctor-patient relationship, to monitor quality of care and cost—or even to demand that physicians certify the necessity of hospitalization before a patient is admitted—have turned a relatively noncompetitive sellers' market for health care into an intensely competitive buyers' market.

F. Kenneth Ackerman, Jr. is the senior vice president and administrative director of Geisinger Medical Center in Danville, PA. Mr. Ackerman was awarded an M.B.A. from the University of Michigan and received a bachelor's degree in biology from Denison University.

In 1950, the United States devoted 4.6 percent of its gross national product to health care [2]. By 1987, in just 37 years, that percentage had nearly tripled to 11 percent of the gross national product, or $500 billion. Government finances 40 percent of all health care benefits. One out of every ten new legislative proposals and regulations introduced in Congress is related to health care. Among the most far-reaching was the introduction in 1982 of prospective payment for the federal Medicare program's share of health care services. That legislation has become a watershed for American medicine and has dramatically reconfigured the role and function of health care administration.

Nearly half of all physicians might characterize their area of medicine as very competitive [3]. The number of physicians in the United States grew from 311,000 in 1970 to 534,800 in 1986 [4]. By the year 2000 that number is expected to be 696,500, and 4 out of every 10 physicians will have trained in the 1980s, or later. By the first year of the twenty-first century, the ratio of physicians per 100,000 Americans will have doubled from what it was just half a century earlier [5].

In 1980, after three years of comprehensive health manpower analysis, the Graduate Medical Education National Advisory Committee reached a number of important conclusions:

— There would be too many physicians in 1990

— There would be substantial imbalances in some specialties

— There would continue to be marked unevenness in the geographic distribution of physicians [6].

By 1987, research surveys found that an increasing proportion of doctors, including specialists, were willing to locate in areas with previously low numbers of physicians, evidence of the oversupply of physicians and an indication of a new preference by physicians for small-town living. More evidence of the oversupply was data showing declines in physicians' real incomes [7]. The fact that the average age of physicians in group practice has dropped indicates that many younger physicians saddled with high medical-legal liability insurance premiums and medical education debts are finding it increasingly difficult to start solo practices because of competition from physicians already established in an area.

According to the health care consultant, Jeff Goldsmith, the turn of the century will find us with

1. Substantially underemployed specialty physicians
2. Strained physician-to-physician relationships
3. More reluctance to seek specialty consultation

4. Physician services that are more accessible to the rural population

5. Physicians who will have more time to spend with their patients, if they choose [8].

In addition to the pressure of market forces, the oversupply of physicians, and competition, such factors as the insecurity of solo practices, the high cost of starting a new practice, the overhead cost of maintaining an existing one in terms of equipment, medical-legal liability insurance, office rental, and personnel expenses became forces motivating physicians to form or join medical group practices.

Medical groups by definition are groups of at least three licensed physicians engaged in a formally organized and legally recognized entity providing health services. They share equipment, facilities, common records, and the personnel involved in patient care and business management. Of 1,700 groups surveyed by the AMA in 1986, 9 out of 10 were physician-owned [9]. Because each physician-owner receives a share of the profits, group practice physicians have strong economic incentives for ensuring that the techniques and outcomes of their colleagues' cases meet high quality standards. The emphasis in group medicine is on ambulatory care, with hospital facilities reserved for those patients having serious medical problems and those requiring major medical procedures.

Medical groups are classified as single or multispecialty, depending on the variety of clinical specialties they have. They range in size from groups of between three and five physicians to large institutions employing hundreds of physicians. The majority of groups are of the single-specialty variety. Single-specialty groups are typically small, often in the range of three to five members, though some primary care and internal medicine groups are exceptions.

The number of physicians practicing in groups and the number of medical groups themselves are increasing and show every indication that they will continue to increase. That fact reflects a major change in the practice of American medicine because group practice was not always looked upon favorably—even though, historically, group practice evolved from the Mayo Clinic concept and its emphasis on quality health care. In 1932, the *Journal of the American Medical Association* referred to group physicians as "medical soviets," and more recently, in other circles, salaried physicians have been disparaged as being unethically involved in the corporate practice of medicine [10]. The group practice concept grew out of the proposition that better patient care would result if physicians could share knowledge and resources. Yet the organization of physicians in group practice was formally ignored until after World War II when the American Medical Association's Commission on Medical Care Plans extended full recognition to medical group practices [11].

Since World War II the growth in the number of medical groups has been exponential. Between 1950 and 1980, the number of medical group practices in the United States increased 20-fold. In 1950, there were about 5,000 physicians in approximately 500 group practices [12]. By 1980, more than 88,000 physicians, or 20 percent of the physicians active in the United States, worked in a total of 10,762 medical group practices. Between 1980 and 1984, the number of group practices increased 43.9 percent, rising from 10,762 to 15,485 [13].

The Medical Group Management Association, in a survey of more than 1,400 medical groups, asked how much they expected to grow over five years. Fifty-six percent expected to add between 1 and 11 new physicians. Fifteen percent anticipated adding between 11 and 45 new full-time physicians [14].

In 1986, the average group practice had 13.2 full-time or equivalent physicians, an increase of 109 percent from the average number of physicians in group practice just six years earlier [15]. Physicians have always placed great value on the autonomy and freedom afforded by independent solo practice. Yet there is now strong evidence that market forces, the capacity to provide improved consumer-oriented services, a more ordered work week, good fringe benefits and the other advantages of group practice have come to outweigh the traditional determinants of physician behavior. In addition, managed-care systems such as health maintenance organizations (HMOs), preferred provider organizations (PPOs), and other forms of managed care are creating new group practice environments.

Who is the medical group practice administrator? Medical group practice administrators support physicians in designing, managing, and improving health care delivery systems. An important part of the administrator's role is developing specific participative methods for solving problems. It is up to the administrator to provide the fiscal expertise physicians need through education in its various forms so that they understand the medical group's finances.

The administrator of a medical group relies on teamwork and involves the physician in management. In nationwide surveys, physicians share the sentiments of other middle managers who feel they need to get help to meet managerial requirements and, in addition, want more and better management training for themselves.

About three out of ten medical group practices are multispecialty groups [16]. They are the largest groups and present a variety of unique challenges and growth opportunities for medical group practice administrators. Administrators of large multispecialty group practices may deal with from 20 to more than 500 physicians. To meet the group's organizational objectives, the administrator must have the direct support of the group's medical leadership. In larger groups, that may include a broad management team composed of the medical director, administrators at various levels, and a board of directors. If a team concept does not exist, then it is a "no win" situation. Figure 1 illustrates a large corporate structure.

Administrators of small medical groups often refer to themselves as generalists. If they were asked to describe their jobs they might write out a long list of tasks beginning in alphabetical order with accounting and ending with travel agent. Physician employers sometimes expect administrators in small group practices to do their own typing, to work at the front desk, or even, in a pinch, to assist in direct patient care. A 1985 survey for the Medical Group Management Association found that 51 percent of the small group administrators who responded did their own clerical work [17].

Surveys show that administrators of small group practices often stay in their jobs for many years, express overall satisfaction with them, and say they would not want to leave for positions with larger groups.

Group practice administrators are unique in health care, because they work so closely day by day with physicians. An important part of their role is to bridge gaps of understanding between medical group physicians and the public, and, when necessary, to pose the tough philosophical and pragmatic questions that revolve around issues of service and quality. The administrators, no less than the physicians, have a responsibility to every patient and to the community.

Medical group administrators have historically been in the precarious position of middlemen between the physician, as owner, and the physician as income producer. Administrators' performances are subject to constant day-to-day scrutiny and evaluation. Each physician represents the "board of directors," and each tends to judge administrators' competence from the perspective of personal experience. Their employers spend almost all of their days in the clinic, in close proximity with the administrators. Like the physicians, the administrators' work is subject to frequent interruptions. Both must respond quickly to a variety of situations. Administrators in small medical groups become more deeply involved in operational details than would their hospital counterparts.

As Austin Ross, a past president of the Medical Group Management Association, has said, "Perhaps the most important advantage [of working in a medical group] is the satisfaction an administrator derives from using management expertise to help physicians accomplish patient-related objectives and goals. In spite of all of its problems, the clinic is one of the most

FIGURE 1:   Geisinger Corporate Structure—1987

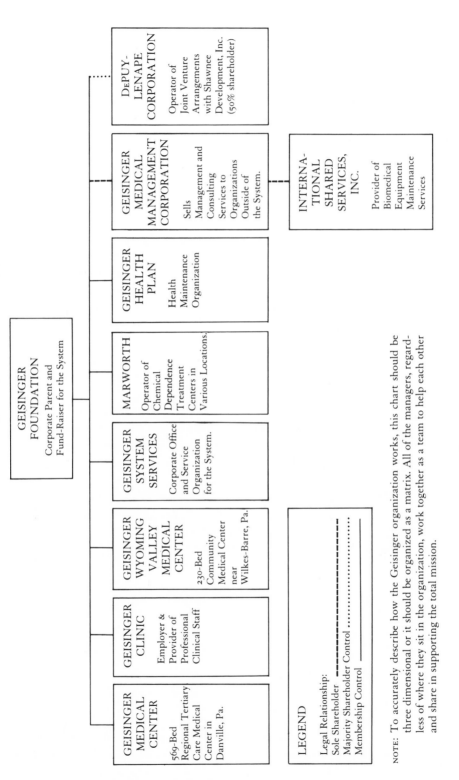

GEISINGER
FOUNDATION

Corporate Parent and
Fund-Raiser for the System

GEISINGER
MEDICAL
CENTER

569-Bed
Regional Tertiary
Care Medical
Center in
Danville, Pa.

GEISINGER
CLINIC

Employer &
Provider of
Professional
Clinical Staff

GEISINGER
WYOMING
VALLEY
MEDICAL
CENTER

230-Bed
Community
Medical Center
near
Wilkes-Barre, Pa.

GEISINGER
SYSTEM
SERVICES

Corporate Office
and Service
Organization
for the System.

MARWORTH

Operator of
Chemical
Dependence
Treatment
Centers in
Various Locations.

GEISINGER
HEALTH
PLAN

Health
Maintenance
Organization

GEISINGER
MEDICAL
MANAGEMENT
CORPORATION

Sells
Management and
Consulting
Services to
Organizations
Outside of
the System.

DePUY-
LENAPE
CORPORATION

Operator of
Joint Venture
Arrangements
with Shawnee
Development, Inc.
(50% shareholder)

INTERNA-
TIONAL
SHARED
SERVICES,
INC.

Provider of
Biomedical
Equipment
Maintenance
Services

LEGEND

Legal Relationship:
Sole Shareholder ——————
Majority Shareholder Control ···············
Membership Control ——————

NOTE: To accurately describe how the Geisinger organization works, this chart should be three dimensional or it should be organized as a matrix. All of the managers, regardless of where they sit in the organization, work together as a team to help each other and share in supporting the total mission.

invigorating and satisfying settings—even if the administrator seems always to be caught between competing and conflicting forces [18].

The group practice administrator must be a facilitator, factfinder, and information broker. The greatest challenge to any medical administrator is to provide high-quality background information and accurate data to those involved in the decision-making process through committees, the board of directors, and the medical staff. Medical group practice administrators must have strategic planning skills to be able to predict access needs, anticipate the next generation of competition, and to evaluate the need for diversifying or vertically integrating their group's services. Administrators also are responsible for marketing, establishing multi-institutional linkages for controlling costs, emphasizing and expanding ambulatory care programs, and searching for innovative alternative methods of delivering health care in response to their communities' changing medical and health needs.

The successful administrator's professional style embraces a wide range of characteristics, including flexibility, sincerity, loyalty, a talent for listening, the ability to communicate, delegate, and innovate. Successful administrators are energetic, healthy, intuitive, patient, and understanding. They care about people. They build networks. They like physicians. They work hard.

Veteran clinic administrator, Clyde T. Hardy, Jr., has noted, "The four primary ingredients that constitute a successful career in group practice management are (1) the ability to understand and deal with physicians, (2) skill in mediating conflicts, (3) willingness to give the necessary time to your job, and (4) fairness and honesty in dealing with others" [19].

As in other health care organizations, the medical group administrator must have an open door. Particularly in large multispecialty groups, administrators need to know what is going on, and they must have strong skills in dealing with people. Administrators often see "people management" as their most difficult responsibilities. Seasoned administrators advise:

— Handle your employees well; that is 90 percent of management.

— Make each employee feel like an individual.

— Be a good leader by setting a good example and by making the environment pleasant and tension free.

— Surround yourself with competent people, give them responsibility, and reward their efforts.

In summary, the challenge of group practice administration is the need to communicate persuasively with many people. The administrator who accepts and meets that challenge earns the respect of motivated and intelligent professionals and has the satisfaction of demonstrating personal and professional competence.

Management consultants Brown and McCool characterize the successful group practice administrator as a "high-performing manager." They point out that such managers welcome the competition of the new health care environment, use all the opportunities available to them, do not take no for an answer, and, even in the 1980s, position their organizations to play major roles in the emerging vertically integrated systems of health services [20].

As the preceding analysis suggests, the ever-increasing trend toward medical group practice offers tremendous opportunities for young administrators. Medical group practice administration embodies a rich tradition of knowledge and service; but, hand in hand with that tradition is a responsibility to the community in which the administrator, as a business leader, lives and works. Whether in government or in the expanding area of voluntarism, the administrator's skills of management, leadership, and decision making count for something. What the individual administrator makes them count for is important, and that responsibility grows and expands as the individual reaches higher levels of professional achievement.

There is a story told of the political columnist George Will who, when he was in high school, was drafted by the cross-country team and found it sheer misery for an entire year. When at long last the season finally ended, his mother thought he would be delighted and relieved, and he was. But he said he intended to go out for cross-country the following year *because the team needed a captain*. He learned early to take on the unpleasant jobs that had to be done. Successful medical group administrators accept leadership responsibility when their skills are needed, in the group and in the community.

In the 1980s, group practice administrators came from a variety of professional backgrounds, and most came to group practices at the age of 30 or older after beginning their careers in other areas of administration [21]. Seasoned administrators advise students interested in medical group management to begin by getting the best education possible. One highly regarded survey found that 70 percent of group practice administrators have baccalaureate degrees. Of those, 62 percent have degrees in business administration. Another 22 percent have master's degrees such as MBAs or graduate degrees in health administration [22].

After college graduation, one of new managers' highest priorities ought to be to continue their education, and the quality and reputation of the graduate school selected is of immense importance. There are few, if any, graduate programs specifically designed for group practice administration but, as leading writers and educators have pointed out, it would be a useful option within health services administration programs. With the number of hospitals declining and the number of health administration program graduates increasing, it is important to expand career options. A general health administration orientation is better than no health administration background, but an MHA with a concentration in medical group management will be especially marketable in the future.

When their formal education is completed, group practice administrators should begin to build a continuing education process into their lives that will help them learn and grow throughout the remainder of their careers. Senior administrators in outstanding medical group practices routinely advise younger associates to broaden their horizons by keeping in touch with other progressive clinic managers, especially those who have demonstrated leadership.

After graduate school, young administrators should look for opportunities for mentoring—administrative residencies and fellowships. New managers should plan to participate actively in at least one high-quality seminar each year on a subject that will renew or increase their basic knowledge in an area of management that needs review and change in their medical group.

Finally, young administrators should learn as much as possible from colleagues and associates. For that reason, it is important as new graduates select their first jobs, to consider carefully the people with whom they will be working as well as where they will be working. In their early careers they will be developing work habits, management skills, and management philosophies. The people with whom they work and from whom they learn will significantly influence their management careers.

New graduates should look for opportunities to assume responsibility as soon as they can, and not put off demonstrating what they are really able to do. At the same time, seasoned administrators often urge patience and counsel their younger colleagues to concentrate on doing each job well regardless of how disagreeable the task.

Medical group practice administrators in the 1990s will need high-technology skills and strong analytical backgrounds. Expertise in health services finance, computer technology, and management information systems will be essential as complex financial systems, planning, and quality assessment require group practices to be completely computerized.

Administrators starting their careers will need to develop strong human relations skills and the ability to work within increasingly complex organizational models. Health care rewards the diligent network builder. As

Montague Brown and Barbara McCool have pointed out, "The network builder is one who weighs and balances perspectives to ensure that all relevant stakeholders know he or she cares and will be there for them just as he or she expects they will be there as needed" [23]. The new health care organization will place a high premium on flexibility, speed of response, and internal reorganization. Administrators must learn to identify with the process of change and to recognize that the health care and economic environments will never be quiet, orderly, tidy, or solid in their lifetimes.

Medical group management has excellent opportunities for women. The number of women in administration has more than doubled in the past ten years. In the 1950s, only about 15 percent of management positions were held by women. Today more than one out of four health care administrators is a woman. Thirty percent of all MBA graduates are women, as are half of all the graduate students in health services administration [24].

Medical groups typically compensate their administrators with a salary arrangement or with a percentage of average physician profits. Entry-level salaries are comparable to those at similar levels of hospital administration. A 1987 survey by the Medical Group Management Association showed that the mean salary of a group practice administrator with more than 15 years' experience was nearly $70,000 a year [25]. Salaries ranged from $21,000 to $120,000 and higher, depending on the medical group's size and the administrator's level of responsibility. Chief administrators in groups with between 6 and 15 physicians earned median salaries of $45,500; in groups with between 51 and 100 physicians, $71,400; and in groups with more than 100 physicians, $78,000. With increasing frequency, a bonus is also a possibility. The benefit package is comprehensive, often including essentially the same benefits that are available to physicians in the group.

The Kiplinger Forecasts predict that by the year 2000 the majority of American employees will be served by some form of prepaid group health program [26]. The swiftness of change in all health services will put an extra premium on agility and quickness of response. Executives, whether in health care or other areas of business, already speak of "issues management" as a recognized specialty and a key area of expertise. Health care authorities recognize that one of the most important areas of the medical group administrator's work is to provide early warning of market trends, community issues, government initiatives—anything that might constitute an issue to be managed or an opportunity to be seized.

We have begun to see a significant movement toward networking in group practices. There are a variety of combinations: clinic to hospital or medical center, clinic to clinic, large clinic to small clinic. These arrangements run the gamut from loose networks, which may be informal agreements to share technology or manpower, to outright mergers and acquisitions. The purpose is to deal imaginatively with increasing competition in an effort to provide market-sensitive—that is, cost-effective—care of the highest quality.

Futurists see medical groups, clinics, outpatient surgery centers, and other efficient organizations providing less expensive alternatives for health care that now requires high-cost hospitalization. Administrators will be called upon to recognize a variety of health care environments and the opportunities for strong alliances that will exist among them. Health services administration graduates who have prepared themselves to recognize and to manage the close relationships of medical group practices, hospitals, and managed care organizations, including HMOs and PPOs, will have exciting futures in management.

Health care organizations are the most complex human institutions we have ever tried to manage. The changes in health care, and particularly in medical groups, offer administrators a real chance to do creative, positive, and exciting things. With ingenuity, and perhaps financing, as the only limits, it is a time for experimentation, for assuming risks in new and promising ventures. New administrators will discover untold opportunities in health care if they have the wisdom and courage to take advantage of the resources and skills they possess. There will always be plenty of grist for the gloomy prophet, but the challenges of the unreadable future will not be different in kind from the challenges that health care administrators have met and conquered in the past.

REFERENCES

1. *The Medical Practice Letter* (January): 5(1), 1985.
2. "Critical Condition: Defying All Expectations, Health Costs Continue to Soar," *Time Magazine*, February 1, 1988: 131(5), p. 42.
3. Moody, T. Competition Among Physicians: Physician Perceptions. *The Marketing Prescription Newsletter* (November 5): 1, 1986.
4. Health Care Spending: Growing Through the Year 2000. *Medicine and Health, Perspectives* (June 22): 1987.
5. Ginzberg, E. The Restructuring of U.S. Health Care. *Inquiry* 22(3), 1985, p. 275.
6. United States, Graduate Medical Education National Advisory Committee. *Report of the Graduate Medical Education National Advisory Committee.* Hyattsville, Maryland, U.S. Department of Health and Human Services, Public Health Service, Health Resources Administration, Of-

fice of Graduate Medical Education, Washington, D.C., Superintendent of Documents, 1981, Vol. 1, p. 99.

7. Freshnock, L. J. and L. E. Jensen. The Changing Structure of Medical Group Practice in the United States, 1969 to 1980. Chicago: Center for Health Policy Research, American Medical Association.

8. Goldsmith, J. C. The U.S. Health Care System in the Year 2000. *Journal of the American Medical Association* 256(24): 3371–72, 1986.

9. Group Practices Flourishing. *Modern Healthcare* 16(26) December 19, 1986.

10. Sommers, A. R. "Factors Affecting Group Practice Growth." *Medical Group Management* 11(2) January 1964, p. 13.

11. Colligan, R. D. and E. Berglund. Changing Roles of Physicians, Nurses, and Administrators. *Medical Group Management* 32(4): 39, 1985.

12. Times of Trial, an interview with C. Rufus Rorem. *Hospitals* 57(1) January 86–90, 1983.

13. Group Practices Flourishing. *Modern Healthcare* (December 19): 30, 1986.

14. *Medical Group Management Association Strategic Plan.* Medical Group Management Association, Denver, CO, 1982, pp. iii–4.

15. Group Practices Flourishing. See 10.

16. Steinhauer, B. W. "Issues Facing Group Practice in the 1990s." *Henry Ford Hospital Medical Journal* 1986: 34(4), p. 237. Article is 237–240.

17. Kerber, R. B. The Small Group Administrator. Professional paper submitted to the American College of Medical Group Administrators, Denver, CO, December 1985, p. 2.

18. Ross, A. Group Practice Administrator. In *The Challenge of Administering Health Services: Career Pathways*, ed. L. E. Bellin, 67. Washington, DC: Association of University Programs in Health Administration, 1986.

19. Hamity, G. I. and J. W. Gauss. A Profile of the Group Practice Administrator. *Medical Group Management* 29(4) (July-August): 30–31, 1982.

20. Brown, M. and B. P. McCool. High-Performing Managers: Leadership Attributes for the 1990s. *Health Care Management Review* 12(2): 74, 1987.

21. Hardy, C. T., Jr. Personal Requirements for Survival. *Medical Group Management* 29(4), (May-June): 22, 1981.

22. Hamity, G. I. and J. W. Gauss. See 14, 30–31.

23. Brown, M. and B. P. McCool. See 15, 71.

24. U.S. Department of Commerce. Female Health Administration Graduates—Sex Roles and Employment Status. Springfield, VA: National Technical Information Service, Report No. HRP-0017379, pp. 1–27. See

also, Sherry A. Babbitt's unpublished professional paper, "Profile of a Woman Clinic Manager—Revisited 15 Years Later": The American College of Medical Group Administrators, Denver, CO, August 1987, p. 5. And "Women in Health Care Administration," *Hospital Forum*, January-February 1981; 24(1), p.8.

25. *1987 Membership Salary and Fringe Benefit Survey Report*. Medical Group Management Association, Denver, 1987, p. 15.

26. *Kiplinger Forecasts: The New American Boom*, The Kiplinger Washington Editors, Inc., Washington, D.C., 1986, p. 106.

PART IV

THE INFRASTRUCTURE OF HEALTH SERVICES

10

HEALTH INSURANCE: MANAGING A VAST AND COMPLEX INDUSTRY TO SERVE THE INDIVIDUAL

DAVID H. KLEIN

The possibility of working as an insurance company executive did not even briefly cross my mind when I was applying for admission to programs in health administration. Health administrators manage, consult with, or regulate hospitals, health maintenance organizations (HMOs), nursing homes, or other medical care organizations. Their mission is to ensure the delivery by clinicians of quality care as cost effectively as possible. Insurance companies only pay the bills! How wrong and naïve were these thoughts!

Upon graduation from The University of Chicago Graduate Program in Hospital Administration in 1972, I found the supply of meaningful assignments in hospitals to be limited. A professor suggested that if I really wanted to have an effect on the delivery system, working for the Blue Cross and Blue Shield organization was a better vantage point than a single hospital. Blue Cross and Blue Shield affect virtually all providers while hospital administrators can affect only their own institutions. His comment that "providers chase dollars" offered an image of significant leverage. Sixteen years later, the advice of that sage professor still rings true.

David H. Klein is senior vice president of Blue Cross and Blue Shield of the Rochester Area, Rochester, NY. He holds an M.B.A. in health administration from the University of Chicago and a B.S. in management from Rensselaer Polytechnic Institute.

In the United States, over 85 percent of hospital and physician revenue comes from private or public sector third party payers, that is, it is paid for by other than the patient or the patient's family. Third party payers is industry jargon for health insurers. Third party payers include the federal government Medicare program, state government Medicaid programs, Blue Cross and Blue Shield Plans, commercial insurance companies, health maintenance organizations, and third party administrators. In paying medical care bills, third party payers must decide

— whether to recognize a provider as a bona fide care-giver
— whether the care provided is covered under a person's health insurance program
— whether the price charged by the provider is fair and reasonable.

If third party payers do not recognize a provider as being legitimate, or if health insurance programs are designed or administered to offer very limited coverage, or the fees allowed are low, eventually care will not be delivered. Conversely, if third party payers are too liberal in their decisions, the cost of health insurance could grow to unaffordable levels.

In this chapter, the health insurance industry is described, the functions found in a typical health insurance company are reviewed, and finally the possible career opportunities for program graduates are discussed.

DESCRIPTION OF THE HEALTH INSURANCE INDUSTRY

In the United States, health insurance companies are a significant component of the health care industry. The key role played by health insurance companies in the U.S. health care industry is exemplified by their

— Provision of group health benefits to about 100 million workers and their families through 2.3 million employers, trust funds, or associations. (In 1986, over $100 billion worth of group benefits were paid to hospitals and physicians.)

— Provision of individual health benefits to about 3 million people. (In 1986, $3 billion of individual benefits were paid to hospitals and physicians.)

— Administration of Medicare benefits on behalf of the federal Health Care Financing Administration for over 31 million older and disabled Americans. (In 1986, $78 billion of Medicare benefits were paid to hospitals and physicians.)

There are many health insurance companies in the United States. The focus of this chapter is on Blue Cross and Blue Shield plans, commercial health insurance companies, and third party administrators. Management of health maintenance organizations and governmentally operated health benefit programs (for example, Medicaid) are related careers.

BLUE CROSS AND BLUE SHIELD PLANS

There are 77 Blue Cross and Blue Shield plans in the United States. Each of the plans is a separate local company which generally limits its operation to a statewide or substatewide area. Each of these companies has its own board of directors. The Blue Cross and Blue Shield Association coordinates the actions of the plans.

Blue Cross plans generally provide hospitalization coverage, while Blue Shield plans generally provide physician coverage. Some of the plans are joint Blue Cross and Blue Shield plans while others provide only hospital or only physician coverage.

Most operate as not-for-profit health service corporations. Most were originally incorporated under special enabling laws that were passed by state legislatures in the 1930s and 1940s. States passed these laws to recognize a societal demand to provide health insurance coverage which was then not being met by commercial health insurance companies. These laws, while making establishment of a Blue Cross and Blue Shield plan easier than creation of a commercial insurance company, also required the plans to be much more highly regulated than commercial insurance companies or third party administrators.

Blue Cross and Blue Shield plans are market leaders with their overall national market share being 34 percent and their market shares in particular localities ranging from about 60 percent in the northeast to about 20 percent in the south and west. Their market leadership is generally attributed to a premium price advantage they offer their customers. This price advantage is derived from contracts negotiated with hospitals and physicians which call for Blue Cross and Blue Shield to pay a lower charge than commercial insurance companies or third party administrators.

COMMERCIAL HEALTH INSURANCE COMPANIES

There are over 1,200 commercial health insurance companies in the United States. Together, their national market share is 37 percent. Most commercial insurers are components of either mutual or stock life insurance companies.

Mutual insurers include such major companies as Prudential, John Hancock and The Equitable. Mutual insurance companies are owned by their policy holders. Mutual insurance companies return their profits to their policy holders as dividends.

Stock insurers include such major companies as Cigna, Travelers, and Aetna. Stock insurers are owned by shareholders like other for-profit general business corporations. Stock insurers distribute their profits to their shareholders per their dividend policy. Mutual and stock insurance companies are regulated by the insurance commissioners of each state in which they write coverage.

The market shares of individual commercial insurance companies are substantially less than those of the Blue Cross and Blue Shield plans. Prudential, which is the largest commercial health insurance company, has a national share of about 3 percent. Most of the commercial insurance companies are relatively small, operating in a single state or region. Of note, the top 25 companies account for over half of all commercial health insurance issued.

THIRD PARTY ADMINISTRATORS

There are at least 125 third party health benefit administrators (TPAs) in the United States. Their market share in total is 7 percent. However, in contrast to Blue Cross and Blue Shield plans and commercial health insurance companies, these TPAs represent a growing segment in the health insurance market.

Third party administrators are for-profit general business corporations which can provide all of the services of a Blue Cross and Blue Shield plan or a commercial insurance company with the exception of the insurance underwriting. Because no underwriting is provided, third party administrators are regulated much less than either Blue Cross and Blue Shield plans or commercial insurance companies. However, because the third party administration market is limited to large employers or trust funds that can self-insure, their share is very limited. The names of major third party administrators include: U.S. Administrators, Alta Health Strategies, American Benefit Plan Administrators, and Gallagher Bassett Services.

FUNCTIONS IN A TYPICAL HEALTH INSURANCE COMPANY

Third party payers—Blue Cross and Blue Shield plans, commercial insurance companies and third party administrators—all share the following major functions:

— marketing

— provider relations

— operations

— finance and administration

Additionally, unique to Blue Cross and Blue Shield plans and commercial insurance companies are the following functions:

— actuarial and underwriting

— regulatory relations

The functional organization chart of a typical health insurance company is shown in Figure 1.

MARKETING

Marketing refers generally to customer relations. In group health insurance, though, there are often two levels of customers—the group and the employee within the group. The creation of the two-level customer is tied to the recent introduction by employers of multiple health insurance options from which employees choose. It has made the industry intensely competitive.

Typically, health insurance options for employees will include one or two traditional plans, one preferred provider organization (PPO) and two to four HMOs. All of these options can be offered through a single health insurance company or through multiple competing companies.

The traditional plans offer complete freedom of choice of provider but require higher levels of employee contribution towards the premium for equal levels of coverage. The PPO is similar to the traditional plan in terms of freedom of choice, but at selected, preferred providers, higher levels of coverage are offered. The HMOs provide no patient choice except for the selection of a "gatekeeper" primary care physician who approves all specialist and hospital care prior to coverage being awarded. However, in return for these limitations in choice, HMOs typically offer more benefits for the same employee contribution.

Thus, selling health insurance involves securing clearance from a group to have your product offered and then using traditional consumer service marketing approaches (for example, presentations, literature, advertising, word-of-mouth endorsements) to entice the employee to choose your option.

This customer relations function is often broken into the following major components:

FIGURE 1:   Functional Organization Chart of a Typical Health Insurance Company

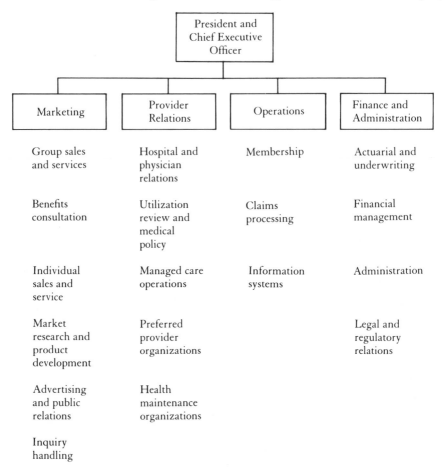

— Group sales and service is responsible for the overall relationship with groups which leads either to acquisition of new business or retention of existing business. Often, the group sales and service staff works with brokers or consultants that employers hire to help in selecting health insurance companies to use for their health plans. Enrollers working in the group sales and service area assist in selling to individual employees through presentations and one-on-one meetings.

— Benefits consultation is responsible for assisting a group as a specialist in designing their health insurance plan. It also prepares reports to explain a group's cost and utilization patterns and recommends actions to reduce cost.

— Individual sales and service is responsible for the overall relationship with those customers not buying their coverage through a group.

— Market research and product development is responsible for conducting research regarding group and individual preferences which will lead to greater sales. It also coordinates product development projects across a health insurance company. Examples of new products being developed by many health insurance companies include long-term care insurance and dental HMOs.

— Advertising and public relations is responsible for developing advertising and literature to assist in selling. It also handles inquiries from the media.

— Inquiry handling is responsible for answering questions posed by the insured about coverage.

PROVIDER RELATIONS

Provider relations refers to the process by which a third party payer will decide which providers should be recognized as bona fide care givers, what health care services should be covered under a given benefit, what price should be paid for those services, and what constitutes an appropriate level of use for those services. The medical policy, provider payment, and utilization review activities conducted by third party payers require extensive interaction with health administrators as well as physicians.

This provider relations function is often broken into the following major components:

— Hospital and physician relations is responsible for the overall relationship with hospitals and physicians. In Blue Cross and Blue Shield plans, this function also negotiates contracts with providers that yield an economic advantage to the plans. Hospital contracts often provide incentives for cost containment, while physician contracts ensure that fees charged are in line with community norms.

— Utilization review and medical policy is responsible for interpreting benefits to decide what services rendered by hospitals and physicians are reimbursable. Recent examples of controversial utilization review and medical policy issues include human organ transplant and mental health services coverage. Many health insurance companies deemed the organ transplant procedures experimental and denied payment. Coverage of care by psychiatric social workers and psychiatric nurses has also been denied by some companies.

— Managed care operations is responsible for operation of second-opinion surgery, preadmission review, concurrent review, and case management programs offered by health insurance companies. Many employers have recently added managed care to their traditional health care plans to assist in reducing unnecessary utilization of health care services. These managed care programs require patients or their families and hospitals or physicians to discuss their plans for treatment with, and sometimes gain approval from, the insurance companies prior to service delivery. Failure to follow the managed care procedures will cause a reduction in coverage for the patient.

— Preferred provider organization is responsible for selecting and contracting with providers to create a panel of hospitals and/or physicians that will deliver services more cost effectively than the norm. It should be noted that hospitals and physicians sometimes self-select into a panel and then market themselves as a PPO to health insurance companies and, occasionally, directly to employers. Examples of these self-selected PPOs are the VHA–Aetna Partners Plan and the HCA–Equitable Equicor Plan.

— Health maintenance organization is responsible for creating and managing captive HMOs or for selecting and contracting to provide marketing and administrative services to freestanding HMOs. There are many types of HMOs. The reader is referred to other chapters of the book for a further description of HMOs. However, it should be noted that about half of all HMOs are either owned by, or affiliated with a health insurance company.

OPERATIONS

Operations generally refers to the handling of the high volume of transactions received by third party payers. There are two major types of transactions: maintenance of membership eligibility data bases, that is, keeping track of who is covered for what type benefit; and adjustment and payment of claims received. Because of the volume of the transactions received, operations are heavily dependent on electronic information systems.

The operations function is often broken into the following components:

— Membership is responsible for processing transactions which add, change, or delete coverage for an individual or a group.

— Claims processing is responsible for adjudicating and paying claims. Adjudication involves encoding of diagnostic and service (procedural) nomenclature presented on hospital and doctor bills into standard classifications; determining if, under terms of a patient's coverage, a provider is "allowed" to render service; calculating a fee payable for the services; and certifying the patient's eligibility for coverage at the time of service. Payment involves issuance of checks and explanation of benefits.

— Information services is responsible for information systems to support the total operation. Major systems include membership, claims, inquiry, billing, and financial reporting.

FINANCE AND ADMINISTRATION

Finance and administration generally refers to the management of a health insurance company's finances and general support areas. Finance and administration in a health insurance company is similar to the same function in a general business corporation. The major exceptions to this description are in the actuarial/underwriting and legal regulatory relationship areas.

The finance and administration function is broken into the following components:

— Actuarial and underwriting is responsible for assessment of the risk presented by a given group or individual using health care services and the establishment of a rate or premium to fund the risk.

— Financial management is responsible for typical treasury and accounting functions but applied uniquely to health insurance companies. Financial management includes the billing and collection of premiums for insured groups and individuals, cash and investments management, and cost accounting.

— Administration is responsible for human resources and building services. Due to the high volume of transactions, key building services in a health insurance company are the mail room and the telephone system.

— Legal and regulatory relations is responsible for general legal services and for maintenance of a positive relationship with regulators and with state and federal legislators. Legal services generally involve corporate or contractual issues. Regulatory concerns include securing approval regarding all insurance contracts from their state insurance commissioners. Health insurance companies must also demonstrate to the commissioners that their premium rates will generate continued financial solvency. Interactions with state and federal legislators are needed to assure that new regulation does not unnecessarily hamper the operation and competitive position of the third party payer. In recent years, many legislatures have mandated that health insurance companies provide coverage or benefits for certain health care services—especially those related to mental illness. It should be noted that TPAs generally do not maintain regulatory relations functions as self-insured health plans fall outside the purview of state insurance commissioner control.

POSSIBLE OPPORTUNITIES FOR PROGRAM GRADUATES

As can be discerned from the above description of the health insurance industry and the functions of a typical company, it is an extremely complex and competitive industry that is comprised of a mix of large and small not-for-profit and for-profit corporations. These corporations have heavy transaction processing and financial management requirements in addition to being material elements in the health care delivery equation.

A career as a third party payer or health insurance executive can begin in almost any of the above functional areas. The ranks of senior health insurance executives have a variety of educational backgrounds.

Graduates of programs in health administration are well suited for careers in health insurance. Typical starting points for a career can include assignments in provider relations or marketing. The basic courses in a health administration program provide knowledge about medical care organizations, medical sociology, health economics and financing, and health care marketing. This information serves as relevant background material for a health insurance executive, often providing insight regarding implications of actions being proposed or taken.

Technical knowledge regarding how a health insurance company actually works as well as a basic understanding of actuarial science, operations management, and information systems disciplines can be learned on the job, though students who avail themselves of courses in these areas would improve their candidacy for entry-level jobs.

Students seeking employment in health insurance would be well served by writing some of their papers and theses about aspects of the industry as well as securing summer or part-time employment at health insurance companies.

The process to be used in securing a job in health insurance is typical of most employment searches. Networking is certainly the most effective means followed by applications to personnel offices. From an employment standpoint, the industry is growing, with the highest need found in functions where program graduates are best suited for placement.

Careers in health insurance can be very rewarding for program graduates. Since graduation in 1972, I have worked for the Blue Cross and Blue Shield Association, Blue Cross and Blue Shield of Illinois and Blue Cross and Blue Shield of the Rochester area. I would estimate that over half of the program graduates with whom I have worked in these three firms are still working in the industry, finding meaningful, interesting, and well compensated assignments.

11

HEALTH MANAGEMENT CONSULTING: SOLVING PROBLEMS AND PROVIDING ADVICE

JOHN S. LLOYD
With the Assistance of Karen M. Kelly

Consulting is an exciting career option—but probably more than some other health care administration career paths, it is clearly not for everyone. There is a lifestyle commitment to consulting that may make it an appropriate career choice for some individuals at some stages of their careers, but not for others.

Consulting may be the right career choice for a period of time, or it may be a lifetime's pursuit. It may be that consulting for a few years will satisfy your desires for new learning, for travel, for ways to influence others, or to see a project get back on track. This is true particularly if you have marketable expertise and are in the right place at the right time. It is one of consulting's virtues that it offers the opportunity to change careers without any loss of expertise or experience.

What *is* consulting, and who are these exotic creatures called consultants? The dictionary tells us that the consultant offers expert professional advice, but that simple definition cannot begin to describe the various types of con-

John S. Lloyd is president of Witt Associates Inc., consultants to health care management, in Oak Brook, IL. He holds an M.B.A./M.S.P.H. degree in health care management and finance and a B.S. degree in business administration from the University of Missouri. *Karen M. Kelly* is director of communications of Witt Associates Inc.

sulting relationships in health care today. Some sources focus on the problem-solving character of the consulting activity, while others highlight its catalytic nature or its results orientation. It is all this, and more.

The first consultants were physicians and accountants and lawyers—people whose professional advice and opinion were sought because they had training and experience in a basic body of knowledge. But the increasing complexity of today's society, and especially of its health care industry, has created opportunities for consultants from a wide variety of disciplines and skills.

Consultants are in demand because they have the special expertise and experience needed to solve problems and the objectivity to see situations clearly. Consultants can expand management capacity at critical times and make easier the organization's passage through a difficult decision or transition.

FIELDS OF EXPERTISE

Itemized in Table 1 are the broad categories of functional and specialized fields of consulting expertise that are recognized by the American Association of Healthcare Consultants. Consulting opportunities are as broad as the health care field. Acute care facilities, long-term care, intermediate care, ambulatory care, managed care, resort/retirement communities, government agencies, financing organizations, DME (durable medical equipment) suppliers, industrial health management, multispecialty clinics, and multi-hospital systems are simply some of the organization types that may require the services of a consultant.

WHAT DOES A CONSULTANT DO?

What does a consultant, regardless of his or her area of special expertise, actually *do*? These are some of the most usual tasks:

— *Problem definition.* The consultant looks beyond the obvious to discern the real problem, and is adept at stating it clearly. Why is management less able to do this? Sometimes, management *is* the problem, but more often it is simply too close to the situation to see it and recognize it. The consultant's fresh perspective is a major contribution to the problem's solution.

— *Research and analysis.* Understanding the problem usually requires additional research and penetrating analysis. Few problems are entirely unique, but there is always a "twist" that keeps things interesting for the consultant and requires analytic skills.

TABLE 1: Fields of Consulting Expertise

Strategic Planning and Marketing
    Strategy development
    Market research
    Marketing plans
    Product-line planning
    Program planning and implementation
    Regulatory assistance

Organization and Management
    Organizational evaluation and structuring
    Mergers and affiliations
    Governance
    Medical staff organization/relationships
    Organization development

Human Resource Management
    Executive search
    Outplacement
    Compensation
    Succession planning

Facilities Programming and Planning
    Facility assessment
    Master planning
    Functional programming
    Design consultation
    Project management

Finance
    Financial planning
    Financial feasibility analysis
    Financial operations analysis

Operations and Information Systems Management
    Operations analysis and improvement
    Labor productivity analysis
    Systems planning and evaluation

Health Specialist
    Equipment planning
    Food service
    Materials management
    Risk management
    Surgical services
    Other services

SOURCE: 1988 Directory of Member Consultants and Affiliated Firms, American Association of Healthcare Consultants, Arlington, VA.

    — *Alternatives for action.* A number of choices are always available for consideration, and the consultant's role is to identify and consider them all when seeking a solution. Sometimes, the best action is to do nothing, but usually a range of interventions can be considered.

    — *Recommendations.* The consultant is expected to make recommendations, which the client is free to accept or not. The consultant may offer a range of possible solutions or lay out a single optimal strategy, but clients usually prefer to act on the consultant's reasonable recommendation.

— *Plan*. Nothing happens unless there is a feasible plan of action, with mileposts, target dates, and clear responsibilities noted for all. In many cases resources must be marshaled and budgets prepared, and sometimes strategies for fund-raising or governmental assistance must also be mapped out. It is the consultant's task to design the plan in consultation with the client.

— *Follow-up methods*. The consultant usually suggests follow-up and evaluation that is to be performed by the client.

You will notice that *implementation* does not appear in this list of consultant's activities. Except in rare instances, the consultant does not play an operational role. By the time the building has been built, or the new system installed, or the new executive hired and in place, or the new product launched, the consultant has moved on. Good consultants will of course stay in contact with their clients to ensure that any questions are answered, but typically the consultant does not have hands-on participation in carrying through his or her recommendations. That is the client's task.

Is it possible to be satisfied with this role? Absolutely—if you are the kind of person who can *let go* of your ideas and allow others to take them to the next stage.

WHAT IS THE CONSULTANT'S OWN INVESTMENT?

How invested is the consultant in the outcome? He or she will not be around when the community expresses its thanks, when the lives are saved or the building is dedicated. There really can be little personal investment in the work. There is a professional pride in a job well done, of course, but perhaps the best measure of a consultant's investment is found in monetary rewards.

Especially in consulting, financial rewards are a good measure of the quality of the work. Some consultants perform the specified tasks for a specified fee. Other consultants are paid in stock that may rise or fall in value, depending on the quality of their advice. For the duration of the consulting assignment, these individuals virtually become members of the staff of the client organization. Their fortunes are tied in to the fortunes of the client.

This issue of "investment" is important to many individuals, especially in health care. It is possible to have a healthy self-interest and still maintain the consultant's objectivity. These differences of degree, not of kind, create a visible spectrum, a range of consulting roles. The person who is engaged for a short time and is paid an hourly wage will obviously have a smaller investment but may still draw satisfaction from consulting work. The person at the other end of the spectrum, who virtually joins the management team for a period of time, is simply a different kind of consultant.

It is important to understand that these two extremes—and all that falls in between—can rightly be called consultants.

A WORD ABOUT ETHICS

Ethics are essential to the quality of work and the satisfaction to be derived from that work. Every consultant will say he or she is ethical, of course. It is a "mom and apple pie" issue that no one is going to buck. But the proof of claims to ethical principles will be found in a consultant's adherence to a code of behavior that has been established by a wide-ranging group of consultants, over a considerable period of time (see Table 2).

This code may seem self-evident, but there are many firms and practitioners who do not subscribe to a code of ethics. Ethics serve as a protection for the client and provide a reasonable framework for guiding the consultant's behavior. To cite one example of how the code is applied: A client used a consultant, and then did not use him again for a period of two years. At that time the consultant was invited by a rival organization to do work for them. The first client objected, saying the consultant had access to all of their key marketing information and was in a position to do them real damage with a competitor. The consultant was censured by the professional organization for violating its code of ethics.

An ethical tenet of our firm says we will check out the educational attainments claimed by a candidate for employment. If they cannot be verified, we tell our client. This has often caused us difficulties because a candidate

---

TABLE 2: Code of Ethics: American Association of Healthcare Consultants

To exercise independence, objectivity, and integrity in all professional engagements
To maintain client confidentiality
To strive continuously to improve their professional skills
To fully disclose to a client any interests or relationships that may affect independent judgment in a specific engagement
To continuously enhance the professional standards of consulting
To fully disclose to clients in advance all financial arrangements related to an engagement
To uphold the honor and dignity of the profession
To maintain the highest standards of personal conduct

SOURCE: American Association of Healthcare Consultants, *The Code of Ethics.*

who has inflated his or her credentials may otherwise be perfect for a client's organization. It could be tempting to keep quiet and simply close the search. Everyone would be happy, right? We would not be happy, and ultimately our client might become unhappy as well. We adhere to the tenet and inform the client, even though we may give ourselves considerably more work to do.

ORGANIZATIONS THAT EMPLOY CONSULTANTS

Consultants work in professional organizations, or firms. These may be solo practices or small or large firms. They may also work in divisions of companies as in-house consultants, but these individuals will not be treated in this discussion, as they are too diverse.

The solo practitioner is an entrepreneur who chooses to call himself or herself a consultant. Remember Paladin, riding into town with his card that said, "Have gun, will travel"? He was a solo practitioner. He hired himself out to solve problems and had no particular overhead except hay for his horse and his bullet inventory. Perhaps one of the most challenging businesses is that of solo consultant, as he or she is responsible both for conducting assignments and for finding and selling new engagements. The solo consultant must have an established ethical framework and be unwilling to take on assignments for which he or she lacks the appropriate qualifications.

Solo consultants can be effective as long as they are not overloaded. The benefit of this type of work is obvious—you are your own boss. The disadvantages may be more subtle: no colleagues to kick an idea around with; no one to give you a hand with an assignment when you are ill or tired or just have too much to do; no one to sell the next job while you perform the current engagement.

The solo consultant negotiates a fee that becomes his or her income, in a way that is similar to the sports star. If a pitcher thinks he is worth $1 million a year, he can ask for it. If the team owner agrees, he pays what the pitcher asks. Another player may ask for a similar amount and be denied. Each one negotiates the best deal possible, and each purchaser pays what he feels the service is worth. This is the situation of the solo consultant as well. The marketplace will dictate what fees are possible.

The *junior consultant* usually works in a large firm for an annual salary, is less likely to have client contact, and is more likely to learn his or her craft by doing the basic tasks of consulting work: research, analysis, interviewing, and data tabulation. The junior consultant may work in accounting, data processing, or other areas of technical expertise. Firms often hire young people out of graduate school for the skills and fresh outlook they can provide.

They perform valuable service while they learn what consulting is "from the ground up." In this way they can also decide whether it is an appropriate career choice.

It is important to distinguish between what an individual is paid and his or her billing rate. The client may be charged $70 to $80 per hour for the time of the junior consultant, but that is not the actual rate of pay received by the individual. According to a salary survey conducted in 1987 by the American Association of Healthcare Consultants, junior consultants in large firms averaged $35,000 annually [1].

The *manager* is a more experienced individual, usually one who has served time in the trenches and has demonstrated a talent for managing people as well as for cultivating client relationships. The manager is likely to be a member of a large- or medium-sized firm. As a means of demonstrating his or her desire for advancement, the manager is often willing to take on particularly challenging assignments. The manager is usually good at problem definition and identifying key ideas and issues, and is skilled in client relationships. While some individuals may choose to remain at a manager level, others seek the risk and reward of status as a partner/owner. The average hourly billing rate for managers is $113 to $133, and the average annual salary was $56,000 in 1986, according to the AAHC's salary survey [2].

The *partner* usually has parlayed a great deal of experience and success in consulting, along with skill in sales and assignment development and management of people, into an ownership position with a mid- to large-sized firm. Partners like to sell and are good at it. Hourly billing rates in 1986 averaged $132 to $185 for a firm owner, with an average annual salary of $86,000. Add to that an average bonus of $23,000 for a total compensation for partners in 1986 of $109,000 [3].

A consulting firm is a very flat type of organization; if you are hung up on titles, then consulting is not likely to satisfy you. Junior people are sometimes given the title of *associates*. More senior people are, predictably, called *senior associates*. Beyond them is the officer level, with titles of *vice president* and *president*. Table 3 depicts another way of looking at the roles, based on the pluses and minuses for each level of consultant.

ENTERING THE FIELD

When is the best time to enter consulting—fresh out of school or after years of practical work experience? The answer is that either time is appropriate, depending on your circumstances. A special virtue of consulting is that it may fit into either career plan.

TABLE 3: Types of Consultants: Advantages and Disadvantages

CONSULTANT TYPE	ADVANTAGES	DISADVANTAGES
Solo practitioner	own boss make own hours take only as much work as you wish	no backups no colleagues no sales force down time between jobs
Junior consultant	work provided learning experience salary assured varied assignments skills valued growth potential	tedious tasks bonus unlikely must serve time in the trenches to move up
Manager	interesting work skills valued growth potential stimulating client contacts	major time commitment still salaried but bonus po- tential must do time in the trenches to move up must sell
Partner	own boss, with others management control excellent compensation selling interesting engage- ments	greater time commitment compensation tied to busi- ness success difficult to leave a firm

Some individuals may not truly be consultants, although they will use the title freely. If you wonder how it is possible for senior officials to leave government service and command huge salaries in private industry as "consultants," consider their superb contacts and insider expertise. As long as they act within the laws that cover their activities, they may perform for a time as consultants, but this is typically a brief tenure. These folks are usually merely salespersons or members of the company's public relations department, serving as conduits rather than as consultants. There are also "consultants" who are really people between jobs. They are not committed to consulting and are using the designation (and perhaps even finding some work in the field) to save face during a job search. The litmus test is whether he or she is still working as a consultant one year later.

TRENDS IN CONSULTING

Consulting is a trend-intensive field. Some areas or issues become "fashionable" for a time, and everyone has to have a consultant who is knowledgeable on those subjects at that time. But fashions may fade and issues can change, leaving the once-sought-after consultant with a silent phone and an empty bank balance. Facilities planning was, for a time, a very "hot" field, but as dollars to build new buildings became scarce, so did the facilities planning consultants. Of course, now that much of our hospital stock is aging, we may need their services again. Some aspects of the business are cyclical, as you can see.

One of the interesting outcomes of this sensitivity to trends is the rise of the technical consultant, whose expertise is of a different type than that of the general consultant. The technical consultant may know a great deal about computer programming or board development or menu selection or sterilization for central supply, or whatever—but may lack the interpersonal skills considered essential for consulting. The technical consultant is hired to solve a technical problem and does it well. A general consultant may subcontract with a technical consultant for a specific piece of work.

Thus, the consultant need not be expert in every facet of the assignment. The consultant's role is often to assemble, like a general contractor, supplier consultants who can provide certain technical expertise. It is the role of the general consultant to define the problem correctly and to prescribe, like a physician, a course of treatment.

WHAT DOES IT TAKE TO BE A CONSULTANT?

If a consultant is something like both a doctor and a building contractor, you may be wondering what mix of skills and abilities is needed to perform this role. The list of qualities, personality traits, and interpersonal skills needed to be a successful consultant may be either brief or extensive, but energy and intellect are always critical. James Kennedy, editor of *Executive Recruiter News*, says you need "good appearance, brains and charisma." That is probably true, but it may be helpful to look at a more detailed listing of descriptors to see the whole picture. These words mean different things to different people, but the sum total they represent should be clear.

As Robert E. Kelley notes in his book *Consulting*: "It is reasonable to expect that a person with these qualities could succeed in any profession" [4]. But these skills are *vital* for success in consulting.

LIFESTYLE ISSUES

A quick test to determine whether you have potential as a consultant is to ask yourself: "Do I really *like* to see the same people every day for coffee?" Some people place great value on the stability that may imply. The consultant's life can take you far from home base, sometimes for weeks at a stretch, and so you need to have not just a high tolerance for change but a real appetite for it.

TABLE 4: Qualities of a Consultant

Objectivity	Outgoing personality
Problem-solving skills	Maturity
Creativity	Lifelong learner
Self-confidence	Professional attitude
Integrity	High energy
Courage	Above-average intelligence
Ability to communicate	Conceptual ability
Understanding of what motivates people	Judgment
Good health	Established ethical framework
Good character	Desire to be on the cutting edge

"Healthy and energetic" are characteristics that must apply to a consultant. A fast, often strenuous pace is required, and individuals with chronic conditions or general poor health will not be successful. Someone has said his health was great until he had to eat airline food for several years, and now his health is only average. The fact is, hot dog lunches on the run in an airport are far more frequent than anyone would wish. Beyond basic good health, it is important to have a healthy lifestyle, with time taken for exercise, meditation, family activities, hobbies, reading, community affairs, and the like. Striking a balance is often difficult, but it is essential to a long and successful career.

And the spouse in a consultant's marriage needs to be an independent soul. There will be many times when he or she will get a call from the meetings that ran too long, or the flights that were canceled, or the dozens of other problems than can arise when you travel for a living. Put bluntly, you will have a somewhat disjointed family/personal life. You will sleep away from home often, and you will probably miss some of the school programs or parent-teacher conferences that others take for granted as part of their lives.

If you have season tickets for the symphony, you will probably miss some or all of the dates. You will catch a baseball game at the last minute rather than as a weeks-ahead plan. You will have plenty of time to read, since you'll be on your own and out of town much of the time. Your family will simply have to get along without you at times. The remarkable thing is how well everyone actually does in handling life's crises.

Your stress-handling mechanisms will need to be well honed and effective. Work as a consultant involves working with a variety of people in a variety of climates and settings, and also long hours of effort. Stress is a natural concomitant of this lifestyle, so you had better have excellent coping strategies.

A final lifestyle issue: consulting can be very rewarding financially. You may be able to make many of your personal dreams of success come true:

house, automobile, vacations, personal possessions. Handling the success well can itself be a cause of stress; it is a happy problem, however.

EDUCATION AND TRAINING

Somebody said the best prescription for a long life is to be very careful when you select your parents and grandparents. Similarly, you should be careful in selecting your college or university, as some of them are more likely to produce consultants than others, because of their theoretical slant or their location near key business markets. Look at the alumni listings of your own school for a measure of the success graduates have in the consulting world.

Your advanced degree in health care administration is an excellent "ticket" to consulting in this industry. It implies that you understand the systems and speak the language of your clients in health care organizations, and these are critically important measures.

THE REWARDS

Aside from the financial rewards, the primary reward for a consultant comes from the satisfaction of seeing an idea take hold and grow, making a difference in the lives of people and in the success of their organizations.

It is possible, as a consultant, to leave a true legacy, to know that because you were there and because you did your job well, change and growth have occurred for many people. This evokes a pride and quiet pleasure that make up for the long days and constant travel, the fast food, the canceled flights and postponed meetings, the intransigent AV equipment, and all the rest of the daily occurrences in the life of a consultant.

THE OUTLOOK

Consulting is a growth industry. Read the business press as well as health care media and you will learn that the role of the consultant is enlarging. We are seeing an increase in specialists, both as solo practitioners and as members of consulting firms.

Increasingly, as organizations pare themselves down and reduce the numbers of senior executives, consultants will be called in to handle projects as "temporary executives." They will be assigned a task, do the work, and then leave the organization. Everyone will be satisfied, and senior management will remain lean. This may appear to fly in the face of our earlier comments on implementation, but note the key point that is always true of a consulting assignment: there is an end point, a conclusion, a finish.

REFERENCES

1. 1987 Survey of Firm Practices, Consultant Compensation and Benefits. Arlington, VA: American Association of Healthcare Consultants, 1987.
2. 1987 Survey of Firm Practices, Consultant Compensation and Benefits. See number 1.
3. 1987 Survey of Firm Practices, Consultant Compensation and Benefits. See number 1.
4. Kelley, R.E. *Consulting*. New York: Charles Scribner's Sons, 1986.

12

EDUCATION AND HEALTH SERVICES RESEARCH: GIVING FUTURE DIRECTION TO ADMINISTRATIVE EDUCATION

SAMUEL LEVEY, Ph.D.
With the Assistance of James Hill, Ph.D., and
Daniel W. Russell, Ph.D.

Health services research has come of age. Within the past 30 years, this young field has acquired the status, resources, and visibility necessary to any legitimate area of study, and now presents career-minded individuals with challenging and rewarding possibilities. Yet the opportunities it offers are by no means as distinct as the traditional health care professions, such as medicine, nursing, and health administration. The identity of health services research and its present and future roles in the furtherance of health care and health policy are frequently matters for debate by researchers themselves. At least two factors account for this irony: (1) the multidisciplinary nature of the field, and (2) the field's vaguely defined boundaries, largely a consequence of its broad scope and brief history.

Samuel Levey is Hartman Professor and head, Graduate Program in Hospital and Health Administration (GPHHA) and Center for Health Services Research, College of Medicine and Graduate College, The University of Iowa, Iowa City, IA. He earned M.A. and Ph.D. degrees in health administration from the University of Iowa. He also holds an S.M. from Harvard University and a bachelor's degree in psychology from Bowdoin College. *James Hill* is a research associate, and *Daniel Russell* is associate director of the Center.

In recent years, health services research has received wide notice. From its obscure origins in the first decades of this century and the privately funded surveys of limited scope carried out in the 1920s, it has expanded to a veritable growth industry financed at local, state, and federal levels. Over 40 university-based and independent centers for health services research and/or health policy are now in operation. Interest is high. Support is significant, although the need for new sources of revenue always exists. Rewards (intellectual, professional, and financial) are considerable and, as one would expect, the number of graduates choosing to make a career of health services research continues to grow. As with any career choice, however, the decision to become a researcher or policy analyst requires careful deliberation. Those considering a career in health services research would do well to examine the nature of the field, as well as its development, demands, rewards, problems, and prospects.

WHAT IS HEALTH SERVICES RESEARCH?

There is no definition of health services research specific enough or of sufficient scope to satisfy all members of its constituency. According to Flook and Sanazaro, it addresses "problems in the organization, staffing, financing, utilization, and evaluation of health services" [1]. In the view of Mechanic, health services research is concerned with the "production, organization, and distribution" of services, and their effect on health status, illness, and disability [2]. Shortell and LoGerfo place the emphasis of health services research on relationships between consumers and providers "as they affect and are affected by health care organizations, technology, financing, and payment systems" [3]. Central to the concerns of health services research is the enhancement of personal and public health services and the promotion of greater efficiency, effectiveness, and equity in the utilization of resources.

Commentators on the nature of health services research distinguish it from biomedical research, the set of activities concerned with the origin, diagnosis, and treatment of disease. Although the distinction between the two is often blurred, the concerns of health services research may be said to begin where diagnosis and intervention end (that is, in the measurement of matters such as patient satisfaction and cost of care). In figurative terms, biomedical research prepares the stage for medical action, while health services research follows with a review of the performance and suggestions for enhancing future presentations. A further distinction applies to the scientific domain of each activity. Whereas the subjects of biomedicine are located in the life sciences, the problems of health services research have solutions primarily in the social sciences, the management sciences, and the engineering sciences. As an illustration of this distinction, DeFriese points out the recent tendency to identify health services research with the economic analysis of health care—he argues for a broadening of emphasis—while Blendon calls attention to its focus on populations rather than individuals [4, 5].

Since health services research is multidisciplinary in nature, it is rarely referred to as a discipline. Rather, it is generally viewed as a field that encourages the synergy of a host of disciplines on the rationale that combined strength is greater than the sum of parts. Within its wide purview, health services research draws upon the concepts, methods, and data of disciplines such as medicine and other health professions; social and behavioral sciences such as economics, sociology, and psychology; applied social sciences such as social work and health services administration; and other areas such as industrial engineering, biostatistics, and demography [6].

Studies in health services research include various levels of complexity, from a description of clinical practice to an issue of concern across the health care industry. For example, a clinical study may examine the influence of physician workload on the quality of care at a particular health care organization, an organizational study may compare the quality of care given by physicians in solo practice and that of a group practice or health maintenance organization, and a systemic study may examine the influence of financing mechanisms on the capital expenditures of various types of hospitals [7].

Examples of the mix of recent studies in just one university-based program include analyses relating to improved diagnosis and treatment of urinary incontinence in the elderly, development of a statewide plan for child health services, and formulation of a national agenda for health policy related to the aged [8]. Perhaps the most dramatically successful and far reaching health services research effort of the past 20 years was the group of cost-related investigations that led to the creation of the prospective payment or diagnosis-related group (DRG) system for Medicare. In the early 1970s, a series of cost-control studies at Yale University, financed by the National Center for Health Services Research, generated the conceptualization and design of DRGs. In 1983, introduction of DRGs on a national scale ushered in a new era of health care financing.

HISTORICAL PERSPECTIVE

The roots of health services research lie deep in the medical care reform movement of the first decades of this century, particularly the emerging liberal-democratic spirit of equality in access to health care. The first research studies, primitive by today's standards, were characterized by observation and description; later studies added dimensions of explanation and analysis. Examples of such early efforts include the 1908 Chicago Medical Society survey of the supply and distribution of physicians and midwives in Chicago and the landmark 1910 Flexner report on the quality of medical education [9, 10]. Such surveys of health care resources, as well as the limited compilations of social and economic data completed before the 1920s, were carried out not at public (that is, government) urging, but through the initiative of philanthropic foundations and other private organizations.

Some historians of health services research see its origins in the working of social consciousness, particularly evident in the descriptive studies of the 1920s that examined matters such as equity of access, prevalence of illness within the population, and the health status of the poor. One observer is more precise, marking its beginning with the creation of the Committee on the Cost of Medical Care in 1927 [11]. Privately financed by six foundations, the Committee carried out 27 field surveys and produced 28 reports between the years 1928 and 1932, representing the most far-reaching health care studies of the time. In the words of a leading authority on health services research, "Never before in this or any other country was such an ambitious attempt made to establish a benchmark of factual information for the consideration of public policy in the health field" [12].

The Committee became a model for collaborative studies that would follow. Comprised of a multidisciplinary group—physicians, economists, social scientists, and other investigators—its areas of study included (1) diseases and disabilities, (2) organized facilities, (3) cost of care, and (4) provider compensation for services. Prominent among the recommendations in the Committee's reports were the encouragement of group practice among providers and the implementation of insurance programs to provide for health care coverage. Among the key proposals, there is a strong recommendation for continued health services research: "The Committee recommends that the study, evaluation, and coordination of medical service be considered important functions for every state and local community, that agencies be formed to exercise these functions, and that the coordination of rural with urban services receive special attention" [13].

On the momentum of the Committee's work, other studies followed, some sponsored by private foundations and others by the federal government. Notable among them was the first national health survey, carried out by the U.S. Public Health Service. Interviews of 700,000 households generated a data base showing the prevalence of illness and its social and economic contexts which served for 20 years as a valuable information resource. The purpose of this research, then as now, was to contribute to the formulation of public policy.

In the 1920s and 1930s, most research was carried out on an ad hoc basis by statisticians, economists, and physicians hired by government or private associations. In subsequent decades, university centers for the study of health management began to offer a base for health services research. For example, research into the economic and social aspects of health care was initiated at the University of Michigan in the early 1940s. Immediately after World War II and into the 1950s, other universities followed suit with the development of programs. Academics from various disciplines (for example, sociologists, economists, political scientists, psychologists) were brought together to conduct studies, and the tentative outlines of contemporary health services research were formed. A body of knowledge for teaching, research, and policymaking began to grow.

During the 1950s nationwide health surveys were conducted with some regularity under the auspices of federal commissions and private foundations. In 1951, the Commission on the Financing of Hospital Care was established for the purpose of analyzing the costs of hospital services and determining the best means for payment of such services; from 1949 to 1956, the Commission on Chronic Illness carried out its large-scale study of illness and hospital costs; and in 1953 and again in 1956, the Health Information Foundation, a not-for-profit organization which supported health research, conducted a national health survey that studied, among other things, differences in utilization of health services by the poor as compared with higher income groups, and solo, fee-for-service practice versus prepaid group practice.

The 1960s and 1970s brought access to and expansion of health care within a context of regulation. Following the passage of Medicare and Medicaid legislation in 1965, steadily rising health care expenditures accompanied by growing public concern about cost and access heightened the need for data collection to guide policy. Economists in particular were attracted to the field of health services research. The sophistication of collecting and analyzing data became vastly enhanced with the availability of computer technology and multivariate applications. Operations research came into vogue in research centers at universities such as Johns Hopkins and Wisconsin. As a consequence of these rapid developments, health services research received the largest federal funding in its history.

Since 1970, at least two major developments have served to strengthen health services research dramatically: (1) the growth of the field within the nation's universities, and (2) the expansion of the federal government's role in health care. The institutionalization of the field in the academic setting has not transpired without dispute, owing perhaps to the divided loyalty of health services researchers. A multidisciplinary activity, it has no "natural" departmental affiliation, and consequently must operate either as a freestanding center with interdepartmental support or—the usual case—within kindred fields such as health services administration and policy. Adding to the problematic identity of health services research is the increasing sophistication of contributing disciplines without a parallel enhancement of the health services research base. As a consequence of this uneven partnership, researchers trained in a discipline must often perform a difficult balancing act between the two.

The second major development is the growth of the federal government's role in the financing and delivery of health care. For years that function has been a topic of debate: How far should the role of the federal government extend as a financier, provider, planner, and regulator of health services for its citizens?

To illustrate this issue, the idea of a government-sponsored health service has been recommended and resisted from the early decades of this century, with the tide shifting according to the prevailing national mood. In the 1950s and 1960s, debate on the subject of health insurance focused on adequate coverage for the elderly and disadvantaged, and by 1965 a nationwide mandate influenced by various health services research initiatives had forced the passage of Medicare and Medicaid legislation. With the passage of this legislation, the federal government became the nation's largest health insurer and, with the development of new programs in the "Great Society" years, the largest spender for health services.

In 1968, the National Center for Health Services Research (NCHSR) was created within the (then) Department of Health, Education, and Welfare to plan and oversee the government's research efforts and to seek ways to enhance the performance of the nation's health care industry. The emergence of NCHSR was the natural outgrowth of a number of trends: (1) a growing direct federal involvement in providing, financing, and planning health services; (2) a growing recognition that problems in the health care industry were due to fundamental organizational deficiencies; (3) a belief that reforms could be achieved and should be based on knowledge derived from systematic, large-scale research and development programs; and (4) the emergence of an identifiable field of health services research [14].

NCHSR became one of the primary sources of support—charged with reviewing and funding grant proposals as well as pursuing its own research agenda. In recent years, however, it has been overshadowed to an extent by the Office of Research and Demonstrations in the Health Care Financing Administration (HCFA), which has also become a major player in government-sponsored health services research.

When federal support began to drop off in the 1970s, private foundation grants proved to be important to the ongoing life of health services research. Sources of funding such as the Robert Wood Johnson Foundation, the Pew Memorial Trust, and the John A. Hartford Foundation continue to provide financial backing not only for research, but also for the maintenance and expansion of training programs for health services researchers.

Giving further support and legitimacy to the field during the 1960s and 1970s was the formation of a number of professional health organizations, and also the introduction of journals that present both health services research findings (for example, *Medical Care, Health Services Research*) and discussions of national health policy issues (for example, *Inquiry, Journal of Health Politics, Policy and Law*). These outward features of professionalism as well as the promotion of dialogue through national conferences are slowly giving health services research a persuasive voice that is able to advance its interests with funding sources and policymakers.

THE NATURE OF THE WORK

The business of health services research is varied, with responsibilities in the generic academic activities of reading, listening, discussing, researching, writing, and presenting. Such duties may be circumscribed by disciplinary activity carried out at "think tanks" such as the Rand Corporation, the Brookings Institution, university institutes, and federal agencies. Or the health services research may be a mix of research, teaching, administration, and outside consultation conducted in the academic setting.

The techniques of health services research range from health statistics and clinical studies to technology assessment and policy analysis. Inquiry tends to be descriptive or analytical, following the stages of empirical procedures, from selection of the problem, formulation of methodology, measurement and data collection, analysis and interpretation, and finally translation and application. Of course, the inquiry need not proceed through the entire sequence to implementation. Indeed, one observer finds examples of health services research in any combination of the following activities:

1. *Description* of institutions, or people's roles within them, their purpose, behavior, and interactions with others
2. *Collation* of statistical data establishing relative orders of magnitude of key phenomena
3. *Interpretation* of 1. and 2. as giving rise to "problems" (and especially policy problems) with rival formulations of such problems usually ensuing from one source or another
4. *Invention* (and promotion) of particular solutions to these alleged problems

5. *Evaluation* of rival solutions (and sometimes of rival problem formulations)

6. *Extrapolation*, or speculation, from what is (sort of) known, to what is not known

7. *Recommendation* about policy, based on any or all of the above [15].

Most studies, however, tend to follow a pattern of inquiry that begins with a problem and proceeds through formulation and adjustment of hypotheses, to the testing of hypotheses. In the view of Klarman, this pattern of health services research includes

> recognizing and distinguishing between the real and apparent problems that occasion a particular study, finding hypotheses that can be tested empirically, selecting the combination of methods to be employed and allocating resources to them, arranging for appropriate statistical analyses of data, comparing the study's findings with related studies reported by others, and drawing conclusions as bases for policy recommendation or as points of departure for further targeted study [16].

For researchers with academic appointments, teaching constitutes an important responsibility. Many researchers would agree, however, that far from being a freestanding activity, teaching is intimately connected with research, with the efforts of one area informing and strengthening the other. Inevitably, to be a senior researcher is to be an educator. In addition to instructing students in the methods of research, educators may lead doctoral students through seminars and direct dissertations; both activities offer stimuli for research since they involve a review of classic studies and the latest developments in the field.

Customarily, then, researchers wear many hats. Not only do they design studies, conduct surveys, and write up results (with the help of colleagues and research assistants) as well as teach, but they often must also raise funds and administer a research budget: grantwriting and management of financial resources are major responsibilities for many health services researchers. Further responsibility may include consultation services with health care organizations.

HEALTH SERVICES RESEARCHERS

To meet the demands and pressures of the work, health services researchers should possess certain habits of mind and strengths of character in addition to the specific relevant knowledge and skills. A temperament strong in self-discipline offers an advantage, as do rational attributes such as patience, logic, and assiduity. An active interest in identifying and resolving human service problems is a further asset. In addition, the engaging, outgoing skills of the manager or entrepreneur are particularly important in today's competitive environment, because health services researchers must frequently "sell" ideas to policymakers prior to funding.

In the view of Blendon, health services researchers should spend more time "in presenting our facts and our results to non-scientific audiences, particularly in regard to current problems facing the nation" [17]. Successfully bridging research and practice requires a talent for public presentation—an ability that combines the virtues of the academic, the manager, and the entrepreneur.

Education for a career in health services research, unlike training for most other careers involving a high degree of specialism and technology, may be achieved by either of two avenues: (1) experience in a traditional field such as finance or systems engineering, followed by training in health services research; or (2) interdisciplinary studies in health care administration. In most cases, an advanced degree (for example, M.A., M.S., M.H.A., Sc.D., Ph.D.) is required.

Doctoral work in a single discipline can be oriented to health services research through cross-disciplinary training, part of which is available through course work, seminars, field work and discussions. If the prospective researcher proceeds via the route of a doctorate in health services research, then the training involves (in most cases) concentration in areas such as the management of health care delivery organizations, and quantitative analysis. The doctoral program in Hospital and Health Administration/ Health Services Research at the University of Iowa, the nation's first doctoral program in the field of health management, is representative: the requirements include a minimum of 90 graduate credit hours, comprehensive examinations, and a dissertation based on original research. Doctoral candidates are expected to develop expertise in three areas:

1. *Health Services Management and Policy.* A core of four required courses covering the specialized knowledge and skills necessary to advanced health management

2. *Research Methodology and Advanced Statistical Techniques.* Three required courses in health services research and one of three statistics sequences

3. *An elective minor field of study.* Examples include sociology, political science, economics, management science, or social psychology [18].

Typically, the doctoral dissertation is the culmination of training for the health services researcher; it presents one with the requirement to demonstrate a full scope of knowledge and skills in addressing a research problem, and also the opportunity to develop a special competence in an area.

In today's health services research center, one does not find a uniformity of interchangeable positions, but a hierarchy of research roles, including senior investigators, junior investigators, postdoctoral fellows, and doctoral and master's students from various disciplines and fields. A center also includes project managers, data and policy analysts, proposal writers, and other support staff. Advancement through the levels of responsibility within the academic research center—as throughout academe—depends on a number of factors, including quality of research, publications, grantwriting and funding, teaching, and service.

Although most researchers are academics employed by universities, many can also be found in applied settings such as government regulatory agencies, insurance companies, independent research organizations, private consulting firms, and a variety of health services settings, such as hospitals, medical centers, and multihospital corporations. Within these arenas, researchers may concentrate on specialties such as planning, financing, and marketing.

REWARDS AND CHALLENGES OF A CAREER

What rewards does a career in health services research bring? To begin, the financial compensations are typically more generous than those available in many traditional academic disciplines and fields. Also, the intellectual pleasure of bringing a project to completion and the emotional gratification of laying the groundwork for some far-reaching social good are in themselves substantial satisfactions, particularly if one is able to see research findings applied to health services management and policy. (This, after all, is the raison d'être of health services research.) To recognize and reward major contributors to health services research and to encourage the highest levels of performance, prizes have been designed for distinguished books, articles, and innovative research efforts. For example, the Association of University Programs in Health Administration with the generous support of the Baxter International Corporation has created the Baxter Foundation Prize to recognize significant contributions to the health of the public through health services research.

Unfortunately, the prompt implementation of even the most distinguished and consequential research findings is not always a likely event. Indeed, one of the frequently cited frustrations among health services researchers is the failure of those who could use research to avail themselves of readily available studies. The reason for this neglect is a matter for ongoing debate. At least part of the cause lies in the methodological complexity of health services research: simply put, greater analytical sophistication has generated greater communication difficulty. One prominent health services researcher asks with obvious dismay, "How can the results of this research reach practical people when these studies are filled with ever-more-complex statistical analyses?" [19]. Manifestly, making research findings accessible to practitioners and policymakers remains a problematic part of the research-er's work.

Most of the questions that are of concern to decision makers in management and government are of a practical nature. For example, what are the risks and benefits of nursing home use among the elderly? Do copayments and deductibles present a barrier for the use of health services? How can HMOs reduce costs without sacrificing quality? Ironically, then, in spite of the fact that health services research is an applied field, much academic research tends to be theoretical, and the orientation of academic researchers is more likely to be toward theory development than practical problem solving. Quite naturally, this may bring disappointment to practitioners whose expectations of research are direct implications for action, and whose response to elaborate theory tends to be either dismissal or slighting of the work.

Perhaps lying at the heart of the problem is the need for a unifying framework for the various participating disciplines. Because many researchers identify themselves with their specific academic specialty, the field often seems split along disciplinary lines (that is, physicians, economists, sociologists, others). As Greenberg and Choi observe, "Health services research is conducted by individuals from different disciplines who vary greatly with regard to perspective, methods, assumptions, and language" [20]. If, as Flook and Sanazaro observe, the goal of health services research is "progressively greater understanding of all relationships in health services to be derived from social, political, medical, financial, economic, legal, organizational, operational, and theoretical perspectives" [21]—then the integration of discipline-focused research into a unified theoretical framework would seem to be as important, and as elusive, as a comprehensive general theory of management.

FUTURE PROSPECTS

As with so many other technologically complex endeavors, the vitality of health services research depends in large part on funding—more precisely, on a dependable flow of dollars. In view of the steadily rising health bill (currently one ninth of our gross national product), one who expects a similar rise in appropriations for health services research may be surprised at its small fraction of the more than $450 billion spent on health care in 1986. Fortunately, however, other funding sources exist. Although federal investment in the National Center for Health Services Research has declined from a high of $70 million in 1972 to $47 million in 1987, a number of public and private funding sources have stepped in to offset the cutbacks. In the opinion of the past president of the Association for Health Services Research, "The field bottomed out for a while. But it's on the way up again. The problems are not getting any smaller, and the policymakers are finally learning how to use our work" [22].

At the federal level, various sources of financing besides NCHSR and the Health Care Financing Administration include the National Center for Health Statistics, and the National Institutes of Health. Private contributors include a growing number of regional foundations. With large, multi-institutional systems becoming more keenly interested in developing applied research programs, stronger links between academe and provider are likely to occur, producing further funding.

What types of current and future research projects are the strongest candidates for appropriations and grants? An indication of the more attractive emphases in research is suggested by the health services research agendas of three organizations: the National Center for Health Services Research, the Robert Wood Johnson Foundation, and a university center for health services research. Current priority areas at the NCHSR are

1. primary care or health promotion and disease prevention
2. technology assessment
3. the role of market forces in health care delivery (for example, economic incentives and the supply of services, alternative delivery systems, quality of care, and barriers to competition)
4. medical practice variation and disease prevention [23]

At the Robert Wood Johnson Foundation the research emphasis of late has focused on projects designed to

1. improve access to personal health care for the most underserved population groups
2. help people maintain or regain maximum attainable function in their everyday lives
3. make health care more accessible, affordable, and effective [24]

The Center for Health Services Research at the University of Minnesota, a representative program, identifies its primary areas of emphasis and expertise as

1. evaluation of alternative delivery systems
2. competition
3. finance or reimbursement
4. long-term care
5. state health policy analyses [25]

As one might expect, health services researchers' concern with health care among the needy elements of the population, the disadvantaged and elderly, is strong. With the aging of the population and the growth of the competitive environment, a keener interest in both long-term care and the uninsured segment of the population, within frameworks of cost, quality, and access is to be expected. As for the current interest in competition, alternative delivery systems, and technology assessment, recent developments in technology and the structure of health care organization, financing, and delivery have brought to the fore issues that received merely passing notice ten years ago. Given the business orientation of health care, one may assume that aspects of competition such as marketing, productivity, and risk management will continue to be key issues in research into the 1990s.

The vital importance of building bridges between the academic and practitioner communities cannot be overstated. According to Altman, "the responsibility for making ourselves and our work known rests very firmly with us—the research community" [26]. Researchers have a duty to make their work available to potential users such as policymakers and practitioners because they share a common goal of improved health services. Toward this end, one prominent commentator calls for researchers to establish stronger links with major user constituencies: "We need to build their confidence in our work and the infrastructure of our field. We need to help identify those really important questions which deserve serious research attention and we need to enlist the collaboration of the user community during the sometimes long process of research project formulation and execution" [27].

The future of health services research looks promising, even within sight of disconcerting facts such as unstable health care resources and rising competitiveness. Federal funding is rising after a decade of decline; the call for focused, applied research has become stronger and researchers are learning to market their findings to the nonresearch community; and within research centers, the demand for enhanced integration of disciplines is slowly bringing about greater cooperation.

Although health services research is relatively young as a field, its place in our health care system is now well established. The operations of hospitals and health maintenance organizations have become extraordinarily complicated matters, with managers now more inclined than ever to be analytical and quantitative in their approach. In the view of one observer, administrators are learning that "data on local markets, productivity, the cost of care, and other topics are common tools of management. Health services researchers created those tools, and now they are being asked to refine them" [28]. At the federal level, policymakers will continue to look to researchers for ways to slow the rising tide of health care costs.

A restrained optimism about the future of health services research prevails. In the view of Mechanic, "a well-structured health services research program is essential to future health care policy and to adequate monitoring of a massive national investment" [29]. Blendon sees the need for research becoming ever more critical, because of a renewed commitment to the country's health care system. Reasons for this renewal include

1. the absence of a solution to rising health care costs
2. the potential of Medicare bankruptcy
3. the need for a new public agenda after defense and deficits [30]

Health services research will remain vital to the future of health management and policy as long as questions of effectiveness and efficiency in the organization, financing, and delivery of health care continue to be posed. For the graduate considering a professional life in a health-related field, health services research offers a career route with substantial rewards. One finds opportunities that present financial compensation and intellectual satisfaction, as well as the emotional gratification of knowing that health policy may be affected for the good of all.

REFERENCES

1. Flook, E. E. and P. J. Sanazaro. Health Services Research: Origins and Milestones. In *Health Services Research and R & D in Perspective*, ed. E. E. Flook and P. J. Sanazaro. Ann Arbor, MI: Health Administration Press, 1973.
2. Mechanic, D. Prospects and Problems in Health Services Research. *Milbank Memorial Fund Quarterly* 56(2): 127–39, 1978.
3. Shortell, S. M. and J. P. LoGerfo. Health Services Research and Public Policy: Definitions, Accomplishments, and Potential. Paper prepared for the Institute of Medicine Steering Committee on Health Services Research, March 1978.
4. DeFriese, G. H. Rediscovering the "Health" in Services Research. Presidential address at the third annual meeting of the Association for Health Services Research. Boston, June 1986.

5. Blendon, R. J. Health Services Research: Future Trends and New Directions. Opening address at the first national meeting of the Association for Health Services Research. Chicago, IL, June 1984.

6. Institute of Medicine. *Health Services Research*. Washington, DC: National Academy of Sciences, 1979, 33.

7. Institute of Medicine. See 6, 18–21.

8. Association for Health Services Research. *Directory: University-Based Health Services and Policy Research Centers*. Washington, DC: The Association, 1985, 46.

9. "Midwives of Chicago," *Journal of the American Medical Association* 50 (17): 1346-50, 1908.

10. Flexner, A. *Medical Education in the United States and Canada: A Report to the Carnegie Foundation for the Advancement of Teaching*, New York: Carnegie Foundation, 1910.

11. Neuhauser, D. Health Services Research, 1984. *Medical Care* 23(5): 739, 1985.

12. Anderson, O. W. Influence of Social and Economic Research On Public Policy In the Health Field. In *Health Services Research*, ed. D. Mainland, 19. New York: Milbank Memorial Fund, 1967.

13. Committee on the Costs of Medical Care. *Medical Care for the American People*. Chicago: University of Chicago Press, 1932. Reprinted 1970, Washington, DC: U.S. Department of Health, Education, and Welfare.

14. Institute of Medicine. See 6, 76.

15. Williams, A. The Practice of Health Services Research. *Community Medicine* 5(4): 317–20, 1983.

16. Klarman, H. Training Requirements for Health Services Research: How Many? At What Skill Level? From Which Discipline? *Health Services Research* 16(3): 263, 1981.

17. Blendon, R. J. See 5.

18. From the 1987 brochure of the Graduate Program in Hospital and Health Administration at the University of Iowa.

19. Neuhauser, D. See 9, 742.

20. Choi, T. and J. N. Greenberg. The Role of Social Sciences in Health Services Research: An Overview. In *Social Science Approaches to Health Services Research*, eds. T. Choi and J. N. Greenberg, 10. Ann Arbor, MI: Health Administration Press, 1982.

21. Flook, E. E. and P. J. Sanazaro. See 1, 81.

22. Friedman, E. Those Wonderful People Who Brought You DRGs. *Hospitals* 58(5): 85, 1984.

23. University of Iowa. Center for Health Services Research. *Guide to Funding Sources*. Iowa City, IA: The Center, 1986.

24. University of Iowa. Center for Health Services Research. See 23.
25. Association for Health Services Research. See 8.
26. Altman, S. H. Health Services Research: Do We Matter? First presidential address at the second annual meeting of the American Association for Health Services Research, Chicago, June 1985.
27. DeFriese, G. H. See 4.
28. Friedman, E. See 20, 88.
29. Mechanic, D. See 2, 131.
30. Blendon, R. J. See 5.

13

FOUNDATIONS: PROMOTING CHANGE THROUGH GIVING

ROBERT A. DeVRIES

The sage Aristotle asserted: "To give money away is an easy matter and in any man's power. But to decide to whom to give it, and how large, and when and for what purpose, and how, is neither in every man's power—nor an easy matter."

Preparation and practice in health administration have proven to be a desirable background for a career in philanthropy. Foundation boards and chief executive officers often seek professionals who are thoroughly knowledgeable of a field or discipline and also possess good management skills.

This chapter describes foundations and charitable trusts; cites an example of a large international foundation; reviews career interests in philanthropy; describes potential professional positions; and discusses preparation, personal traits, and compensation in this field.

FOUNDATIONS AND PHILANTHROPY—PRIVATE GIVING FOR THE PUBLIC GOOD

The Foundation Center defines a private foundation as "a nongovernmental, nonprofit organization having a principal fund of its own, managed by its own trustees and directors, and established to maintain or aid charitable, educational, religious, or other activities serving the public good, primarily by making grants to other nonprofit organizations" [1]. There are at least

Robert A. DeVries is program director at the W. K. Kellogg Foundation in Battle Creek, MI. He holds an M.B.A. in health administration and a B.S. in physiology from the University of Chicago.

four types of foundations: independent (private) foundations, company-sponsored foundations, operating foundations, and community foundations.

Independent foundations, which make up the largest group, are grant-making organizations whose funds generally come from an individual, a family, or a group of individuals. These foundations might be operated under the direction of the donor or the donor's family members or the foundation may have an independent board of trustees that manages its activities. In most cases, independent foundations have broad charters but frequently limit their giving to a few selected fields. Because of their broad charters, they may move from time to time into new fields in response to changing societal priorities. While these private foundations are largely concerned with grantmaking, some may also directly operate demonstration or fellowship programs. Other names that may be given to independent foundations are "general purpose" or "special purpose" foundations. Examples of such foundations are the Ford Foundation, John D. and Catherine T. MacArthur Foundation, W. K. Kellogg Foundation, Robert Wood Johnson Foundation, Pew Memorial Trust, and the Rockefeller Foundation.

Company-sponsored or corporate foundations are separate legal organizations established and supported by a business for the purpose of making grants and carrying out other philanthropic functions. These foundations are usually managed by a board of directors, often composed of corporate officials, but which may also include persons with no connection to the supporting business. Not uncommonly, company-sponsored foundations involve local plant managers and officials in setting policy and establishing grant-making programs. The giving programs of company-sponsored foundations often focus on communities where the business has operations and on activities or fields related to the company's objectives. Corporate foundations are distinguished from corporate contributions or direct giving by a business, since the latter are provided by and administered within the corporation itself. A company-sponsored foundation makes it possible for a business to put aside funds for use in future years when company earnings may be reduced and the needs of charitable organizations might be greater. Examples include the Atlantic Richfield Foundation, General Motors Foundation, Exxon Education Foundation, Amoco Foundation, and the AT&T Foundation.

Operating foundations are, as the name implies, organizations established to operate charitable programs, research, educational activities, or human services which are determined worthy by the governing body or donor. While some grants may be made outside the foundation, the majority are spent for its own charitable programs. For some operating foundations, endowment funds may have been provided, although most also receive some contributions from the general public. Examples include the J. Paul Getty Trust, Norton Simon Foundation, Robert A. Welch Foundation, and the Russell Sage Foundation.

Community foundations are generally supported by and operated for a specific community or region. Their funds are derived from a variety of donors and in many cases they are composed of a number of different trust funds, some of which bear the donors' names. Investment funds are generally managed professionally, usually by trustee banks. A governing board or distributions committee are typically representative of the range of community interests and professions. Examples include the San Francisco Foundation, New York Community Trust, Cleveland Foundation, Chicago Community Trust, and the Communities Foundation of Texas.

Overall, there are approximately 23,000 U.S. foundations. About 350 have annual outlays of between $1 million and $10 million and approximately 20 provide $10 million or more in annual grants. In 1984 the distribution of grants by subject categories or fields was about 14 percent to cultural activities, 17 percent to education, 24 percent to health, 2 percent to religion, 8 percent to science, 8 percent to social science, and 27 percent to welfare.

At least 60 percent of U.S. foundations have no professional staff, and only 1 percent have three or more. In a 1985 staffing patterns of foundations survey conducted by The Foundation Center involving 4,402 foundations, of which 2,425 responded, only 48 percent reported employing full-time or part-time staff. These 1,163 foundations together employ 5,724 staff members, including 1,831 full-time and 712 part-time professional staff.

Future outlook for private grant-making foundations and charitable giving looks positive. There is a generally favorable regulatory environment and, when the U.S. economy grows, new foundations of all types are seen. Community foundations are the fastest growing segment of the grant-making foundation community. As additional foundations are established and existing ones increase their assets and grantmaking, additional professional and support staff will be needed.

W. K. KELLOGG FOUNDATION—AN EXAMPLE OF A LARGE, INTERNATIONAL PHILANTHROPIC ORGANIZATION

The W. K. Kellogg Foundation, Battle Creek, MI, was established in 1930 by the ready-to-eat cereal pioneer "to help people to help themselves." Will Keith Kellogg was both the founder and president of the Kellogg Company and the founder of the philanthropic organization which bears his name. In his later years he echoed Aristotle's sentiment saying, "it has been much easier to make money than to spend it wisely."

Since its inception 58 years ago, the Foundation has been managed independently by its own board of trustees and administration. Since 1930, it has expended more than $1 billion and in its 1987 fiscal year distributed $95 million in grants in support of more than 869 active projects in 24 countries in the fields of agriculture, education, and health. It is numbered among the largest philanthropic organizations in the world.

Recognizing society's difficulty in using available knowledge for human benefit, Mr. Kellogg gave to his foundation its distinctive commitment, "for the application of knowledge to the problems of people." Today the Foundation addresses significant human issues with direct, pragmatic answers obtained through pilot programs and demonstrations. As a private grant-making foundation, it provides seed money to organizations and institutions that have identified and analyzed problems and have designed constructive action programs aimed at practical solutions. Current program priorities concentrate grants in the United States, Latin America, the Caribbean, and southern African countries. The Foundation also operates a National Fellowship Program and recently began Kellogg International Fellowship Programs in food systems and in primary health care or health administration.

As part of its commitment to support the most promising projects, the Foundation gives special recognition to grantmaking which involves the physically handicapped, the elderly, women, children and youth, and minorities.

Like many other human service organizations, the Foundation has three organizational levels: (1) a 10-member board of trustees responsible for overall policy; (2) Foundation administration comprised of the chairman and chief executive officer, president, and vice presidents responsible for finance and administration; and (3) program staff who are responsible for program development, proposal review, award recommendations, grants administration, evaluation, project visibility; and the office of communications and dissemination.

The Kellogg Foundation employs about 90 full- and part-time professional and support staff, including officers and 12 program directors (2 of whom operate the Kellogg National Fellowship Program), and 8 associate program directors. Of these 20 professional staff members, 3 have backgrounds and experience in health administration. In health, other disciplines represented are medicine, nursing, sociology, and science education.

The responsibility for hearing and reviewing about 350 proposals per month falls to the program directors and their staffs and consultants. Current program interests of the Foundation include adult continuing education; community-based, problem-focused health services; a wholesome food supply; leadership; youth; economic development in Michigan; and several emerging or exploratory areas such as development of rural America, water resources, management of information systems, philanthropy and volunteerism, and science education.

CAREER INTERESTS IN PHILANTHROPY

At high school graduation or even when finishing college, few people would ever think about becoming a foundation officer, except for the handful who grew up with wealth or were in some way exposed to the opportunities and challenges in private giving. While there are relatively few new positions available in any year, these positions do offer highly challenging, creative, rewarding, and broadening professional experiences which are well worth seeking.

In addition to the position of chief executive officer of a foundation, the larger philanthropic organizations employ program directors or program officers who are well-regarded professionals with sound experience in one or two fields or disciplines. Their responsibilities are to recommend awards, manage active grants, monitor projects, and suggest new program opportunities. Beyond this, public agencies (U.S. Department of Health and Human Services, state health departments, federal agencies and centers) and leading consulting firms attract persons with like preparation for distributing public funds, for counseling organizations, and for providing reports of findings and recommendations for institutional growth and development.

In the medium to large foundations that are committed to programming in health services delivery, health professions education, and health policy, opportunities exist for employment of individuals prepared and experienced in health administration. Positions would include those of the chief executive officer, program director, consultant, and general grants officer. Examples of foundations that have employed graduates of master's programs in health services administration include the Robert Wood Johnson Foundation, the Duke Endowment, The Pew Memorial Trust, W. K. Kellogg Foundation, and the Cleveland Trust.

THE POSITIONS OF FOUNDATION EXECUTIVE AND PROGRAM DIRECTOR

The position of president or chief executive officer (CEO) of a regional or national foundation making grants in the health and human services field requires a seasoned professional, usually with a master's or doctoral degree. This professional must possess excellent personnel and communications skills, demonstrate general management ability, and knowledge of the fields of medical care organization and health professions education. In most cases, the individual is expected to have published books or articles and be experienced in public speaking and teaching. In addition, the CEO must have a sound grasp of budgeting and financial management, personnel relations, and communications.

The position of program director in a health foundation also demands that the professional be a capable manager with a good personality for working with prospective grantees and project leaders of active awards. Unlike the CEO, the program director should possess special in-depth expertise in several areas in which the foundation makes grants, such as community health services planning, epidemiology, health professions education, health services administration, medical care organization, medical economics, and health promotion or disease prevention. This professional may work in all of these, using personal training and experience as a base.

Recognizing that the program director's responsibility is more an art than a science, this professional should be well attuned to changes, new technology, innovations, and future trends. At the Kellogg Foundation, program directors commit about 30 percent of their time to program development and future opportunities for foundation investments, 40 percent to grants management and the administration of active awards, 15 percent to program (a cluster of like grants) and project evaluation and communications and dissemination, and 15 percent to foundation representational responsibilities including community service.

Preparation for the program director position requires a minimum of a master's degree in health services administration or the equivalent M.P.H., M.B.A., and preferably a doctorate in one of the applied disciplines. In most cases, one does not apply for the program director position; rather talented individuals are "discovered" by the board or management of the foundation and invited to interview. Very often they are successful grantees or authors of outstanding, thoughtful articles.

In many cases, the selected individual has served as a consultant to the foundation, has been involved with a grant or project supported by the foundation, or has served on an advisory committee for a grant or the foundation itself. Some program directors begin with a limited contract as research assistant, project evaluator, or as a fellow of the foundation (where fellowships are given).

Visibility to foundation senior staff and officers is important so individuals should watch for evaluator, researcher, project assistant, and fellowship notices in journals, *Foundation News*, and health association newspapers. Also, selectively sending curriculum vitae to appropriate foundation staff you have met can be helpful. Historically, health program directors at the

Kellogg Foundation have a minimum of 10 years of professional experience before being invited to an interview. All had made a number of professional acquaintances in a range of disciplines such as medicine, nursing, the allied health professions, health administration, and health governance before joining the foundation staff.

Financial compensation for the program director is generally equal to that of a CEO of a medium to large hospital or medical center. Unlike the rest of the health management field, it is rare to move from one foundation to another.

Individuals who will be successful in the position are those who are willing to "keep sharp," continue to write and teach, be creative and risk taking, and display an ability to conceptualize new, unique combinations for advancing both health services delivery and health professions education. The professional in this line of work must have a high tolerance for change and ambiguity and should be an excellent writer and an appropriate representative of the foundation. To help develop these skills, continuing education programs are offered by Grantmakers in Health and the Council on Foundations—professional organizations for foundation professionals.

The position of program director requires much listening, learning, information gathering, and questioning. The program director should be a good estimator of character and should be tolerant and sympathetic to the causes that are addressed by prospective grantees. One of the best experiences for foundation program officers is to work on the "other side of the desk"—and successfully direct a grant.

Clearly, advantages of the position include travel and exposure to creative people who are leaders in their fields and to new ideas. Some disadvantages include long hours (60 to 80 per week are common) of listening, evaluating, writing, and having to say no, politely, many more times than yes. Depending upon one's view and family situation, travel also can become a burden.

SUMMARY

Especially within the last 15 years, the philanthropic world has employed a number of health administration graduates as program representatives and senior officers. Foundation health management professionals have contributed much to foster creative demonstrations for improving health services delivery and health professions education, for evaluating new practices and procedures in the health and higher education fields, for networking health care leaders, and for the framing of public policy.

Unlike government resources that are largely categorically committed, private foundation and company resources can be used effectively on the pressure points of health and human services as the essential risk capital to effect change. Foundation executives and senior program staff who have effective skills and knowledge of medical care organization and general management can and will continue to make key contributions to this relatively small but rewarding public service field.

SOURCES ON PHILANTHROPY

Council of Michigan Foundations. Information for Seeking Foundation and Corporate Grants: How to Research, How to Prepare a Proposal, Where to Get More Information. Grand Haven, MI: The Council.

The Foundation Center. *The Foundation Directory, 10th Edition*. New York: The Center, 1985.

Grantscene, Newsletter of Grantsmaker in Health.

W. K. Kellogg Foundation. *1986 Annual Report and Program Information Brochure*. Battle Creek, MI: The Foundation.

14

PROFESSIONAL ASSOCIATIONS: A POWERFUL INFLUENCE ON PEOPLE AND INSTITUTIONS

JEAN-CLAUDE MARTIN

William H. Whyte Jr. said, in *The Organization Man*, "The whole is always greater than the sum of its parts. . . . Through interaction, we can produce ideas beyond our capabilities as individuals [1]. Human beings have always felt a need to associate. They joined forces to defend themselves against attack and to protect their land and families. Culture, language, and geography all led to the formation of these kinds of associations. Sociologists have done extensive studies on the need to associate, and have commented that "associations are organizations which combine both formal and informal, more rational and less rational, forms of behavior [2].

Associations can be defined in a number of ways; for the most part, these definitions are dependent on the author's field of expertise. I have chosen a simple, well accepted definition:

Associations are organizations which are more formal than collectivities, which perform specialized functions for their members, and which combine in complex ways elements of both less rational and more rational forms of human behavior. They are small societies made up of workers, rank and file members, leaders, and patrons. Thus, when we refer to an organization as an association, we are singling out a type of social group which performs crucial functions, particularly in

Jean-Claude Martin is president of the Canadian Hospital Association in Ottawa, Ontario. Mr. Martin received an M.H.A. and a B.Pharm. from the University of Montreal.

modern societies. Associations may range in size from relatively small social or recreational clubs to large-scale organizations [3].

Health care associations must define their specific mission, their raison d'être. The individuals or institutions that form the association decide why they are getting together and exactly what objectives they want to pursue. This first task is often a long and difficult one which requires skilled leadership, as the mission must be clear and well understood by all concerned. It is often the result of considerable compromise on the part of the individuals participating in the process. In general, the mission of a health care association is to represent the interests of its membership and to provide services that will enhance the membership's common interests or goals.

The pursuit of common interests and goals is the essential ingredient to make an association work. Improving relationships with governments and other health organizations, better financial support for services, and improved quality of care are ultimate goals of most health care associations. On the more practical side, the formulation of objectives and policies (based on consensus of the membership) such as definition of types of care, access to care, funding of care, quality of care, and so on, and the promotion of these policies, are essential to the proper functioning of the health care system. The planning, organizing, and providing of services such as education, information dissemination through publications, and research, are a few of the many practical roles that health care associations must play.

HEALTH CARE ASSOCIATIONS

My aim is to describe the types, characteristics, activities, and funding of health care associations. New associations, with new missions, are created every day in our rapidly changing society.

Health care associations can be broadly divided into four different types:

— Personal membership
— Institutional membership
— Disease-specific
— Services only

The professional personal membership association is by far the largest category. In the health sector, every profession has one or more associations; generally, their role is to set professional standards, provide educational services, and promote the interests (professional or financial) of their members. Physicians, nurses, administrators, pharmacists, dentists, and dietitians all rely on such associations. Some examples are the Canadian College of Health Service Executives, American College of Healthcare Executives, American College of Medical Group Administrators. Virtually all of those with full-time professional staffs are national in scope. State and provincial personal membership associations also exist to serve specific or local purposes.

Associations based on institutional membership (corporations or organizations which run and manage institutions) have as their main activity advocacy or representation but also may be extensively involved in services. In this categtory are associations of general, long-term care, teaching, psychiatric, pediatric, for-profit and denominational hospitals, nursing homes, home-health services, and many others. This group includes many provincial, state, metropolitan (city), and regional associations, some of which have professional staffs as large as or larger than national associations. Examples include the hospital associations of Ontario, New York State, and California, city associations in Chicago and Cleveland, and regionals such as South Florida and the New England Hospital Assembly. National examples include the Canadian and American Hospital Associations, Catholic Health Association, Federation of American Health Systems, Group Health Association, and the National Hospice Association.

The disease-specific association exists for a number of specific missions or goals, for example:

— To attract public attention

— To promote education

— To raise funds to provide specific types of patient care

— To promote and stimulate research

This group is well known for their creative fund-raising activities. There are associations concerned with heart, lung, and kidney diseases, cancer, cerebral palsy, arthritis, and so on. The involvement of volunteers in these associations is extremely important to their success and an important dimension of management's role.

A number of associations or organizations in the health care field are operated solely for the purpose of providing one or more services. They are generally not involved in advocacy or representation. The focus of activities of these organizations is usually well defined and requires special knowledge and expertise from its staff. Examples of such activities are accreditation, planning, shared services, negotiations, education, specific services in health care such as nursing, laboratory, and blood bank. Organizations such as the Red Cross, nursing services, regional planning councils, national or regional labor negotiation, and group purchasing organizations are examples of this type of association or organization.

One of the main characteristics of a health care association, as in any other type of association, is that it operates on a consensus based on the views and opinions of the majority of its members. This consensus is often precarious and changes from time to time as the membership, environment, and issues evolve. For instance, more emphasis may be put on representation to the public or government if one or more issues which affect most of the membership emerge. On other occasions and for different reasons, emphasis may be placed on services. The environment and processes of health associations are dynamic, so mission and objectives are under constant review. The association that does not formally facilitate this process will be rapidly repudiated by its membership.

Another important characteristic of health care associations is their usually high political profile, as their representation function—to inform or influence others—is basically in the domain of political science. This characteristic often greatly influences the management of the organization which has to be well informed and ready to adapt itself to the political environment of the day.

The association based on membership views and opinions must develop policies on which its representation strategy is built. Having achieved this first step, the association must develop a network of relationships with the view that, at the proper time and under proper circumstances, it will try to influence others to accept its views or opinions.

The size of an association is another important characteristic. Although there are a few large health care associations, most of them are relatively small organizations in terms of staffing and funding, particularly when compared to health care institutions. They also have a tendency to fluctuate in size as objectives are adapted to the needs of the membership. In addition, the size of the membership and its capacity to support the association through fees and purchased services greatly influences the scope of the activities and projects in which it becomes involved. In recent years health associations have become very creative in expanding revenue sources in order to be less dependent on member dues and fees.

The issues which associations deal with and the activities of associations are also very diversified. Even a small association may be involved in a wide variety of activities. Because issues may change quickly and membership service needs also change, the mix of activities is in flux. In many cases, associations must be prepared to run crash programs or projects to meet the needs of the moment. Flexibility, mobility, and responsiveness are all essential elements of a good health care association and are the responsibility of management.

In summary, associations (groups of individuals or institutions pursuing common interests or goals) are mostly small organizations which operate according to consensus of their memberships to represent their interests (political and otherwise) in a very diversified range of issues and services.

The activities of health care associations can be grouped under three general headings: representation or advocacy, services, and general management.

The advocacy or representation process involves identifying a problem, proposing a solution, and encouraging acceptance of that solution. Advocacy or representation is the most important activity of an association and the most volatile and difficult activity to evaluate. The need to influence the process of public policy making is the fuel for advocacy or representation activities. Advocacy is the function of an advocate—in support of a particular objective or proposal. Representation is the action of placing a formal position, reasons, or arguments before others to influence opinion or action to effect some change. Depending on the circumstances, the targets of such action may include politicians, civil servants, the media, health care providers, other health care associations and organizations, and the public.

Input for advocacy or representation activities usually originates from

— Policy positions developed by the board of directors

— Resolutions proposed by the membership and approved by the board of directors

— Priority setting exercises undertaken periodically in consultation with the membership

Operating from this base, the association staff develops an advocacy or representation strategy which defines target audiences, the method by which the message will be delivered, and the outcomes against which effectiveness will be assessed.

For health care associations, audiences can be broken down into the following broad categories:

— Government authorities involved in health care legislation or regulations

— Other health care associations

— Other organizations which become involved in health care issues from time to time

— Occasionally the general public on major issues

The message can be delivered in a variety of ways:

— Official policies describing the association's views on an issue or problem are formulated for approval by the membership and board of directors

— Position briefs giving the association's views, opinions, and recommendations are prepared for approval by the membership and board of directors

— Communications (including special reports), meetings (including lobbying) with appropriate individuals or organizations, speeches to selected audiences, published messages or interviews, and any other way that will achieve the advocacy or representation goal of the organization

Advocacy or representation is probably the one association activity for which the typical graduate of a program in health administration is least prepared. To be successful, those considering a career in the health care association field should seriously consider taking courses in political science, public relations, public speaking, and marketing to complement their professional education.

Services offered to their members by health care associations can be manifold. The most common activities are in education, publications, and research and development. Many institutional membership associations also offer assistance with fundraising, group purchasing, labor negotiations, computer services, biomedical engineering, other specialized consulting services, employment placement bureaus, electronic information networks, and more.

The broad range of possible association services is another indication of the diversity of expertise which association management requires. The rationale for developing such services is that the quality is going to be as good or better than that produced by individual members or institutions, but the main factor is that—from a financial point of view—it is a better, more efficient way to use financial resources. Many of these services produce revenue which is used to underwrite needed but unprofitable activities, or to planning, finance, and other business skills.

The following activities are usually considered general management:

— Corporate affairs, which deal with the responsibilities of the board of directors, such as bylaws, policies, programs, budget, committees, and strategic planning

— Internal administration, such as finance, personnel procurement, offices and equipment, and public relations

— Membership relationships, such as meetings, correspondence, and information on activities

There are four primary sources of association financial support: membership fees or dues; income from services or revenue from projects; donations, grants, and subsidies; and investments.

The main source of association funding is membership fees. Fees are set by the board of directors, who often use complex formulas to spread the costs fairly among the members. Although there is no firm rule, it is generally agreed that membership fees should represent at least 30 percent to 50 percent of the total operating budget of the association. It depends greatly on the type of association and the mission it is pursuing, and the mix of revenue sources will often change from year to year.

Donations, grants, and subsidies are mainly used for research, demonstration, or other special projects. These funds can fluctuate tremendously and cannot be viewed as a solid base on which to build the future of an association. They are often called soft money and help get a project started, or fund a specific research project. Government health grant programs, foundations, corporate donors, and special fundraising organizations are the main sources of funds in this category.

Periodically, associations may have a surplus. Usually surpluses are invested on a medium- or long-term basis in relatively secure stocks, bonds, or bank certificates. Associations also invest in real estate to provide adequate office space at a reasonable cost. Extra space can be rented to generate revenue. Real estate often appreciates in value over a period of time, allowing the association to increase the value of its investment. Generating a surplus for investment is wise association management which allows an association to stabilize its financial situation. Again the need for sound management skills is obvious.

HEALTH ASSOCIATION EXECUTIVES

Having described some of the general characteristics of health care associations, along with their different types and functions, let us now look at some of the requirements, suggested training, and career opportunities for individuals wishing to make a career in these organizations.

Association executives must have a clear understanding of and commitment to the mission of their organization. Usually mission statements are very specific and require the development of goals and objectives that will lead to the achievement of the mission. Executives who are not totally committed to the mission of the association would do better to look for another job, as one can predict that within a relatively short period of time they will run into difficulty with the association's membership and governing body. A clear mission is fundamental to the effectiveness of a health association and the chief executive officer is its chief advocate 24 hours a day.

Association executives must adapt to their environment and in the health sector, as in many other spheres of activity, the environment is changing rapidly. The nature and types of membership change, the political and legislative situations change, services must be adapted constantly. Essentially, health associations deal with people and projects and must always respond to the needs of the membership. Association staff, at whatever level, must be frequently prepared to adapt to a new working environment.

Most of the time the activities of a health association, whether it is in the advocacy or representation field or the services field, is project-oriented. A brief on a specific subject, a set of policies on an issue, research on a particular problem, seminars or conferences dealing with current issues or to upgrade membership knowledge, publication of reports or news stories represent some of the continuing projects of a health association. To be project-oriented means being prepared to work with new or different methodologies to resolve issues.

An important characteristic for health association administrators is that, from time to time, and within reasonable and calculated parameters, they are willing to take risks. They should be no different, and behave no differently, than normal entrepreneurs, with one exception—they must realize that an association is not in business to make a profit for its shareholders, but rather to defend the individual, professional, or institutional interests of its membership. Therefore association executives have to walk a very narrow line—on the one hand being entrepreneurs and risk takers, while at the same time never losing sight of the mission of the association, nor offending the sensitivity of the members.

One of the main activities of association management is working with people. Individuals considering a career in health association management should keep in mind that beyond the nature of an association (people oriented) the health care sector itself is people oriented; health association administrators, of necessity, must deal with people at every level of operation.

Creativity is another important characteristic of successful health association executives. Solutions to problems (old or new) have to be found rapidly and frequently. Individuals with imagination and a good knowledge of the health care system will usually have the ability to develop policies, structures, or methodologies to address difficult issues.

Health association executives work in a nonstructured environment. This encompasses office environment, size of the association, exercise of control, working hours, and the need to travel. Health associations often have a high rate of staff turnover. As issues and projects change, so, often, does the staff. The majority of health associations are, from the point of view of staff numbers and budget, relatively small, thus requiring each staff member to be a generalist with a frequently changing job description. Individuals are also given great autonomy in their work, the control function being limited to essential and crucial activities.

Meetings, deadlines for projects, and availability of individuals or resources dictate the working hours; one must recognize that work schedules must be adapted to needs, often resulting in long hours and weekend work. Association work also entails travel. While this may be viewed by some as a perk of the job (and it sometimes is), there is a difference between traveling for pleasure and traveling on business. Association administrators are often more familiar with hotels, meeting rooms, train and bus stations or airports, than any other feature of a city or country.

It puts a strain on family life. Social functions can also be a problem. Many association executives have found themselves in deep trouble due to overindulgence. Working long hours, traveling extensively, and constantly meeting with new people in new and different environments create a lot of stress. Personal discipline and a good mix of work, play, and rest are essential to survival.

The job description in Figure 1 represents the span of functions of a typical health association executive.

In addition to the chief executive officer's position, depending on the type, size, and function of the association, there are many other positions that offer opportunities to graduates in health services administration.

In all associations (small and large) there is a need for expertise in the representation or advocacy area. Policy development and writing, preparation and presentation of briefs, meetings with representatives of other associations, governments, and pressure groups are but a few of the functions performed. This stream of activity will often lead individuals to more senior positions, such as the CEO of an association or to a similar role in a larger association with more complex representation or advocacy activities.

The services provided by health associations are in specialized sectors and require some expanded and specific knowledge, such as in education, labor relations, fundraising, and so on. This stream also offers potential for growth. Great opportunities also exist in general management. Accounting, human resources, and system design are examples. The experience acquired in these areas can also lead to promotion in the health association network.

FIGURE 1:   Health Association Executive Job Description

POSITION	PRESIDENT
DEPARTMENT	ADMINISTRATION
REPORTS TO	BOARD OF DIRECTORS

Must have a thorough knowledge of the principles of organization and management, as well as legislation affecting health care institutions; must be particularly adept in the areas of human relations and public relations.

MAJOR RESPONSIBILITIES

1.   Implement Board of Directors' policies and decisions.
2.   Represent the association.
3.   Assume final authority and responsibility for all matters pertaining to the operation of the association.

SPECIFIC DUTIES

1.   Plan, administer, direct and coordinate, in conjunction with senior staff, all activities of the association to carry out its objectives.
2.   Report results to Board of Directors and committees.
3.   Ensure that policies approved by the Board of Directors are interpreted and carried out.
4.   Represent the association, as necessary or desirable, in its dealings with members, governments and government agencies, allied and other health organizations, and any other body to whom representation is directed.
5.   Perform any other duty that may be necessary and in the best interests of the association.

JOB RELATIONSHIPS

All employees of the association report through the senior executive staff.

EDUCATION REQUIRED

Graduate from an accredited university course in administration or equivalent experience.

EXPERIENCE REQUIRED

Five years' experience in a senior position with demonstrated success in the field of health administration. Demonstrated leadership qualities. Good communicator.

SOURCE: Taken from Canadian Hospital Association Job Description

So depending on an individual's interests, training, and ability, health associations offer a wide spectrum of possibilities for growth, and competitive remuneration.

While a number of paths may lead to a career in health association management, it is essential to have a sound education and training in management. In some small associations, a college degree might be optional, while in larger associations university level education is an absolute requirement. An individual can also acquire experience and further training by working in a health care setting, thus becoming thoroughly familiar with the health care system. Later, more specific knowledge about association management may be acquired through specialized courses.

The following are topics with which individuals should be familiar: administrative theory, social and political science, health care organization, public relations, marketing, and personnel administration. As the types and activities of associations are wide-ranging, and as numerous positions are usually available, candidates with specialized qualifications, such as law, education, research, communications (print or electronic), finance, economics, labor negotiations, purchasing, fundraising, and so on, are also in great demand.

On-the-job training is also valuable. Many associations offer residency programs of limited duration or the possibility of working under supervision to students enrolled in programs in health administration. Individuals interested in a career in health association administration should consider this avenue which will allow them to familiarize themselves with the work and environment before finalizing any decision.

In conclusion, a good education in health services administration is the best foundation for a career in health association management. Graduates from university programs in health services administration are increasingly recognized as candidates of choice, because they do have most of the prerequisites for the job.

To sustain interest, to provide a code of ethics, and to further education, health association administrators have access to a plethora of professional organizations. One association groups together association executives. There are presently six large national associations of association executives in the world. As an example, Figure 2 gives the mission and goals of the Institute of Association Executives.

The same national association gives the following perspective on the "executive challenge":

> The Association executive's job has never been easy. Running what is often a complex and challenging organization, keeping the members interested and involved, ensuring stimulating and relevant meetings is difficult enough. However, as we moved into the 1980s, Association boards began to look for a new kind of Association manager.
>
> The Association manager was suddenly expected to become an effective government relations advisor, handle an interview on television as effortlessly as the professional commentator, predict the growth of

FIGURE 2:   Mission Statement

MISSION

To enhance the role of association executives and their associations to better serve their members and society.

GOALS

—   To enhance the role of association management.
—   To promote the Institute or Society as a forum for the interaction of association managers.
—   To develop educational opportunities as a means of upgrading and maintaining the skills and professionalism of association management.
—   To develop and maintain meaningful relationships with industry, government, academic groups and the media at appropriate levels to improve and promote the profession of association management.
—   To promote the development of a profession which will offer rewarding career employment to association managers.
—   To promote the purposes and effectiveness of voluntary and professional associations by any and all means that are consistent with the public interest.

SOURCE: Institute of Association Executives. Mission of the Institute. *Annual Report 1986–87.*

new or emerging issues without the assistance of an accurate crystal ball, and build coalitions with voluntary groups with often conflicting and hidden agendas.

As we move towards the 1990s, these skills and abilities are likely to become more rather than less important. The Association executive will be expected not only to function with confidence and ease in complex external environments, but will be required to assist his or her own volunteer board to gain similar expertise and to identify necessary action steps.

Obtaining an understanding of the external world and how it is changing is an important first step in maintaining professionalism as an effective Association manager. An update of the latest in "how-to" techniques in the tools of effective public affairs management—issues management, stakeholder coalition building, media relations and crisis management, government relations, the importance of opinion polls and effective communications will reinforce this understanding and provide new skills to meet this changing and challenging environment [4].

The above statement gives a good flavor of what is needed to become an effective health association administrator.

WHY A CAREER IN HEALTH ASSOCIATION MANAGEMENT?

Having described health associations and the role and functions of those involved in these organizations, here are my reasons why health association management is an attractive career.

— Health associations offer very *diversified* and *challenging* goals to their executive staff. The range of issues dealt with can be as wide as those faced by the health care sector as a whole. Finance, quality of care, human resources, efficiency, information, and education are some of the broad topics that are addressed.

— Health associations *work with people and for people*. The human factor in day-to-day activities is very important.

— Health associations try to *influence people* so that the services rendered are of the utmost quality. Health associations are at the forefront in the development and the shaping of the health care system.

— Health associations provide the *forum where the exchange of ideas* among all those involved in the health care sector takes place. Health associations should always be the main source for information.

All these factors make working in a health care association extremely interesting and rewarding. As many have said before me, "There is never a dull moment in a health association."

I am a pharmacist by profession and hold a graduate degree in health services administration. My career has led me into a variety of areas: pharmacist in the armed forces, junior to senior administrator in small to large teaching hospitals, a brief career as professor of hospital administration at the university level, and five years in a health care shared services organization. At no point in my career had I ever considered a career with a health association. My broad and diversified experience in the hospital sector was probably the decisive factor in my selection for my present position.

As you can see, I had extensive experience in the health institution sector, and some experience in the management of services. On the other hand, my knowledge and training in political science, sociology of organizations, marketing, and public relations was rather deficient. Through reading, coaching, and seminars I was able to expand my knowledge and complement my training but I had enough at the beginning to get started.

The most important thing I have learned is that solutions to problems can always be negotiated. By nature, an association is a consensus reaching organization, so its staff must be prepared to work in this type of environment. Another thing that I have learned is that associations must have the facility to change and adapt; this is the basis of their survival.

I have been with the Canadian Hospital Association for ten years, and have enjoyed tremendously the diversity of the work and the people involved within and outside of the organization. If I could turn the clock back ten years, there is only one thing I would do differently—I would take a course in political science. It would have made me more productive sooner.

In summary, a career in health association administration can be very interesting and rewarding. The problems you work with are wide-ranging and the environment is often unstructured; it is always challenging and the results are commensurate with the effort you expend. It is a growing field in terms of the number of associations. I am always amazed at the number of new associations being established, so the requirement for well trained, well motivated health association administrators is bound to increase.

REFERENCES

1. Whyte, W. H., Jr. *The Organization Man*. New York: Doubleday & Co., Inc. 1956.
2. Lowry, R. P. and R. P. Rankin. *Sociology—The Science of Society*. New York: Charles Scribner's Sons, 1969, p. 364.
3. Lowry, R. P. and R. P. Rankin. See number 2, p. 310.
4. Institute of Association Executives. Executive Challenge, Information Brochure. Toronto, Ontario, 1987.

PART V

PUBLIC SECTOR

15

CANADIAN GOVERNMENT: MAKING THE MOST OF THE PUBLIC INVESTMENT

AMBROSE M. HEARN

In Canada, since government is deeply involved in the health care system, new graduates of health services administration programs considering employment with government need to be aware of some key features of the structure of government. Canada is a federal state consisting of ten provinces and two territories. It was created in 1867 when the British North American Act (BNA Act) was passed by the British Parliament uniting several of the British North American colonies. This act and subsequent amendments to it comprised much of the constitutional framework of Canada. The BNA Act granted provincial governments primary jurisdiction over most health services, although the federal government is not completely excluded from the field by this act.

Canada has a parliamentary system of government. At both the federal and provincial levels, the people elect a legislature. The party with the majority of elected members usually forms the government. The leader of the government is the first minister (called the prime minister at the national level and the premier at the provincial level). The first minister appoints additional ministers, most of whom are responsible for a particular department or ministry (for example, health, agriculture, or finance). The mem-

Ambrose M. Hearn is executive director of the Canadian Council on Health Facilities Accreditation in Ottawa, Ontario. He holds a diploma in health administration from the University of Toronto and a bachelor's degree in commerce from Memorial University of Newfoundland.

bers who comprise the cabinet are elected members of the legislature. The cabinet determines government policies. Thus health policy in Canada is set by the federal government for those areas under its jurisdiction and by individual provincial and territorial governments for those areas under their jurisdictions.

ROLE OF PROVINCIAL GOVERNMENTS

The provincial governments have primary jurisdiction over health services so they play an extremely important role in the provision of health services in Canada. The role of the provincial government, as set out in the constitution, provides that each provincial legislature may exclusively make laws in relation to the establishment, maintenance, and management of hospitals, asylums, charities, and eleemosynary institutions in and for the province, other than marine hospitals. The constitution also gives the provinces jurisdiction over all matters generally of a merely private or local nature in the province.

ROLE OF FEDERAL GOVERNMENT

The BNA Act (confirmed by the recently approved constitution) has not prevented the federal government from being involved in health services. Section 91 of the act gave the federal government jurisdiction over quarantine, the establishment and maintenance of marine hospitals, and the quality of food and drugs. It also enabled the federal government to provide health services for the military, Indians, the Royal Canadian Mounted Police, and inmates of penitentiaries. The federal government is also responsible for providing health services in the Northwest Territories and the Yukon.

FUNDING OF HEALTH SERVICES

Health services in Canada are funded by the provincial and federal governments on a negotiated cost-shared basis. Constitutionally, the federal government has the power to tax and borrow money, and it has agreed to share its revenues with those provinces willing to establish certain health and other programs that meet federal standards. Provincial governments also have the power to tax and borrow money and fund a portion of the health services. As a result of these two arrangements, provinces have been persuaded to establish hospital and medical insurance programs that comply with agreed-upon federal and provincial standards, the cost of which is partially met by the federal government.

ORGANIZATION OF THE DEPARTMENT OF HEALTH AND WELFARE

In order to meet its mandate, the Department of Health and Welfare has organized itself into the following seven distinct branches.

HEALTH PROTECTION BRANCH. The Health Protection Branch carries out a wide range of activities intended to protect Canadians from hazards that may contribute to untimely illness or death. Among these activities are ensuring the safety and nutritional quality of food, the safety and effectiveness of drugs and medical devices, and controlling the availability of drugs that may be used improperly. Other responsibilities of the branch are programs to reduce the presence of dangerous chemicals in our environment and to monitor exposure to radioactivity. The branch also has a continuing program to monitor trends in the incidence of communicable and noncommunicable diseases in Canada.

MEDICAL SERVICES BRANCH. The Medical Services Branch provides services for prospective immigrants and Canadian public servants and their dependents serving around the world. As well, the branch is responsible for providing services for Indians and Inuit throughout Canada and the provision of health services to the residents of the Yukon and Northwest Territories. Services are provided through a network of hospitals, nursing stations, and community health centers throughout Canada.

The Medical Services Branch also operates occupational health services covering public servants at home and abroad. It is responsible for medical examinations and investigations conducted in the interest of aviation safety.

SOCIAL SERVICES BRANCH. The Social Services Branch promotes and supports programming directed to those Canadians in greatest need; it ensures that there is a safety net to assist those who would otherwise risk poverty, isolation and dependency to meet their basic economic needs. The branch also supports those involved in the development, coordination, and delivery of services in the academic and voluntary sectors by funding research, fellowships, and national voluntary organization activities in the field.

Contributions are provided to groups of retired persons to encourage utilization of skills, talents, and experience for the community. The branch provides funding for provincial and municipal welfare departments, voluntary agencies, citizen groups, universities, and other organizations to carry out research. The branch operates a national daycare information center, an adoption desk, and a clearinghouse for family violence.

HEALTH SERVICES AND PROMOTION BRANCH. The Health Services and Promotion Branch has two main responsibilities: to encourage and assist Canadians to adopt a way of life that enhances their physical, mental, and social well-being, and to provide leadership and coordination in assisting the provinces and territories to improve and maintain their health services and national standards. In the field of health promotion, the branch works closely with provincial governments and nongovernment organizations to develop and deliver health information and educational programs in such areas as smoking, alcohol use, nutrition, drug use, accidents, personal health care, and family and child health.

The branch is also responsible for payments concerning provincial programs covering hospital, diagnostic, medical, and extended health care services, as provided by legislation, and for monitoring provincial compliance with the program conditions associated with federal payments.

It is the responsibility of the Health Services and Promotion Branch to support scientific activities to the concerns and objectives of the department and to provide for the training and maintenance of needed research personnel in the area of health services and public health.

CORPORATE MANAGEMENT BRANCH. The Corporate Management Branch is responsible for providing a full range of financial, personnel, information, and administrative services for the effective integration of planning, resource allocation, and expenditure control activities throughout the department.

POLICY, PLANNING AND INFORMATION BRANCH. The objective of the Policy, Planning and Information Branch is to provide authoritative advice to the minister, deputy minister, and program branches on trends, issues, policy requirements, and information needs relative to departmental objectives, priorities, and programs.

The branch has three main roles designed to meet the objective. First, it undertakes research analysis and gives advice on health and social policy issues. Second, it furnishes support for policy development activities to program branches. Finally, it provides the department, its provincial counterparts, and national and international organizations efficient access to information on health and welfare related matters.

INTERGOVERNMENTAL AND INTERNATIONAL AFFAIRS BRANCH. This branch coordinates Canada's participation in matters involving international, federal, and provincial liaison in the area of health and social affairs.

OPPORTUNITIES FOR EMPLOYMENT FOR NEW GRADUATES WITHIN THE FEDERAL GOVERNMENT

There is a limited number of employment opportunities for new graduates of health services administration programs within the federal government. These opportunities are primarily as health systems analysts, program analysts, and budget analysts.

ORGANIZATION OF PROVINCIAL HEALTH DEPARTMENTS

Generally, provincial health departments are organized into six main branches in order to fulfill their roles. These branches are as follows:

1. Institutional Services
2. Medical Services
3. Public Health Services
4. Policy, Planning and Information
5. Support Programs
6. Administrative Services

INSTITUTIONAL SERVICES. The Institutional Services branch in any provincial government is responsible for ensuring that hospital and nursing home services are provided to all citizens within its jurisdiction. This branch is responsible for hospital and nursing home services planning, approval of new programs for hospitals and nursing homes, approval of all hospital or nursing home budgets within a province, approval of construction programs for hospitals and nursing homes, and institutional consulting services. The largest percentage of any health budget within a provincial jurisdiction is handled by this branch.

MEDICAL SERVICES. The Medical Services branch in a provincial government is primarily responsible for ensuring that physicians are paid in accordance with an approved and negotiated fee schedule within a province. The main work of this branch involves a processing function for claims submitted by individual physicians for services rendered to residents of the province. A very interesting aspect of the work undertaken by the Medical Services branch involves the negotiation of fee schedules with associations representing physicians. A particularly intriguing aspect of this activity relates to the potential for effecting trends in medical practice and medical services through funding mechanisms.

PUBLIC HEALTH SERVICES. The Public Health Service in each provincial government is responsible for ensuring that public health services, including public health nursing, public health inspection, and health promotion and education programs, are provided to individuals and residents throughout the province. These services are provided either directly by the Public Health branch in each province or through public health units governed by community boards and funded through the Public Health branch of the provincial government. This branch will provide policy direction and research into public health issues within a provincial jurisdiction.

POLICY, PLANNING AND INFORMATION. The Policy, Planning and Information branch in a provincial jurisdiction is primarily responsible for analyzing trends in health services, developing a policy framework to deal with emerging health issues, and providing advice to ministers and other senior public servants regarding health issues. As well, this branch is responsible for ensuring that health information is collected, analyzed, and displayed in a useful and meaningful way.

SUPPORT PROGRAMS. The Support Programs branch in a provincial government setting is responsible for those programs which the health department provides to residents in need within a provincial jurisdiction. These programs primarily relate to provision of drugs, prosthetic appliances, hearing aids, eyeglasses, and so on.

ADMINISTRATIVE SERVICES. The Administrative Services branch of provincial governments provides support services—financial management, personnel services, logistical support, for example—for all programs of the health department.

Many health departments have a separate branch for long-term care services independent of the Institutional Services branch mentioned above. This branch may include nursing homes, home care programs, and personal care homes. An alternative organizational arrangement which exists in a number of provincial governments is that long-term care services are included under a hospital services branch.

ENTRY-LEVEL POSITIONS FOR NEW GRADUATES OF HEALTH ADMINISTRATION PROGRAMS

The kinds and types of positions in government services that are available to new graduates from health services administration programs are as follows:

— Health or hospital consultants—many health departments throughout Canada hire new graduates in entry-level positions in their hospital consulting divisions. These divisions which are usually under the Institutional Services branch (hospitals and nursing homes) within a ministry, provide advice and guidance for the ministry on institutional administrative issues, as well as analysis of problem areas in individual institutions or groups of institutions throughout a province. Such positions provide a superb opportunity for the new graduate to develop a full understanding of the global dimensions of the institutional services program within a province. As well, such positions provide an excellent opportunity for the new graduate to gain experience and credibility within a ministry.

— Program analysts—opportunities exist within provincial health ministries as well as federal health and welfare for new graduates to be employed as program analysts. These positions may exist in any branch of the health departments and involve analysis of specific programs with a view to revising existing policies or developing recommendations regarding operational improvements in such programs.

— Financial analysts—ministries often hire new graduates (particularly those with a commerce or financial management background) as financial analysts in their Institutional Services branch, Medical Services branch or Administrative Services branch. These positions primarily involve analyzing budgets.

— Planning officers—ministries also offer positions to new graduates in planning and policy divisions. These positions, called program planning officers at the entry level, involve the individual in a review of existing programs and development of a policy framework for changes in programs or for new programs.

— Executive or administrative assistants—all ministries have positions for administrative or executive assistants to senior managers within ministries. These positions offer excellent opportunities for new graduates to establish important and powerful contacts within ministries to develop a better understanding of how specific programs operate, and to appreciate the role such programs play in provincial health systems.

ATTITUDE OF GOVERNMENT MANAGERS

The attitude (or posture) of many government managers is extremely conservative. The orientation of such managers is one of caution; to move forward slowly building on past experience and knowledge while keeping a watchful eye on "the political winds of the time." Given this attitude, which is prevalent in almost every bureaucracy no matter what the political stripe of the party in power, new graduates are wise to try to understand that the environment will not be conducive to moving forward quickly with ideas that are experimental and revolutionary in nature and may substantially disrupt the status quo.

Despite the tendency of most bureaucracies to be conservative in their approach to issues, there is, nevertheless, in many situations a real willingness to be innovative and creative in developing solutions to complex problems. The level of complexity of such problems is compounded by the need to balance solutions between what is the "right" thing to do based on expert advice and what is "politically saleable" to the party in power.

New graduates interested in employment in a government setting must understand that decisions are sometimes based on political initiatives rather than needs. When such situations occur, one must recognize that the nature of our political process is such that the elected representatives to government make the decisions on behalf of the population. The rightness or the wrongness of these decisions will be judged by the people at the next election, and while this may sometimes seem to be a fickle and unrealistic way of decision making, the alternative to such a democratic system is not very palatable.

CONCLUSION

Splendid opportunities exist within provincial and federal government health services in Canada for new graduates of health services administration programs. These opportunities, some examples of which are outlined above, provide new graduates with a solid introduction to the health care system in a province or the country. The experience gained in such positions will stand them in good stead when they wish to seek other employment opportunities, either outside government or at a more senior level within government.

New graduates must bear in mind the conservative nature of health services administration in government settings, take a long view of these opportunities, and expect to "pay their dues" in order to succeed.

While opportunities exist in all governments for new graduates, small governments provide better opportunities for broad experience. This is due to the fact that in a small provincial government setting there is more opportunity to become involved with decision making at a senior level because there are fewer levels and senior staff have fewer support staff to depend on.

BIBLIOGRAPHY

Evans, R.G. *Strained Mercy, the Economics of Canadian Health Care*. 1984.

Soderstrom, L. *The Canadian Health System*. London: Croom Helm, Ltd., 1978.

Courchene, J., D.W. Conklin, and G.C.A. Cook, eds. *Ontario Economic Council, Ottawa and the Provinces: The Distribution of Money and Power*. Vols. 1 and 2. Toronto: Ontario Economic Council, 1985.

Task Force on the Allocation of Health Care Resources. Health: A Need for Redirection. Canadian Medical Association, 1984.

16

GOVERNMENT IN THE U.S.: MANAGING FOR POLICY AND POLITICAL ACCOUNTABILITY

MALCOLM RANDALL

"The health of the people is really the foundation upon which all their happiness and all their powers as a State depend" [1].

Disraeli

The federal government contributes to meeting the nation's health needs by financing and providing health care services, promoting disease prevention, and supporting research, training, and consumer and occupational health and safety. The *Budget of the United States Government for Fiscal Year 1988* indicates that projected FY 1987 outlays for health care amount to approximately $130 billion.

Of this amount, the largest outlay is for Medicare, with slightly over $71 billion. Forty billion dollars fund programs budgeted under health care services, which include Medicaid grants, federal employee health benefits, the Indian Health Service, research and block grants to states. Health research, funded principally through the National Institutes of Health, accounts for $5.9 billion. The agencies delivering the major portion of direct health care services account for $21.7 billion. Of this amount, $10.2 billion is for the Veterans Administration (VA) health care system, and $11.5 billion is for

Malcolm Randall is the director of the Veterans Administration Medical Center in Gainesville, FL. Mr. Randall earned an M.H.A. from Saint Louis University and an A.B. from McKendree College.

the programs of the Air Force, Army, Navy and Department of Defense (DOD). This amount includes approximately $4.0 billion for the Army, 2.2 billion for the Navy, and 2.8 billion for the Air Force. The government share of the Civilian Health and Medical Program of the Uniformed Services (CHAMPUS) program is estimated at $2.0 billion, the medical information system $142 million, $68 million is for the Uniformed Services University of the Health Sciences, and $324 million for the Defense Medical Facilities Office.

Americans now spend 10.7 percent of the gross national product on medical care, more than any other industrialized nation. Federal spending for health care is growing faster than medical spending generally. According to projections in the FY 1988 budget of the U.S. government, it will more than double in this decade unless present trends are reversed. Figure 1 shows the increase in health costs as a percent of the gross national product for the years 1975 to 1984. Figure 2 shows the outlays for major medical programs starting with the FY 1976 and projected to FY 1992.

Because of the concerns of federal planners and federal decision makers about the costs of health care, repeated calls are being made for more effi-

FIGURE 1:   Health Costs as Percent of GNP, 1975–1984.

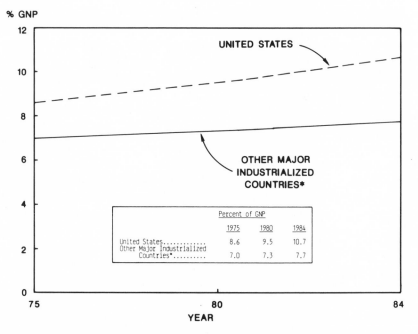

	Percent of GNP		
	1975	1980	1984
United States.............	8.6	9.5	10.7
Other Major Industrialized Countries*..........	7.0	7.3	7.7

*AUSTRALIA, CANADA, FRANCE, WEST GERMANY, ITALY, JAPAN, NETHERLANDS, AND UNITED KINGDOM

FIGURE 2:   Outlays for Major Medical Programs

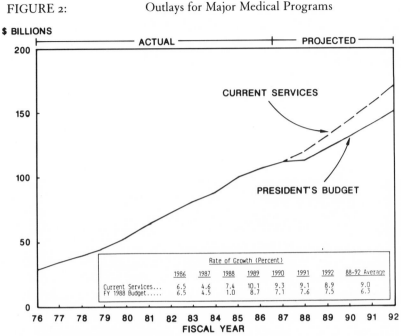

*INCLUDES MEDICARE, MEDICAID, FEDERAL EMPLOYEE HEALTH BENEFITS, HOSPITAL AND MEDICAL CARE FOR VETERANS, AND INDIAN HEALTH CARE.

cient use of health resources. Well trained professional health care administrators can make a positive impact. This means that trained, competent health care administrators are going to be in increasing demand. This chapter focuses on those federal units that are involved with the direct delivery of health care and that use the largest number of health services administrators. These are principally the Department of Defense through the Departments of the Air Force, Army, and Navy; the Veterans Administration; the Public Health Service; and the Indian Health Service. There are also career opportunities for health care administrators in smaller federal agencies involved in administering portions of a $130 billion annual federal health care outlay.

In the federal government, health service administrators are classified as civilian employees or as members of the uniformed services. The positions in the armed forces are as commissioned officers in the Medical Service Corps, in the Veterans Administration as civilian employees under the policies of the federal Office of Personnel Management, and in the Public Health Service and Indian Health Service either as commissioned officers or civilian employees, depending upon the individual assignment.

There are a number of opportunities and rewards in the role of the health care administrator in the federal service. First, there is the overriding opportunity to make an important contribution. Second is the opportunity to make a difference. Federal health care administrators are in a position to provide input into shaping policies that will shape future health care delivery systems. Third is the opportunity to help make these services meet the needs of the people in a concerned, compassionate, considerate, and responsive manner. One of the dangers in any large service organization, and certainly in the federal government, is the danger that that service will become rigid, bureaucratic, unconcerned, and unresponsive. This need not be so. The evidence is that responsive, concerned, and compassionate care is being delivered daily by the practitioners and the operating units of the federal services. It requires constant care and nurturing and the dedicated health care professional can make an important contribution in this area.

With the concerns about the costs of health care and the demand that care be provided in an efficient and effective manner, the opportunities for administrators to participate in providing quality and compassionate care in a cost effective and efficient manner are unlimited. In fulfilling this responsibility, young administrators have an opportunity to contribute not only to the people they serve, but also to the organization, to the people at large, and to this country. Finally, and not the least, there is the opportunity for young health care professionals to carve meaningful lifetime careers in a field dedicated to helping others, and careers which enable them to progress through graduated positions of increasing responsibility. The only limits on advancement will be placed by individuals who start a career in health services administration in the federal service. Advancement will depend solely on preparation, competence, level of dedication, and commitment.

There are also more tangible rewards. The health services administrator in either the uniformed services or the federal civilian sector will never become wealthy but can be assured of a comfortable income which will increase with advances in seniority and responsibility. There is an attractive benefits package, including a sound retirement program. There is the opportunity to work in a variety of interesting and challenging assignments, both in the United States and abroad. The exposure to a variety of assignments, positions, and geographical locations enriches the individual, enhances growth, and contributes to a well-rounded, cultured individual, who also enriches society. Opportunities for the federal health services administrator outlined in this chapter will increase. Similarly, the rewards of today will increase. For those interested in careers in federal health services administration, there is a rich mosaic of opportunities, rewards, and deeply satisfying professional and personal experiences.

To provide a visual concept of the far-flung geographical locations of federal health care facilities, Figure 3 depicts the location of VA and DOD medical treatment facilities. Figure 4 shows major Public Health Service

FIGURE 3:   Veterans Administration/Department of Defense Medical
Treatment Facilities

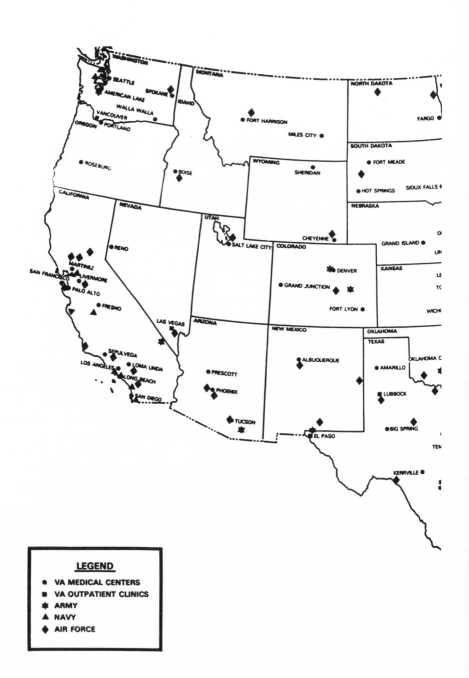

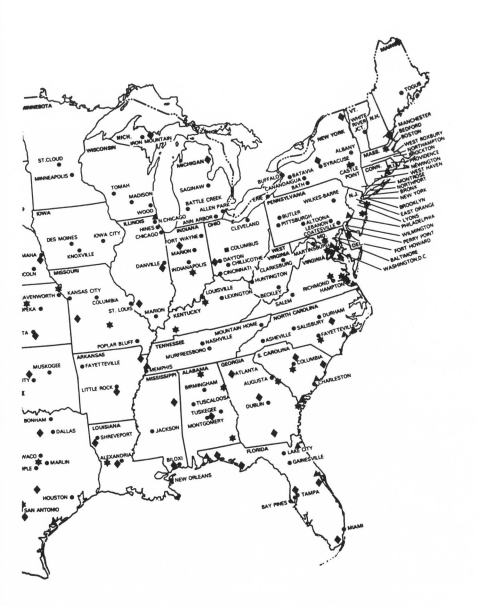

FIGURE 4:   Major Public Health Service Assignment Locations.

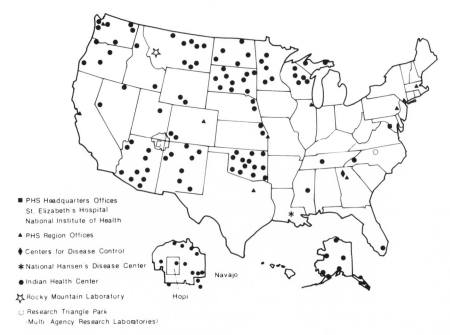

PHS Headquarters Offices
   St. Elizabeth's Hospital
   National Institute of Health

▲ PHS Region Offices

◆ Centers for Disease Control

✳ National Hansen's Disease Center

● Indian Health Center

Rocky Mountain Laboratory

Research Triangle Park
   (Multi Agency Research Laboratories)

assignment locations and Figure 5 gives the location of uniformed services hospitals in the United States. In addition, of course, are the many overseas assignments in facilities operated by the armed forces.

OFFICE OF THE ASSISTANT SECRETARY OF DEFENSE FOR HEALTH AFFAIRS

The assistant secretary of defense for health affairs is responsible for supervision and policy guidance over the medical activities of the military and is the principal staff adviser to the secretary of defense in military health policy and management matters. These include medical readiness, medical program management, preventive medicine, health promotion, quality assurance, professional incentive special pay, drug abuse control, medical information systems, and medical construction projects. As a staff officer, however, the assistant secretary has almost no directive authority over the military departments or any medical program elements.

The military health care system has two purposes: to provide medical support to combat forces during war and to provide a quality health benefit to active duty and retired members of the armed forces, their dependents, and survivors. The military system is comprised of 168 hospitals, over 300 freestanding medical clinics, and 436 dental clinics located in the United States and at military installations throughout the world. These facilities are staffed by approximately 41,400 health professionals, of whom about 36,000 are active duty military personnel. This includes 13,222 physicians, 502 dentists, and 12,255 nurses in addition to veterinarians, optometrists, podiatrists, psychologists, nurse practitioners, and physician assistants. Active duty military personnel in health services administration are a part of the Medical Service Corps, which consists of approximately 8,410 individuals. It is in this latter field that the professional health care administrator has an opportunity for a meaningful career.

The beneficiary population of the military health care system is approximately 8.6 million. This includes 2.1 million active duty personnel, their 2.4 million dependents, 4.1 million retired, and their dependents, all of whom are eligible for health care in military facilities. When care is not available or accessible in a military facility, it is purchased in the private sector. For dependents and retirees, the cost of this care is financed through payments shared by the Civilian Health and Medical Program of the Uniformed Services (CHAMPUS) and the beneficiary. For active duty members, it is purchased by the service under a supplemental payment program.

In addition to these major elements of the military system, each military service has medical units that are integral to the combat unit itself, such as medical facilities aboard ships, battalion aid stations, and air transportable clinics. Hospitals and clinics are administered individually by the Air Force, Army, and Navy. There is no central administrative authority. Each service budgets and administers its medical programs differently. For example, in the Air Force the base commander has direct authority over the clinic or hospital. In the Army, facilities in the continental United States are under the direction of a central health services command; in the Navy, facilities worldwide are under the control of regional divisions of a central naval medical command. The CHAMPUS program is administered directly by the office of the assistant secretary of defense for health affairs. Although it is a major element of the military health care system, it is not directed by the services.

The major concern in the military health care system is medical readiness, and the principal mission is to be medically ready for combat. Medical readiness for the combat mission is defined by the armed forces as the ability to provide life-saving care, including surgery, to wounded U.S. forces within six hours of injury. This requires prepositioning stockpiles of medical equipment in locations throughout the world. It also requires a large reserve of trained military physicians, nurses, dentists, and corpsmen; complete pre-

FIGURE 5:   Location of Uniformed Services Hospitals in the United
States.

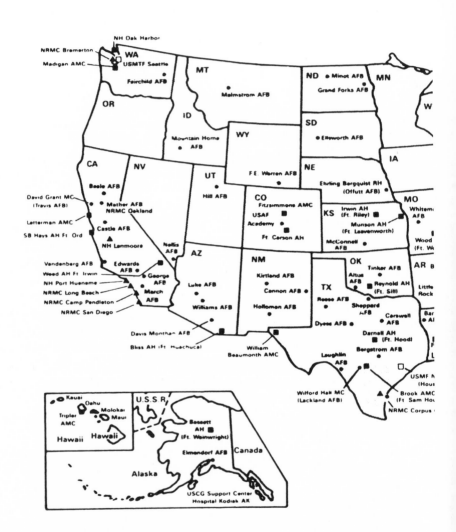

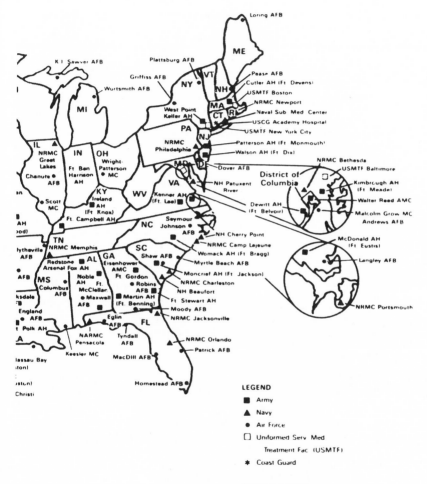

packaged medical units, ranging from small clinics to 1,000-bed hospitals, ready for immediate deployment; and the necessary logistical and transportation support.

The military health care system also has a peacetime mission. This is to provide quality health services to active duty personnel, their dependents, retirees and their dependents. During extended periods of peace, the balance of program and budget tends to tip toward enhancement of the peacetime health care delivery program and away from preparedness for war. Although this does not, in the classical sense, constitute a state of readiness to support troops medically in war on foreign soil, it does provide a professional base for the development and maintenance of the skills of the people in the military health care system and it further provides for the continuity of the system.

The twofold purpose of the military health care system of providing medical support to combat forces during war and providing a quality health service to beneficiaries during peacetime is a task of considerable magnitude and requires competent and dedicated professionals, including trained health care administrators.

AIR FORCE

The Air Force is responsible for nine specific activities which support national security. These are strategic aerospace offense, space operations, strategic aerospace defense, airlift, close air support, air interdiction, counterair, aerospace surveillance and reconnaissance, and special operations.

The U.S. Air Force Medical Service was established in July of 1949. This was an outgrowth of the transfer of the U.S. Army Air Corps to the newly created U.S. Air Force in 1947.

The Air Force Medical Service is organized to carry out a number of functions. The first is to operate a health service to maintain the active forces in the highest possible state of physical and mental health. An equally important function is to provide medical support integral to combat and support forces operating around the world. An important supporting function is the training of health personnel to deal with the medical problems imposed by war.

The Air Force Medical Service also operates a system of medical centers, hospitals, and clinics capable of meeting the needs of beneficiaries. The provision of health care services for beneficiaries as well as the provision of care for active duty personnel provide a benefit that enhances recruitment and retention of personnel to meet Air Force requirements. To carry out all of these responsibilities, the Air Force must attract and maintain a sufficient number and variety of health care personnel to meet both peacetime needs and the immediate manpower requirements imposed by an outbreak of hostilities.

The Air Force direct care system consists of 82 hospitals and 40 clinics. These facilities are staffed by, among others, approximately 3,900 physicians, 1,600 dentists, 5,250 nurses, and 450 physician assistants. There are currently 1,260 Medical Service Corps officers functioning in assignments in the area of health care administration.

The total beneficiary population of the Air Force is approximately 2.6 million living near Air Force bases. This number includes active duty personnel and their dependents, retirees and their dependents, and survivors of deceased military personnel.

Medical research and education are important activities designed to support the mission and the functions of the Air Force health care system. They are carried out through formal education and training programs and through residencies which are established in Air Force facilities.

Air Force medical facilities are integral to the mission performance and organizational structure of the wing or base they support. Wings are organized in peacetime for war, with emphasis on their primary mission, and are structured for rapid decision making. The medical facility commander is responsible to the wing commander or the highest echelon exercising command over the installation. In most cases, the medical facility commander also serves as director of base medical services. Base medical services include medical centers, hospitals, clinics, medical aid stations, and related functions. An installation may have tactical medical units in addition to the fixed medical centers, hospitals, and clinics. Tactical units include air transportable hospitals, air transportable clinics, and aeromedical staging facilities. These units are the responsibility of the medical facility commander unless they are specifically assigned to combat tactical units. All Air Force medical resources are located on an Air Force installation or at a satellite facility and are managed by the director of base medical services. The organizational chart of a representative Air Force hospital is shown in Figure 6.

Entry into the Air Force Medical Service Corps is through direct commission, the Reserve Officer Training Corps (ROTC) program, line transfers, or through the enlisted route. Approximately 70 percent of Medical Service Corps officers come through direct commission of civilians who have master's degrees. Approximately 30 percent come through the ROTC program, transfer of line officers, or the enlisted ranks. The Air Force also sends officers to universities to pursue either master's or doctoral degrees. The rank structure is similar to that found in the Army and the Navy and the opportunities are similar. The young person who decides to make a

FIGURE 6:   Representative Air Force Hospital.

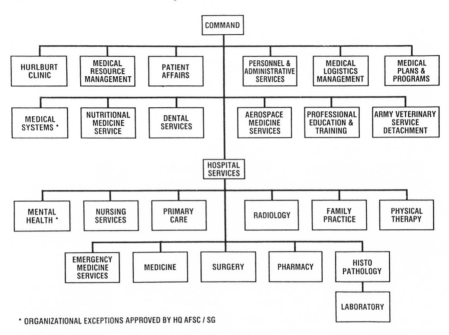

* ORGANIZATIONAL EXCEPTIONS APPROVED BY HQ AFSC / SG

career in the field of health care administration in the Air Force has an opportunity for steady advancement through positions of increasing responsibility. In fact, the Medical Service Corps officer can move through the ranks to become the commander of a hospital. Future plans call for about 70 percent of Air Force hospitals to be opened to command for all medical service corps officers.

ARMY

The primary purpose of the Army Medical Department is to provide support to combat forces during war, and to provide quality health care to active duty and retired members of the armed forces, their dependents, and survivors.

In 1947, the Congress established the Medical Service Corps as a component of the Army Medical Department. The new corps absorbed the existing Pharmacy Corps, Sanitary Corps, and Medical Administrative Corps. In 1973, as part of the general reorganization of the Army, the United States Army Health Services Command was established at Fort Sam Houston, Texas. This provided a single manager for the entire health care delivery and educational system within the continental United States. In 1974, this command assumed responsibility for Army health care in Alaska, Hawaii, and the Canal Zone.

This health care system of the Army is one of the larger systems in the nation. It serves its beneficiaries through 50 hospitals, dispensaries, health clinics, and related medical treatment facilities. Thus, the Army Medical Department needs a number of trained individuals in health care administration. These positions range from field medical assistant to deputy commander for administration of some of the foremost teaching hospitals in the country. The organizational chart for a representative Army hospital is depicted in Figure 7.

Because the primary mission of the Army's health care delivery system is mobilization preparedness, the majority of health care administration positions are for Army officers who could be deployed in the event of a national emergency. There are, however, additional career opportunities in civil service positions in Army hospitals. These civilian administrators are normally located in teaching hospitals and may be assigned in various positions from clinical administrator to assistant administrator. Because of the relatively few positions available, however, the greatest opportunity for career development exists as commissioned officers in the Medical Service Corps. The

FIGURE 7: Representative Army Hospital.

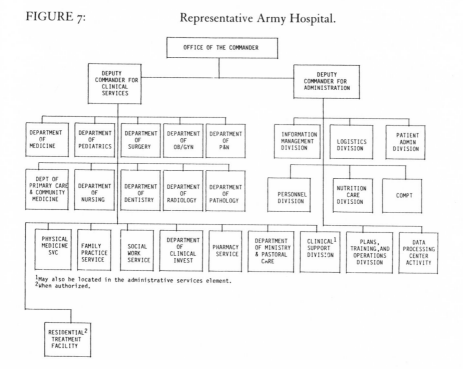

civilian positions are in civil service grades GS-9 to GS-11. Health care administration positions in the Officers Corps begin at the rank of second lieutenant. There is opportunity for promotions through all ranks up to and including general officer.

The primary entry as an officer in the health care administration field is through the Army Reserve Officer Training Corps. College students participating in the Army ROTC program select a specialty branch in terms of their long-term goals. Those students who desire a military career in health care administration may request branching in the Medical Service Corps.

A limited number of additional opportunities for entrance into the Medical Service Corps are available either through Army Officers Candidate School or through direct commission. These two mechanisms, however, provide only a small minority of the total number of Medical Service Corps officers entering active duty. The direct commission route, in particular, is limited to those with preparation at the graduate level in specific disciplines. Undergraduate degrees are appropriate for entry level positions in the Medical Service Corps. However, many positions of increased responsibility require graduate level preparation. Officers are encouraged to complete an accredited master's degree. In addition, the Medical Service Corps provides a limited number of opportunities for sponsored training in a graduate program in health care administration.

In 1951, a formal educational program in hospital administration was started at the Army Medical Field Service School. Through an affiliation with the graduate school of Baylor University, the first master of hospital administration degree was awarded to Army Medical Department officers in 1953. The U.S. Army-Baylor University Graduate Program in Health Care Administration provides midcareer education for officers. This program is for officers who have five to seven years of active commissioned service. The program requires 60 graduate semester hours in the didactic phase and a 52-week residency leading to a Master of Health Administration degree from Baylor University. At the end of this two-year assignment, graduates return to positions in the Medical Service Corps.

NAVY

Since the activation of the first commissioned warship and the establishment of the Navy by the Continental Congress in 1775, health care professionals have made an indispensable contribution to the Navy's fulfillment of its national defense mission. In 1842, the Bureau of Medicine and Surgery was established within the Navy Department. The first hospital ship was commissioned during the Civil War. Organizational development increased rapidly after 1900.

World War I brought expansion of treatment facilities at home and abroad, commissioning of more hospital ships, and conferring full military titles on all staff corps officers. More than in any previous era, the medical department was integrally involved in the operational arena, most conspicuously ashore with Marine Corps forces in Europe. Authorization of a two-ocean Navy in 1940 introduced new requirements in logistics and medical supply, mobility, and casualty evacuation. Mobile field units, from 10 to 3,000 beds, were developed, and hospital ships were made functionally equivalent to fixed facilities ashore. All major ships were given a substantial medical capability, and even the smallest vessels carried at least one hospital corpsman specifically trained for independent duty.

It was in 1947 that legislation was passed recognizing the need for a permanent commissioned officer corps for professional allied health scientists and medical administrators by establishing the Medical Service Corps. This legislation established the pathway for the trained health care administrator to achieve a career in the Navy.

Prior to 1982, virtually all commanding officers in medical facilities were physicians. They were appointed on the basis of their competence as clinicians, with little management training or experience. In 1982, the pool of potential managers was expanded by providing highly qualified dentists, nurses, and Medical Service Corps officers the opportunity to compete for assignment to command or to assume other positions of organizational responsibility. A system of leadership and management training and a stepwise progression of experience through positions of increasing responsibility were established. The Surgeon General is responsible for the development of policy for Navy Medicine, while the Commander, Naval Medical Command, is responsible for the execution of those policies and for all activities in the Medical Department.

Naval hospitals are typically organized into five directorates, as shown in Figure 8.

Officers in the health care administration section of the Navy are assigned positions of graduated responsibility at naval hospitals, dental centers, and with the operating forces of the Navy and Fleet Marine Force. Successful practitioners in health care administration can look forward to gradual advancement, including command of health care and research facilities or various schools. The Navy health administration field includes management positions in the areas of financial and material resources management, and health facility and operating services management. Health care administra-

FIGURE 8: Representative Naval Hospital.

■ **IHS AREA OFFICES**

ABERDEEN AREA
Aberdeen, South Dakota
ALASKA AREA
Anchorage, Alaska
ALBUQUERQUE AREA
Albuquerque, New Mexico
BILLINGS AREA
Billings, Montana
NAVAJO AREA
Window Rock, Arizona
OKLAHOMA CITY AREA
Oklahoma City, Oklahoma
PHOENIX AREA
Phoenix, Arizona
PORTLAND AREA
Portland, Oregon

☐ **IHS PROGRAM OFFICES**

BEMIDJI PROGRAM
Bemidji, Minnesota
CALIFORNIA PROGRAM
Sacramento, California
NASHVILLE PROGRAM
Nashville, Tennessee
TUCSON PROGRAM
Tucson, Arizona

ABERDEEN AREA

● Hospitals

NEBRASKA
1 Winnebago
NORTH DAKOTA
2 Belcourt
3 Fort Yates
SOUTH DAKOTA
4 Eagle Butte
5 Pine Ridge
6 Rapid City
7 Rosebud
8 Sisseton
9 Wagner

▲ Health Centers

NEBRASKA
10 Macy*
NORTH DAKOTA
11 Fort Totten
12 New Town
13 Williston*
SOUTH DAKOTA
14 Fort Thompson
15 McLaughlin
16 Wanblee

✳ School Health Centers

NORTH DAKOTA
17 Wahpeton
SOUTH DAKOTA
18 Flandreau
19 Pierre

ALASKA AREA

● Hospitals

ALASKA
1 Anchorage
2 Barrow
3 Dillingham*
4 Kotzebue
5 Mt. Edgecumbe
6 Nome*
7 Bethel

▲ Health Centers

ALASKA
8 Fairbanks
9 Fort Yukon*
10 Juneau*
11 Ketchikan

12 Metlakatla
13 St. George
14 St. Paul
15 Tanana

ALBUQUERQUE AREA

● Hospitals

NEW MEXICO
1 Albuquerque
2 Mescalero
3 Santa Fe
4 San Fidel
5 Zuni

▲ Health Centers

COLORADO
6 Ignacio
7 Towaoc
NEW MEXICO
8 Isleta
9 Jemez
10 Dulce
11 Taos
12 Ramah*
13 Canoncito
14 Laguna
15 Magdalena*

BILLINGS AREA

● Hospitals

MONTANA
1 Browning
2 Crow Agency
3 Harlem

▲ Health Centers

MONTANA
4 Lame Deer
5 Lodge Grass
6 Poplar
7 Box Elder
8 St. Ignatius
9 Wolf Point
10 Poison
WYOMING
11 Arapahoe
12 Fort Washakie

✳ School Health Center

UTAH
13 Brigham City

NAVAJO AREA

● Hospitals

ARIZONA
1 Chinle
2 Fort Defiance
3 Ganado*
4 Tuba City
NEW MEXICO
5 Crownpoint
6 Gallup
7 Shiprock

▲ Health Centers

ARIZONA
8 Dilkon
9 Kayenta
10 Leupp
11 Rough Rock*
12 Teec Nos Pos
13 Toyei
14 Winslow
15 Tsaile*
16 Inscription House
NEW MEXICO
17 Tohatchi
18 Huerfano

✳ **School Health Centers**

ARIZONA
19 Many Farms
NEW MEXICO
20 Fort Wingate

OKLAHOMA CITY AREA

● Hospitals

OKLAHOMA
1 Ada
2 Claremore
3 Clinton
4 Okmulgee*
5 Lawton
6 Tahlequah
7 Talihina

▲ Health Centers

OKLAHOMA
8 Anadarko
9 Oklahoma City*
10 Jay
11 Eufaula*
12 Hugo
13 Broken Bow
14 Carnegie
15 McAlester
16 Miami
17 Okemah*
18 Pawhuska
19 Pawnee
20 Sapulpa*
21 Shawnee
22 Tishomingo
23 Watonga
24 Wewoka
25 Ponca City
26 Stilwell*
27 Concho
KANSAS
28 Holton
29 Lawrence

PHOENIX AREA

● Hospitals

ARIZONA
1 Kearns Canyon
2 Parker
3 Phoenix
4 Sacaton
5 San Carlos
6 Whiteriver
7 Yuma
NEVADA
8 Owyhee
9 Schurz

▲ Health Centers

ARIZONA
10 Bylas
11 Cibecue
12 Peach Springs
13 Second Mesa
NEVADA
14 Sparks*
15 Stewart
16 Washoe*
UTAH
17 Roosevelt

✳ School Health Center

CALIFORNIA
18 Riverside

PORTLAND AREA

▲ Health Centers

IDAHO
1 Fort Hall
2 Lapwai
OREGON
3 Salem
4 Warm Springs
5 Pendleton

WASHINGTON
6 Nespelem
7 Bellingham
8 Auburn
9 Neah Bay
10 Puyallup*
11 LaConner*
12 Taholah
13 Marysville*
14 Wellpinit
15 Toppenish
16 Inchelium

BEMIDJI PROGRAM

● Hospitals

MINNESOTA
1 Cass Lake
2 Red Lake

▲ Health Centers

MICHIGAN
3 Kincheloe
MINNESOTA
4 Cloquet*
5 White Earth
WISCONSIN
6 Lac du Flambeau*
7 Oneida
8 Keshena*
9 Hayward*
10 Bowler*
11 Odanah*

NASHVILLE PROGRAM

● Hospitals

MISSISSIPPI
1 Philadelphia*
NORTH CAROLINA
2 Cherokee

▲ Health Centers

FLORIDA
3 Clewiston*
4 Okeechobee*
5 Hollywood*
6 Miami*
MAINE
7 Perry*
8 Princeton*
9 Old Town*
NEW YORK
10 Salamanca*
11 Cattaraugus*
12 Hogansburg*
RHODE ISLAND
13 Kenyon*

TUCSON PROGRAM

● Hospital

ARIZONA
1 Sells

▲ Health Centers

ARIZONA
2 Santa Rosa
3 San Xavier (Tucson)

CALIFORNIA PROGRAM

◆ Rural-Tribal
Health Program

CALIFORNIA
1 Trinidad
2 Hoopa
3 Anderson

4 Burney
5 Covelo
6 Ukiah
7 Oroville
8 Santa Rosa
9 Auburn
10 Tuolumne
11 Bishop
12 Clovis
13 Porterville
14 Banning
15 Valley Center
16 El Cajon
17 San Bernadino

■ **URBAN INDIAN
HEALTH PROGRAMS**

ARIZONA
1 Tucson
2 Phoenix
CALIFORNIA
3 Bakersfield
4 Compton
5 Fresno
6 Sacramento
7 San Diego
8 San Francisco
9 San Jose
10 Santa Barbara
COLORADO
11 Denver
ILLINOIS
12 Chicago
KANSAS
13 Wichita
MASSACHUSETTS
14 Boston
MICHIGAN
15 Detroit
MINNESOTA
16 Minneapolis
MONTANA
17 Anaconda
18 Billings
19 Butte
20 Great Falls
21 Helena
22 Miles City
23 Missoula
NEBRASKA
24 Omaha
NEVADA
25 Reno
NEW MEXICO
26 Albuquerque
NEW YORK
27 New York City
OKLAHOMA
28 Oklahoma City
29 Tulsa
OREGON
30 Portland
SOUTH DAKOTA
31 Pierre
WASHINGTON
32 Seattle
33 Spokane
WISCONSIN
34 Green Bay
35 Milwaukee
TEXAS
36 Dallas
UTAH
37 Salt Lake City

As of 4/1/84

*Tribally Operated

tion Medical Service Corps officers fill responsible management positions similar to those of hospital administrators in large civilian hospitals.

The Navy offers an attractive and challenging career for the health care administrator. The competent Medical Service Corps officer can advance through the commissioned ranks in increasingly responsible billets, up to and including flag rank.

PUBLIC HEALTH SERVICE

The Public Health Service, a component of the Department of Health and Human Services, is the largest public health program in the world. It is directed by the Assistant Secretary for Health who is appointed by the President. The assistant secretary serves as the principal adviser to the Secretary of Health and Human Services on health related matters and is assisted in the planning and administration of Public Health Service programs by the Surgeon General of the Public Health Service, by deputy assistant secretaries, and by the heads of the five Public Health Service agencies. They are The National Institutes of Health; The Food and Drug Administration; The Centers for Disease Control; The Alcohol, Drug Abuse, and Mental Health Administration; and The Health Resources and Services Administration. The Public Health Service employs about 42,900 civil service workers, and 5,000 officers of the Public Health Service Commission Corps. Major Public Health Service assignment locations are shown in Figure 4. The Public Health Service budget is approximately $8 billion per year.

Certain important programs and special health initiatives are carried out within the office of the Assistant Secretary for Health. Among these are the following: The National Center for Health Statistics, The Office of Disease Prevention and Health Promotion, The National Center for Health Services Research, The Office of Adolescent Pregnancy Programs, The Office on Smoking and Health, The President's Council on Physical Fitness and Sports, and The National Toxicology Program.

The mission of the Public Health Service is to protect and advance the health of the people by working with other nations and international agencies on global health problems and their solutions; conducting and supporting medical research and communicating research results to health professionals and the public; preventing and controlling disease, identifying health hazards, and promoting healthy life styles for the nation's citizens; monitoring the adequacy of health manpower and facilities; assisting in the delivery of health care services to medically underserved populations and other groups with special health needs; ensuring that drugs and medical devices are safe and effective, and protecting the public from unsafe foods and unnecessary exposure to manmade radiation; and administering grants to the states for preventive health and health services, alcohol, drug abuse, and mental health services, maternal and child health services, and primary health care.

The Public Health Service began in 1798 as the Marine Hospital Service, a part of the Treasury Department, when President John Adams signed into law an act providing for "the care and relief of sick and disabled seamen."

In 1870, the medical officer in charge was given the title Surgeon General. In 1889, Congress officially established the Public Health Service Commission Corps. It was established along military lines with titles and pay corresponding to military grades and members subject to duty wherever assigned. In 1912, the service's name was changed to its present designation, United States Public Health Service. With the passage of the National Cancer Act in 1937, the National Cancer Institute was established and set a national pattern for support of biomedical research, conducting research in its own laboratories, awarding grants for research to nongovernment scientists and institutions, and providing fellowships for the training of medical scientists.

The Public Health Service Act of 1944 realigned the service into the Office of the Surgeon General, the Bureau of Medical Services, the Bureau of State Services, and the National Institute of Health. The act also gave the service broad powers to conduct and support research on the diseases and disabilities of man, authorized training fellowships, and made the National Cancer Institute a division of the National Institute of Health. In succeeding years, a number of other institutes were established, and the name of the National Institute of Health was changed to the National Institutes of Health.

In 1953, the Public Health Service became part of the newly created Department of Health, Education and Welfare. The responsibility for the health care of American Indians and Alaska natives was transferred from the Department of the Interior to the Public Health Service in 1955. The Emergency Health Personnel Act of 1970 created the National Health Service Corps which recruits physicians and other health professionals and places them in areas with critical shortages of health manpower. When the new Department of Education was formed in 1979, the Department of Health, Education and Welfare was renamed the Department of Health and Human Services. The Public Health Service became a major component of that department.

The Public Health Service, through its agencies, provides broad opportunity for a career in health care administration. Opportunities exist in both the Commissioned Corps and in positions which are filled under the Health Care Administration Series of the federal Civil Service. Whether or not a position is filled by a commissioned officer or a civil service appointee depends on the particular position. There are approximately 645 positions that may be filled by health care administrators in the Commissioned Corps and approximately 2,800 positions that may be filled by civil service employees. Salaries in the Commissioned Corps are paid at the same level as officers in the military services. Entrance into the Commissioned Corps requires a master's level degree. The civil service series provides entry-level positions at the GS-5, GS-7, and GS-9 grade levels with progressively responsible positions up to and including the GS/GM-15 Series.

Thus, it can be seen that the Public Health Service offers a wide range of opportunities for the professional in health care administration across a broad range of programs that touch all facets of health care. There is no question that the Public Health Service has a major impact on health care. The young administrator who elects to pursue a career in health care administration in this significant organization can have the satisfaction not only of a rewarding career, but also of playing an important role in the health of the people.

INDIAN HEALTH SERVICE

The Indian Health Service (IHS) is a part of the Health Resources and Services Administration of the U.S. Department of Health and Human Services. It provides inpatient, outpatient, and preventive health services to American Indians and Alaska natives through a system of nearly 50 hospitals and 100 clinics operated directly by the Indian Health Service and under contractual arrangements with Indian tribes, Alaska native corporations, or urban Indian organizations. It is the primary federal health resource for more than 960,000 Indians and Alaska natives.

The health care program for Indians traces its origins to the early 1800s when Army physicians began treating contagious diseases among Indian tribes living near military posts. The program of today grew out of negotiated treaties which frequently included provisions for medical services. The goal of the Indian Health Service is to raise the health status of American Indians and Alaska natives to the highest possible level. There are three major objectives that support this goal. These are to deliver the highest quality health services possible, to assist tribes and native corporations to develop their capacity to manage health programs, and to act as the federal Indian advocate in health related matters.

Members of 487 federally recognized Indian tribes live primarily on Indian reservations and in small rural communities. The reservations are principally located in the western half of the country and are found in 28 states. The Alaska natives live predominantly in remote, isolated villages. Many of the reservations and communities are located in areas where climatic conditions are often harsh, and transportation is often difficult. In many areas of Alaska, roads simply do not exist and ill or injured persons have to be airlifted to health facilities.

In addition to those hospitals and clinics that are operated directly, the

Indian Health Service also contracts with tribal and Alaska native health organizations to operate five hospitals and numerous clinics and with state and local health departments and private practitioners for services it cannot provide. The Indian Health Service also provides funding for 37 urban programs that operate outpatient facilities in 20 states. One of the major objectives of the Indian Health Service, as previously indicated, is to assist tribes and native corporations to develop their capacity to staff and manage health programs.

The passage of two laws, the Indian Self Determination and Education Assistance Act (P.L. 93–638) and the Indian Health Care Improvement Act (P.L. 94–437), has dramatically increased Indian participation in health service provision. The first act provides tribes with the option of managing health programs in their communities. The second authorized higher resource levels in the Indian Health Service program and established new programs for health professions training and for the provision of services to Indians living in urban areas. This legislation strengthened the long-standing policy of the Indian Health Service of giving Indian people maximum opportunity to become meaningfully involved in the program serving them and was intended to elevate the health status of Indians and Alaska natives. The impact of these acts and of the efforts of the Indian Health Service is striking. Twenty years ago, Indian Health Service staff did almost all the planning and operating of services. The current environment finds tribes and native corporations playing a leading role in planning their health services and in carrying out other health activities.

Considerable progress has been made since the Public Health Service became responsible for the health care of Indians in 1955. Mortality rates have decreased markedly. The infant death rate is down 81 percent, the pneumonia and influenza death rate is down 80 percent, gastrointestinal diseases death rate is down 92 percent, and the tuberculosis death rate is down 96 percent. Environmental health has been improved through the provision of running water and sanitary waste disposal facilities, new hospitals have been built and new health centers, health stations, and satellite clinics have been opened. Physicians assigned to the Indian Health Service increased from 125 to approximately 600, dentists from 40 to approximately 260, and graduate nurses from 798 to approximately 2,000. Since 1955, hospital admissions have more than doubled from 50,000 to 103,000 a year, and outpatient visits have increased more than eight times from 455,000 to 4,232,000 per year.

The Indian Health Service is organized with a headquarters and 12 geographical regional offices called area and program offices. These are shown in Figure 9. The location of Indian Health Service offices and facilities is shown in Figure 10. The headquarters, area, and special assignment offices are staffed with a variety of administrative positions in finance, procurement, contracting, personnel, facilities management, and general administration and management. The hospitals and clinics are staffed with directors, administrative officers, and a number of other administrators in finance, personnel, supply, and similar positions.

The Indian Health Service uses both the Commissioned Corps of the U.S. Public Health Service and the federal civil service system. The requirements of each personnel system are available from the area offices listed in Figure 9 or from the Indian Health Service headquarters in Rockville, Maryland. Those who want to work in specific parts of the country can contact the directors of the various hospitals and clinics. The Indian Health Service operates under guidelines that give preference to American Indians and Alaska natives in job placement. The opportunities for careers in health care administration for American Indians and Alaska natives are, therefore, particularly good.

The IHS is playing a little known but important role in the federal government's broad involvement in health care delivery. As the programs of the Public Health Service continue to evolve, trained health care administrators will be needed to assist the Indian Health Service in reaching its objectives of delivering high quality services, assisting tribes and native corporations in developing their capacity to staff and manage health programs, and in acting as a federal advocate in health related services. This is a unique organization. It is involved not only in the provision of health services but also in assisting the federal government in meeting its social contract with American Indians and Alaska natives.

VETERANS ADMINISTRATION

In 1951, the U.S. Senate reported that "the medical care program of the Veterans Administration is one of the largest in the world. Obviously, a program of this magnitude is one of considerable and continuing interest to the Congress and the people of the United States. ... That interest ... is considerably heightened by the fact that during the last few years, the quality of the medical care available to the beneficiaries of the Veterans Administration has been raised to a point where it unquestionably represents the best medical care available anywhere in the world at any time in the world's history" [2]. The report acknowledged the remarkable revitalization of Veterans Administration (VA) medicine engineered by General Omar N. Bradley as administrator of veterans affairs, General Paul R. Hawley as chief medical director, and Dr. Paul B. Magnuson as assistant chief medical director for research and education. The leadership of these three men led

FIGURE 9:   Major Health Facilities for Indians and Alaska Natives.

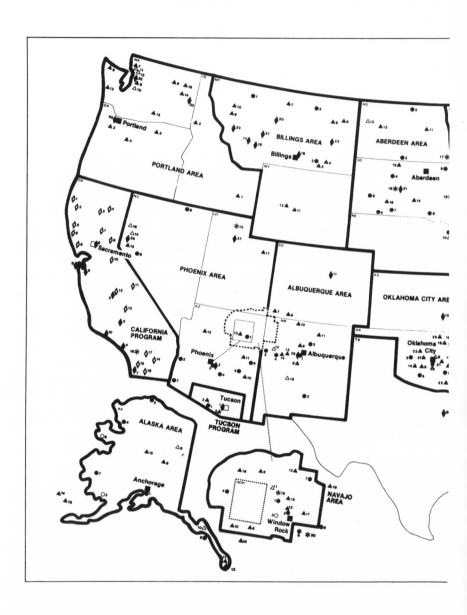

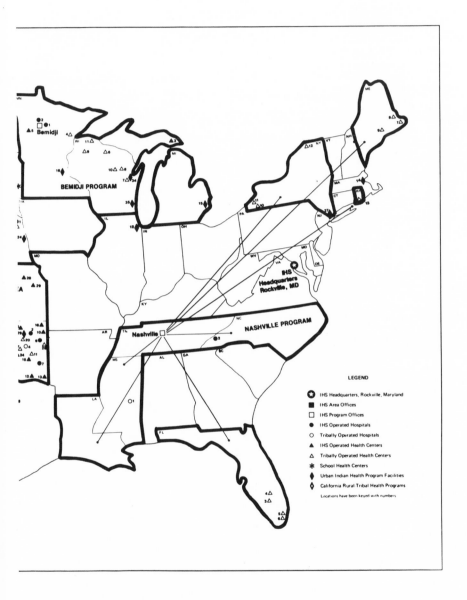

LEGEND

⬤ IHS Headquarters, Rockville, Maryland
◼ IHS Area Offices
◻ IHS Program Offices
● IHS Operated Hospitals
○ Tribally Operated Hospitals
▲ IHS Operated Health Centers
△ Tribally Operated Health Centers
✳ School Health Centers
⬥ Urban Indian Health Program Facilities
◇ California Rural Tribal Health Programs

Locations have been keyed with numbers

FIGURE 10:   Locations of Indian Health Services Offices and Facilities.

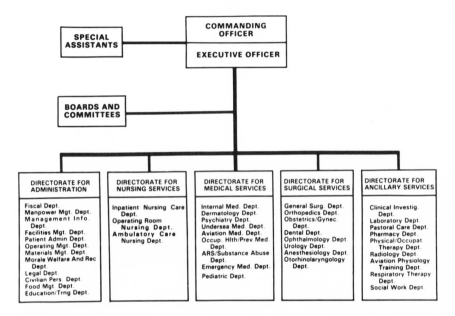

to the establishment of the present-day Department of Medicine and Surgery. At their urging, the Congress passed Public Law 293 which became the "Magna Carta" of the Department of Medicine and Surgery of the Veterans Administration. It placed physicians, dentists, and nurses under a separate system for selection and appointment and established a separate pay system. It made possible the affiliation of Veterans Administration medical centers with medical and other professional health schools.

In 1930, the Congress authorized the President to bring together under a single agency responsibility for providing federal benefits to veterans and their dependents. This brought about the establishment of the Veterans Administration. Fifty-seven Public Health Service hospitals became the nucleus of the present-day Department of Medicine and Surgery. The VA's hospital system has grown to include 172 medical centers, 228 outpatient clinics, 115 nursing home care units, and 16 domiciliaries, the largest medical care system in the country. The location of these facilities is displayed in Figure 11. There is at least one VA medical center in each of the 48 contiguous states, Puerto Rico, and the District of Columbia. These medical centers treat 1.3 million patients on an inpatient basis each year in 78,000 beds. The outpatient program registers more than 19 million visits a year and VA nursing homes and domiciliaries care for 33,000 veterans a year. The Department of Medicine and Surgery employs over 7,000 full-time physicians, over 5,000 part-time physicians, over 10,000 residents, almost 36,000 registered nurses, approximately 11,000 practical nurses, some 16,800 nursing assistants, and about 130,000 other health care specialists and personnel.

The Department of Medicine and Surgery has a four-part mission: patient care, research, education, and provision of backup medical contingency support to the Department of Defense in the event of war or national emergency. Little is known of the role of the Veterans Administration in health care education, training, and research; however, the Veterans Administration makes an important contribution to the health care of the nation as a whole. One hundred one of the nation's medical schools and 59 dental schools are affiliated with VA medical centers. About one-third of U.S. trained medical residents and medical students receive training in VA medical centers and one-half of all physicians in practice in the United States have received some portion of their training in VA health facilities. The educational programs extend to other health professional schools and formal affiliations are in effect with over 1,000 schools and campuses in 49 states, the District of Columbia, and Puerto Rico. Approximately 98,000 students and trainees receive all or part of their supervised clinical and administrative experience in VA medical centers during any given year.

At the same time, the VA is conducting a broad array of research activities. Thus, the triad of clinical care, education, and research not only strengthens the VA health care system and its ability to deliver quality patient care but also enables the Department of Medicine and Surgery to make a significant contribution to health care at large. Approximately 145 VA health care facilities conduct medical research programs, almost 6,000 principal investigators participate in over 11,000 research projects, and approximately 9,000 reports are published annually. VA research has helped to conquer tuberculosis, to develop a heart pacemaker, to perfect kidney transplants, and to develop a laser cane for the blind. The VA has also been a leader in the research and development of prosthetic devices. VA researchers have been recognized nationally and internationally, including the conferring of two Nobel Prizes in medicine on VA scientists.

The Veterans Administration employs approximately 1,750 individuals in positions which would fall under the general umbrella of health care administration. For the most part, these appointments would be made through the civil service system and would be in the General Health Science Series, the Health System Administration Series, or the Health System Specialist Series. In addition, there are approximately 1,700 administrative positions at the service chief and assistant service chief levels in hospitals to which course graduates can advance, after entering the system at the GS-5 to 7 entry level. The vast majority of the positions are in VA medical centers.

FIGURE 11: Locations of Veterans Administration Facilities.

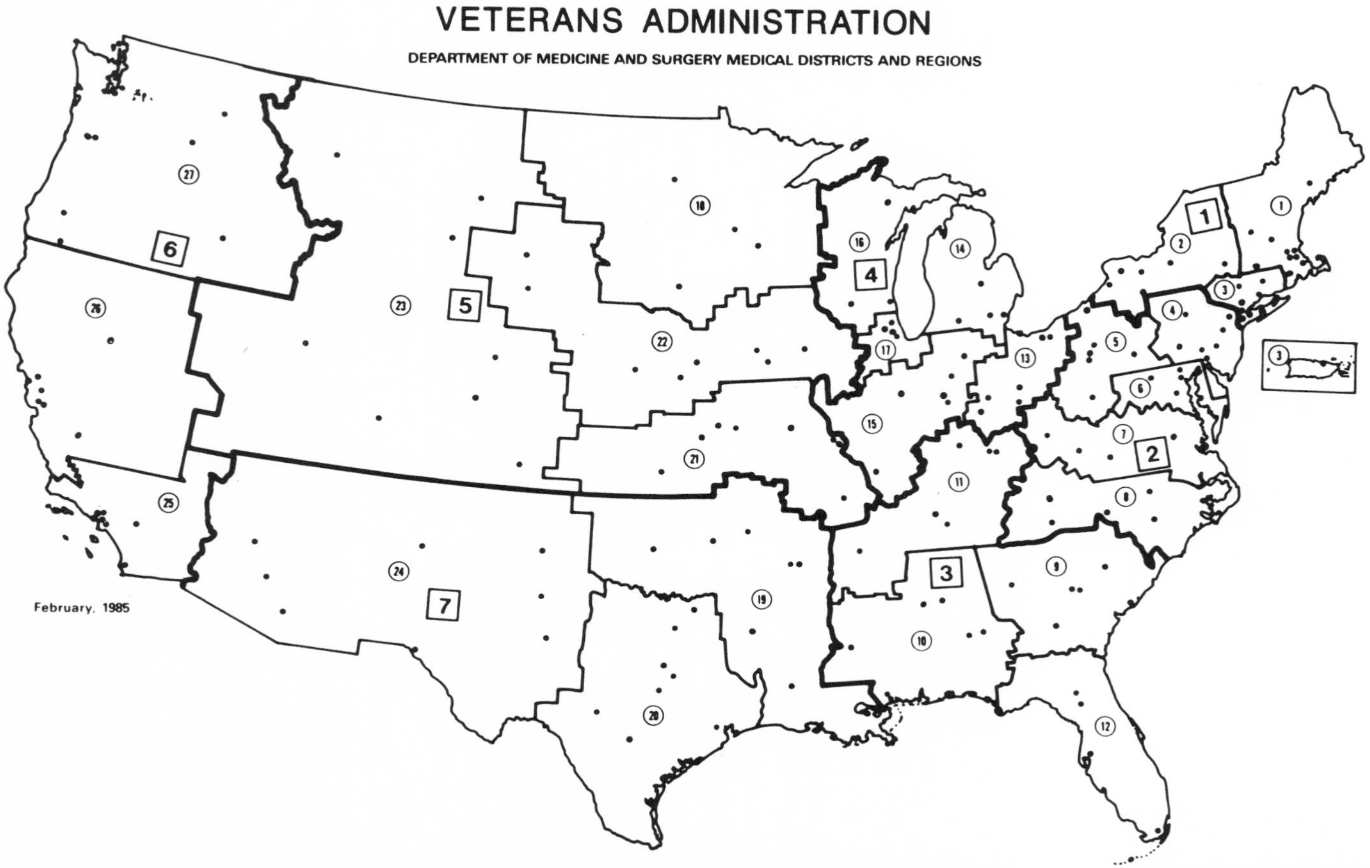
VETERANS ADMINISTRATION
DEPARTMENT OF MEDICINE AND SURGERY MEDICAL DISTRICTS AND REGIONS
1
2
3
4
5
6
7
February, 1985

Medical District 1
Bedford, MA
Boston, OC MA
Boston, MA
Manchester, NH
Northampton, MA
Providence, RI
Togus, ME
White River Junction, VT

Medical District 2
Albany, NY
Batavia, NY
Bath, NY
Buffalo, NY
Canandaigua, NY
Syracuse, NY

Medical District 3
Bronx, NY
Brooklyn, NY (CONS)
Castle Point, NY
Montrose, NY
New York, NY
Newington, CT
Northport, NY
San Juan, PR
West Haven, CT

REGION 2

Medical District 4
Coatesville, PA
East Orange, NY
Lebanon, PA
Lyons, NJ
Philadelphia, PA
Wilkes Barre, PA
Wilmington, DE

Medical District 5
Altoona, PA
Butler, PA
Clarksburg, WV
Erie, PA
Pittsburgh, PA (CONS)

Medical District 6
Baltimore, MD
Fort Howard, MD
Martinsburg, WV
Perry Point, MD
Washington, DC

Medical District 7
Beckley, WV
Hampton, VA
Huntington, WV
Richmond, VA
Salem, VA

Medical District 8
Asheville, NC
Durham, NC
Fayetteville, NC
Mountain Home, TN
Salisbury, NC

REGION 3

Medical District 9
Atlanta, GA
Augusta, GA
Charleston, SC
Columbia, SC
Dublin, GA

Medical District 10
Biloxi, MS (CONS)
Birmingham, AL
Jackson, MS
Montgomery, AL
Tuscaloosa, AL
Tuskegee, AL

Medical District 11
Lexington, KY
Louisville, KY
Memphis, TN
Murfreesboro, TN
Nashville, TN

Medical District 12
Bay Pines, FL
Gainesville, FL
Lake City, FL
Miami, FL
Tampa, FL

REGION 4

Medical District 13
Chillicothe, OH
Cincinnati, OH
Cleveland, OH (CONS)
Columbus OC, OH
Dayton, OH

Medical District 14
Allen Park, MI
Ann Arbor, MI
Battle Creek, MI
Saginaw, MI

Medical District 15
Danville, IL
Fort Wayne, IN
Indianapolis, IN (CONS)
Marion, IL
Marion, IN

Medical District 16
Iron Mountain, MI
Madison, WI
Tomah, WI
Wood, WI

Medical District 17
Chicago Lakeside, IL
Chicago Westside, IL
Hines, IL
North Chicago, IL

REGION 5

Medical District 18
Fargo, ND
Minneapolis, MN
Sioux Falls, SD
St Cloud, MN

Medical District 21
Columbia, MO
Poplar Bluff, MO
St Louis, MO
Kansas City, MO
Leavenworth, KS
Topeka, KS
Wichita, KS

Medical District 22
Des Moines, IA
Fort Meade, SD
Grand Island, NE
Hot Springs, SD
Iowa City, IA
Knoxville, IA
Lincoln, NE
Omaha, NE

Medical District 23
Cheyenne, WY
Denver, CO
Fort Harrison, MT
Fort Lyon, CO
Grand Junction, CO
Miles City, MT
Salt Lake City, UT
Sheridan, WY

REGION 6

Medical District 25
Las Vegas, NV
Loma Linda, CA
Long Beach, CA
Los Angeles OC, CA
San Diego, CA
Sepulveda, CA
West Los Angeles, CA (CONS)

Medical District 26
Fresno, CA
Honolulu OC, HI
Livermore, CA
Manila OC, PI
Martinez, CA
Palo Alto, CA (CONS)
Reno, NV
San Francisco, CA

Medical District 27
Anchorage OC, AK
Boise, ID
Roseburg, OR (CONS)
Seattle, WA
Spokane, WA
Tacoma/American Lake, WA
Walla Walla, WA
White City, OR

REGION 7 (NEW)

Medical District 19
Alexandria, LA
Fayetteville, AR
Little Rock, AR (CONS)
New Orleans, LA
Shreveport, LA
Muskogee, OK
Oklahoma City, OK

Medical District 20
Bonham, TX
Dallas, TX
Houston, TX
Kerrville, TX
Marlin, TX
San Antonio, TX
Temple, TX
Waco, TX

Medical District 24
Albuquerque, NM
Amarillo, TX
Big Spring, TX
El Paso OC, TX
Phoenix, AZ
Prescott, AZ
Tucson, AZ
Lubbock OC, TX

FIGURE 12:   Representative VA Medical Center.

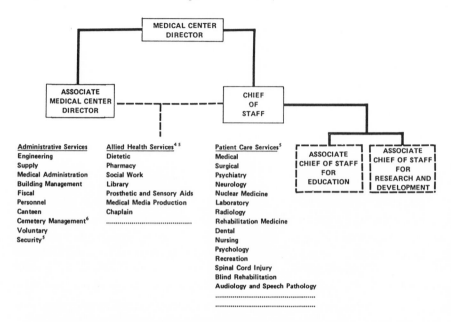

Administrative Services
Engineering
Supply
Medical Administration
Building Management
Fiscal
Personnel
Canteen
Cemetery Management[6]
Voluntary
Security[5]

Allied Health Services[4][5]
Dietetic
Pharmacy
Social Work
Library
Prosthetic and Sensory Aids
Medical Media Production
Chaplain
....

Patient Care Services[5]
Medical
Surgical
Psychiatry
Neurology
Nuclear Medicine
Laboratory
Radiology
Rehabilitation Medicine
Dental
Nursing
Psychology
Recreation
Spinal Cord Injury
Blind Rehabilitation
Audiology and Speech Pathology
....
....

[1] Each hospital organization is subject to approval by Chief Medical Director. The Medical Center Director will submit proposed organization, including assignment or distribution of jurisdiction over Allied Health Services, Regional Director.
[2] The Associate Medical Center Director will routinely serve as the Acting Medical Center Director in the absence of the Medical Center Director unless the Medical Center Director designates otherwise.
[3] Subject to approval by the Chief Medical Director.
[4] Subject to approval by the Chief Medical Director, any or all Allied Health Services may be placed under the Associate Medical Center Director, or the Chief of Staff either directly under him/her or through an Assistant Chief of Staff (Physician).
[5] Only services required to carry out the mission of the medical center will be provided for the organization. Services may be consolidated and additional services may be established when authorized and directed by the Chief Medical Director.
[6] Subject to agreement with DMA. The Medical Center Director will be responsible to the Chief Memorial Affairs Director for this function.
[7] Associate or Assistant title will be utilized as appropriate.

The organizational chart for a representative VA medical center is found in Figure 12. The entry level for most of these positions would be at the GS-5 or GS-7 levels, with higher positions of responsibility found at the GS-15 level.

It has been the policy of the Veterans Administration to assign trained health care administrators to serve as directors of the medical centers and independent outpatient clinics, although there are usually a few medical centers that have physicians as directors. Those individuals entering the VA system under the general schedule of the civil service system at the entry level grades of GS-5 or GS-7 will be assigned to staff positions. From these entry levels there are opportunities for advancement to section chiefs in the medical centers, assistant service chiefs, service chiefs, members of the management team, and associate directors. There are also a number of important line and staff positions in the central office.

The Veterans Administration, as the largest health care system in this country under single management, presents a challenging opportunity for a career in health care administration. Contrary to the misconceptions that some may have about large federal agencies, the VA health care system provides an innovative, stimulating environment. It is a system that is providing quality care in a fast-paced, dynamic, ever-changing setting. The management philosophy of the Department of Medicine and Surgery calls for setting broad policy at the central office, with the authority and responsibility for the operation of the medical centers delegated to the directors. This philosophy provides maximum flexibility, encourages the use of ingenuity and strategic planning to develop programs to meet the needs of each medical center's primary service area, and enables local management to get the maximum mileage out of the dollars allocated to the individual medical center. The VA medical centers operate on a prospective budget, giving the director and the staff, through the strategic planning process, the opportunity to inaugurate program changes to meet changing needs and to prepare a budget plan to support approved program changes. Thus, much more flexibility is provided in the VA system than is commonly thought and this reinforces the need for trained administrators with management skills.

With its wide-ranging clinical care, education, and research programs, the Veterans Administration is at the cutting edge of medicine. A nationwide system of hospitals and clinics provide services ranging from outpatient care to sophisticated tertiary care. Its facilities encompass outpatient clinics, domiciliaries, nursing homes, secondary hospitals, and complex teaching institutions similar to those found in the private sector. The Veterans Administration is committed not only to providing quality care, but to doing so in an effective and efficient manner. This requires the attraction and retention of trained, skilled management people. The opportunity, therefore, for those seeking a career in health care administration has never been greater. For those individuals who are completing programs in health care administration at the university level, and who come into the Veterans Administration system at the entry level, a clear career pathway exists for advancing to positions of increasing responsibility. For the individual who is willing to make a commitment to providing health care to the veterans of this country and who is also interested in making a significant contribution to the health of all of the people, the Veterans Administration offers an exciting and rewarding career.

SUMMARY

Disraeli was right! There is no issue that is as important to the people as their own health. It is an issue which touches the lives of every man, woman, and child. It is, therefore, an issue of concern to government and, particularly, the federal government. Although there is wide debate about the future of health care in this country, many thinkers believe that this country will continue to have a pluralistic health care system with many different approaches being followed in providing that care. Whatever the shape of the health care system of tomorrow, it can be stated with some certainty that the federal government will play an important role. Service in the federal government, therefore, in the field of health administration offers an exciting, challenging, and rewarding career. It offers an opportunity to play a key role in the provision of health care to millions of people and an opportunity to contribute to the shape of the health care system of the future. There are few settings where one can have such a significant impact.

ACKNOWLEDGEMENTS

Julian Barber, Special Assistant, Assistant Secretary of Defense, Health Affairs

Marylyn Gresser, Library Consultant

General Walter F. Johnson III, MSC, U.S. Army

Philip M. Kaplan, Media Consultant

Lt. Commander William K. Knox, MSC, U.S. Navy

Captain Rice C. Leach, Indian Health Service, U.S. Public Health Service

John L. Maddy, Program Analyst, Office of Assistant Secretary of Defense, Health Affairs

Lt. Colonel Timothy C. McKee, U.S. Air Force, MSC

Captain James McTigue, MSC, U.S. Public Health Service

Colonel Richard E. Meiers, MSC, U.S. Army

Geraldine W. Meyers, Consultant

Colonel John E. Murphy, U.S. Air Force, MSC

Christine S. Randall, Ed.D., Consultant

Colonel Herbert Rosenbleeth, MSC, U.S. Army

Rear Admiral Donald E. Shuler, MSC, U.S. Navy

REFERENCES

1. Disraeli, Benjamin, Earl of Beaconsfield. Speech, July 24, 1877.
2. U.S. Congress, House. Medical Care of Veterans. Washington, DC: Government Printing Office, April 17, 1967.

BIBLIOGRAPHY

American College of Hospital Administrators. *Competence, Character, Commitment: Today's Health Care Executive. 1981–1982 Annual Report*. Chicago: The College, 1982.

American College of Hospital Administrators. *Guidelines for Post-graduate Fellowships and Management Development Programs in Health Services Administration*. Chicago: The College, 1984.

American College of Hospital Administrators. *Report of the Task Force on Beginning and Early Career Development*. Chicago: The College, 1984.

Armstrong, H. G. The Air Force Medical Service: 1 July 1949–1 July 1954. *Medical Service Digest* 20 (7): 11–16, July 1969.

Crosby, W. H. The Golden Age of the Army Medical Corps: A Perspective From 1901. *Military Medicine* 148(9): 707–11, September 1983.

Engleman, R. C. *Two Hundred Years of Military Medicine*. Washington, DC: Government Printing Office, 1975.

U.S. Executive Office of the President. *Budget of the United States Government, Fiscal Year 1988. Supplement*. Washington, D.C. Government Printing Office, 1987.

U.S. Department of Health and Human Services. *A Comprehensive Health Care Program for American Indians and Alaska Natives*. Indian Health Service, n.d.

U.S. Department of Health and Human Services. *A Comprehensive Health Care Program, 1955–1985: Thirty Years of Progress*. Indian Health Service, n.d.

National Institutes of Health Began 100 Years Ago, One-Room Laboratory. *ARA Newsletter* 6(2): 1987.

U.S. Department of Health and Human Services, National Institutes of Health. NIH Data Book: Basic Data Relating to the National Institute of Health. NIH Publication No. 87–1261. December 1986.

U.S. Office of Personnel Management. *Federal Civilian Workforce Statistics: Occupations of Federal White-Collar and Blue-Collar Workers, Oct 31, 1985*. Washington, DC: Government Printing Office, 1986.

U.S. Office of the Federal Register. *The United States Government Manual, 1986–87*. Washington, DC: Government Printing Office, 1986.

U.S. Department of Defense. *An Overview of the Military Health Care System*. Office of the Assistant Secretary of Defense for Health Affairs, n.d.

U.S. Public Health Service. Office of Public Affairs. *The Public Health Service*. Public Health Service, n.d.

Bowen, O. R., M.D. Secretary, Department of Health and Human Services, Statement Jan. 5, 1987.

U.S. Congress, House. *Medical Care of Veterans*. Washington, DC: Government Printing Office, 1967.

U.S. Department of Labor. *Occupational Outlook Handbook*, 1986–87 ed. Washington, DC: Government Printing Office, 1986.

U.S. Department of the Navy. *Navy Medical Service Corps*. Washington, DC: Government Printing Office, 1984.

Veterans Administration. Annual Report 1985. Washington, DC: Veterans Administration, 1986.

Veterans Administration. Department of Medicine and Surgery. *Hospital Administration Residency Training Program*, Washington, DC: Veterans Administration, TP 10–27, September 14, 1982.

Veterans Administration. *Facts about the Veterans Administration*. (News Feature) Washington, DC: VA Office of Public and Consumer Affairs, 1986.

The World Almanac and Book of Facts. New York: Newspaper Enterprise Association, Inc., 1986.

17

INTERNATIONAL HEALTH: RESPONDING TO THE GLOBAL CHALLENGE

WILLY De GEYNDT, Ph.D.

In order to meet the objectives of this book, the discussion of international health administration activities focuses on the management or administration of health services and programs as the primary reason of employment and deliberately excludes clinical practice even though some clinicians may perform management tasks as a corollary to their clinical functions. International refers to work carried out by U.S. and Canadian citizens in developing or third world countries. Health refers to activities designed to improve the health conditions in a country and to enhance the health status of its citizens. Health includes activities in the fields of family planning and nutrition which are considered integral parts of the health sector, and in water and sanitation as an important component of environmental health. International health care is not an academic discipline in its own right, as all disciplines in the field of health have international ramifications.

WHO WORKS OVERSEAS?

Data on the number, type, and employers of health professionals working overseas are sketchy. A survey of international health agencies was carried

Willy De Geyndt is a public health specialist at the World Bank, Washington, DC. He holds a Ph.D. in health services administration, a master's in management from the University of Minnesota, and a bachelor's degree in education from the University of Brussels. The opinions expressed in this chapter are those of the author and not the World Bank.

out in 1969 by Johns Hopkins University (JHU) and was updated in 1981. The update concentrated on employers, U.S. institutions and firms, and did not include self-employed health professionals. The 1981 JHU survey showed that about 8,700 persons were working in international health care of which 44 percent were long-term, 19 percent short-term (mainly consultants), and 37 percent volunteers who can be short-term or long-term. Almost half of the total were physicians and nurses and 14 percent were classified as health and hospital administrators, managers, or planners [1].

The roughly 1,200 professionals in the health services administration category consisted of 55 percent long-term employees, 30 percent short-term, and 15 percent volunteers and they were concentrated in corporations and businesses. This concentration reflects the growing market in the last two decades for health services managers in oil-exporting Middle East countries (mainly long-term employees) and the increase in the number of small consulting firms in health-related activities and the addition of health divisions to large consulting firms (both long-term and short-term employees). Volunteers are nonsalaried persons who may receive transportation costs, a living allowance, and a stipend. In the government sector, volunteers are usually in the Peace Corps; in the private sector, they work for church-related organizations and private voluntary organizations (PVOs).

If international health care is not a discipline per se for health administrators, it also does not have a clear educational career track that leads directly to a career in international health care. Although there are courses and programs of study offered in the subject area, there is no pattern of studies that would lead one in an organized fashion to a position in the field as would be the case in accounting, law, nursing, medicine, and so on. If this is so, then how do the people who work in international health care get there and who are they? A first group consists of people with a strong technical background and marketable knowledge and skills who are invited or successfully compete for overseas assignments or consultancies. These health specialists usually have years of relevant experience to their credit and may range from the creative researcher to the noted academician to the well-known lecturer to the seasoned manager. Most of these people work in the developing countries and in oil-exporting nations and return to their home country where their professional roots are. Knowledge of foreign languages is not always an important criterion because English is the accepted scientific language at that level.

The second group of people working in international health care are those who face the catch-22 problem; they want to work internationally but do not have the requisite experience and the language base which is more frequently required at the entry level. Therefore, they cannot get hired, but how does one acquire the experience to qualify for the coveted position? As observed through knowledge of the field, personal experience, and interviews of colleagues, a common thread runs through the motivation of those who aspire to work overseas but do not yet have marketable skills. A large majority have some familiarity with foreign countries directly or vicariously because their parents served in the foreign service, in the military stationed overseas, or in church-related missions. They may have a spouse of a different culture or parents of different cultural or ethnic backgrounds and be immigrants themselves. Some have acquired experience in international affairs through service in the Peace Corps or through missionary or proselytizing work either out of religious conviction or as a requirement of their religion.

This group has a predisposing background and a conscious or unconscious desire to enter the field of international health care. This desire is realized by a small percentage of aspirants and unless they fall within the first category of highly skilled researchers, academicians, or managers, their entry into the area of international health care seems to be partly by coincidence and happenstance, partly through personal contacts, and partly through high motivation and persistence but generally less through a predictable career pattern. Almost all will work in a developing country at the grass roots level or in nongovernmental organizations (NGOs), bilateral and multilateral organizations in the development community that deal with developing countries. Language skills are important to be able to communicate with beneficiaries of development aid and with the various levels of the governments of less-developed countries.

If one has the skills of a generalist, limited or no international experience, and limited language skills, how does one acquire them to be able to qualify for a position in the international community? U.S. entry points are mostly through self-financed or volunteer activities in the Peace Corps, missionary work, North American Indian reservations, refugee camps, or one of the many volunteer organizations. The Peace Corps has traditionally been a source of developing country experience and a training ground for learning foreign languages. In 1978 there were 1,700 Peace Corps health volunteers working overseas but this number has now dropped to 487 volunteers active in 49 countries, in spite of the fact that the number of requests from U.S. nationals to join has increased. The decrease in the number of volunteers posted is mainly due to demands by developing countries for more qualified—that is more highly skilled—volunteers and partly to a reduction in funding levels. Thus, the Peace Corps as an entry point into international health care for the generalist is less promising in the 1980s than it was in the 1960s and 1970s.

Missionary groups are also becoming a less important entry point, partly because their size is shrinking and partly because they are using more nationals and fewer expatriates. Furthermore, church-related organizations are often involved in direct service delivery and recruit mostly physicians and nurses. The practice of recruiting nationals has spread rapidly in the past decade and most bilateral and multilateral organizations are now relying more on local and third world consultants. A number of factors account for this trend: the availability of qualified health professionals in middle-income countries; the local consultant's knowledge of culture, customs, and language; the lower cost of travel, subsistence, and salaries; and the eagerness and motivation of locals to gain additional experience and to enhance their income.

EDUCATION FOR INTERNATIONAL HEALTH

As mentioned earlier, there is no academic or formal training career path leading to a career in international health administration. Much work in international health care has a component of health administration, and the master's degree in public health (MPH) attempts to provide part of that component. A master's degree in health services administration usually does not cover this subject area. The MPH in international health is offered by a small number of U.S. universities (The Johns Hopkins School of Hygiene and Public Health, The Sparkman Center for International Public Health Education in the School of Public Health at the University of Alabama at Birmingham, University of Hawaii, University of Texas, and the University of California in Los Angeles) albeit with great variability in course content, program emphasis, and past experience. It is a leveling degree which provides a common knowledge base to individuals with a wide variety of backgrounds. Having an MPH degree does not guarantee a job in international health care. Combined with another discipline-based degree and overseas experience it may provide the competitive edge in a job search.

A number of colleges and universities offer courses in international health care as part of their regular curricula in, for example, medicine, pharmacy, nursing, epidemiology, health services administration, maternal and child health, family planning, and nutrition. Very often these are elective courses and attract a mix of foreign and American or Canadian students.

The U.S. Agency for International Development (USAID) offers an in-house training program, the International Development Intern Program, which attracts a number of generalists in the age range of 30 to 35 years, most of whom have international experience and an MPH or equivalent degree. All USAID interns receive intensive language training prior to an overseas assignment if they do not already possess language skills upon entry.

ORGANIZATIONS ACTIVE IN INTERNATIONAL HEALTH CARE

Bilateral organizations are governmental agencies from developed countries that provide development assistance to Third World countries. This is the case of the U.S. Agency for International Development and the Canadian International Development Assistance (CIDA). Similar agencies exist in other Western countries, such as Denmark (DANIDA), Sweden (SIDA), Norway (NORAD), and the United Kingdom (ODA). These bilateral institutions, supported by tax monies, restrict hiring of staff to nationals of their countries.

Multilateral organizations are intergovernmental institutions made up of more than one country and their membership usually includes developed and developing nations. The largest in terms of membership (158 countries) is the World Health Organization (WHO) headquartered in Geneva, Switzerland, with six large regional offices in Africa (Brazzaville), the Americas (Pan American Health Organization in Washington, DC), South-East Asia (New Delhi), Europe (Copenhagen), Eastern Mediterranean (Alexandria), and Western Pacific (Manila). Staff are recruited for their technical skills and represent a balanced mix of nationals from member countries. Large-scale international lending agencies active in all sectors of the economy have begun funding health activities in the last decade. The largest multilateral bank is the International Bank for Reconstruction and Development (World Bank) headquartered in Washington, DC having 151 member countries. Regional banks with similar objectives have been established for countries in the Americas (the Inter-American Development Bank), in Asia (the Asian Development Bank), and in Africa (the African Development Bank). Lending for health activities is a very small part of their lending program which focuses mostly on the so-called productive sectors (agriculture, energy, transportation, mining, industry) and staff are recruited from all member countries for their specific skills and international experience.

Philanthropic foundations have long been active in international health activities. The best known and most significant one is the Rockefeller Foundation, established in 1909. Others that are known for their involvement in specialized areas of international health are, inter alia, the W. K. Kellogg Foundation, the Carnegie Corporation, the Aga Khan Foundation, the Milbank Memorial Fund, Pew Memorial Trust, and the Ford Foundation. The

1981 JHU survey reported that endowed foundations represent only 3.5 percent of all organizations reporting international health activities and employ only 38 U.S. health professionals [2].

Private voluntary organizations include church-related organizations and secular groups. Religious groups are by far the largest number of PVOs and represent a highly diverse group of institutions with an equally diverse range of health activities. Bryant described the situation as follows: "There are over 1,200 medical institutions related to Anglican, Orthodox and Protestant churches in developing countries, and they have combined operating budgets in excess of $100 million per year. The Roman Catholic church has more than 2,000 such institutions with expenditures of over $200 million. In some countries, these mission programs account for more than 40 percent of all health care" [3]. Among nondenominational groups, the better known are Project Concern, Project HOPE, International Planned Parenthood Federation, Save the Children, Oxfam, Population Council, and CARE/ MEDICO. As the importance of narrow health programs of some PVOs has decreased in the past two decades, such as those involved in mission hospitals, leprosaria, and orphanages, activities have expanded in areas of community development, integrated rural development, and agriculture. The decrease in specific health activities is a result of governments assuming more responsibility for the health of their people, increasing their scope of action through ministries of health, and training more indigenous personnel. PVOs are the largest employers of volunteers, especially church-related groups, and conversely, employ the smallest proportion of long-term employees. Religious groups tend to employ more physicians and nurses [4].

Commercial companies span a wide range of activities. Best known and present in every country in the world are transnational pharmaceutical companies, and medical supplies and equipment manufacturers and distributors. Of more recent origin are the multinational management companies purchasing, constructing, or managing hospitals, especially in oil-exporting countries (Saudi Arabia, Bahrein, the Persian Gulf Emirates, Venezuela, Mexico, Ecuador), upper-middle-income countries (Singapore, Hong Kong, Taiwan, Brazil) and developed countries (Switzerland, United Kingdom). Also more recently, large and small consulting companies offer a broad range of health care consulting services ranging from broad areas such as strategic planning to very specialized areas such as medical records management and quality assurance programs. Some large transnational companies have company-sponsored health plans. Commercial companies are the largest employers of health services managers, planners, and specialists in specific areas of health care management. Prior international experience is often not a requirement, but a premium is put on technical skills and a proven track record [5].

SOURCES OF INFORMATION

International health services administration is to a certain extent an opportunistic business with people entering it both by design and by accident. As a result a number of information sources are informal, through word of mouth, informal contacts, or being at the right place at the right time. There are, however, a number of formal sources providing information on current job opportunities for U.S. nationals in international health care. Sources usually list job opportunities for all specialties in the field of health care. The common denominator is that the positions deal with overseas programs and are related to health. The New Transcentury Foundation (1724 Kalarama Road N.W., Washington, DC 20009) publishes once every two months a Job Opportunities Bulletin ($15 per year) listing openings in international development with private and voluntary organizations. The National Council for International Health (1101 Connecticut Avenue, N.W., Suite 605, Washington, DC 20036) is a professional association of about 2,000 individuals and about 155 organizations involved in health activities with special emphasis on the third world. It holds an annual conference, organizes technical workshops, publishes periodically a directory, and announces job openings in its monthly newsletter. Many schools of public health have job bulletins. The American Public Health Association's International Health Program (1015 Fifteenth Street, N.W., Washington, DC 20005) and the United Nations Volunteers Program are useful sources of information.

SUMMARY AND CONCLUSIONS

From a skills and knowledge point of view, the small group of U.S. nationals working in international health care can be divided into specialists and generalists. The former group are professionals in all health disciplines with specific marketable skills needed and requested by developing countries. These people are often academicians, researchers, managers, and lecturers who accept short-term consulting assignments or longer-term (one year or more) overseas postings. The generalist has difficulty breaking into the field for lack of experience and of sought-after skills. Cultural sensitivity, languages, and specific program experience are usually acquired in the Peace Corps or with church-related groups or private voluntary organizations on a volunteer basis with minimal financial rewards. There is no established and accepted educational career track that leads to a job in international health care. Courses in international health, usually in one of the major schools of public health, combined with developing country field experience and language skills may provide the competitive edge in a job search. Above all, the pursuit of a career in international health care requires a high degree of motivation to serve and patience and persistence to succeed.

Health services administration is a special case in the field of international health care. Management of health services has often not been viewed by officials and program heads of developing countries as a special skill. Management is still seen as a matter of putting someone in charge who sounds authoritative because he has strong vocal chords or is physically big, or who is revered for having concrete people-helping skills such as the physician. This perception of management is slowly changing, partly due to fiscal constraints or public sector spending and a search for greater efficiency in health services delivery. However, a career in international health administration as it is defined and presented in other chapters of this book is still not promising. The most attractive package may be a combination of an applicable language and solid management skills with credentialed people-helping skills in one of the many health professions.

REFERENCES

1. Baker, T.D., C. Weisman and A. Piwoz. United States Health Professionals in International Work. *American Journal of Public Health* 74 (5): 438–41, 1984.
2. Baker, T. D. et al. (see number 1).
3. Basch, P. F. *International Health*. New York: Oxford University Press, 1978.
4. Bryant, J. *Health and the Developing World*. Ithaca, NY: Cornell University Press, 1969.
5. Taylor, C. E. Changing Patterns in International Health: Motivation and Relationships. *American Journal of Public Health* 69 (8): 803–08, 1979.
6. The White House. *New Directions in International Health Cooperation*. Washington, DC: U.S. Government Printing Office, 1978.

PART VI

CAREER DEVELOPMENT

18

PHYSICIANS IN ADMINISTRATION: WORKING AT THE MEDICINE AND MANAGEMENT INTERFACE

JOHN T. ASHLEY, M.D.

Many physicians have the basic traits to be capable managers. Most physicians have a high level of intelligence demonstrated by the rigorous screening required for admission to medical school. The medical school and graduate training experience prepares physicians to understand the spectrum of health and illness conditions. Most physicians are trained to make difficult decisions affecting individual patients while working with a team of health professionals concerned with caring for individual patients. Some physicians recognize that their independent clinical decision making can only be effective if supported by organizations and systems designed and managed to integrate with the clinical care process but others are not concerned about the functioning of the system.

Not every physician is prepared or oriented to be a successful manager. The physician with concern for institutional functioning needs certain competences that will prepare an individual for success in the field of management. Physicians are prepared to make important human observations throughout their clinical training. The training of physicians prepares them to make decisions with incomplete information and to judge the value of

John T. Ashley is the executive director of the University of Virginia Hospitals in Charlottesville. Dr. Ashley earned an M.D., an M.B.A. in health services management, and a B.A. degree from the University of Missouri—Columbia.

obtaining additional information. Physicians are the informal leaders of the health care system in almost every organizational arena. Until recent years, with few exceptions, physicians have eschewed a formal management role and have preferred to use their informal power in influencing the direction of the health care system.

Changes in the health care system in the past 25 years have shifted it from a cottage industry of small practices to a more structured and organized emerging system for providing services and managing the process of providing medical care. These changes create the opportunity and need for physicians who are willing and prepared to assume a more direct leadership role to participate in the management of changing organizations or, increasingly, to manage physician practice within organizations which are emerging. Major changes have occurred in the management structure of hospitals, nursing homes, physician practices, managed care systems, services for industry, and many other organizations where expanded physician participation in management is crucial to institutional success. Physician leadership is valuable to assure an institutional balance among the competing demands of quality care versus cost containment, prevention versus medical intervention, technology application versus primary care, and conflict over professional domain.

While most physicians are not formally prepared to be managers, or to be managed, the growth of health care organizations, the complexity of interaction among medical disciplines, the demands for management of the medical care process by third parties, and the blurring of the distinction between management and medical care decision making mandates that physicians assume a high level of responsibility for administration of health care institutions and systems.

Medicine has been described as the "queen of professions resistant to management." Physicians have always maintained a role of preeminent power in the system, and that power is being challenged on many fronts. Decisions about medical care for patients are challenged by third party payers, by lawyers, by institutions, and by patients themselves. Decisions about technology acquisitions and use are challenged by regulators, insurers, other institutions, and other professionals. Physicians have the opportunity to transform their latent power into organized management positions with responsibility and authority for leadership and management. Organizations with trained physician administrators should attain greater responsiveness to professional expectations and a more effective response to community health care needs.

The history of the health care system focuses on the private practice of medicine and on hospitals. The earliest hospitals were institutions created for the care of the very poor. These early organizations were dominated by their benefactor board of directors and physicians. With the improvement of science, physicians achieved a dominant role in the management of hospitals. Most large hospitals had designated a physician superintendent to provide the leadership of the institution. Only as medical practice became more complex and specialized did the role of physician in management of hospitals diminish. The need for obtaining funding for hospitals through billing of patients and their insurers led to the expansion of the separate profession of hospital administrator in the 1930s and 1940s [1].

The next five decades saw a continued dominance of physicians in the clinical decision making in hospitals and in private practice but a growing role for the separate board of directors and separate hospital administrators in hospitals. Physicians eschewed a major role in hospital administration because of the inherent conflict between an independent profession and the management prerogatives inherent in hospital administration. Hospitals grew up with a tripartite organizational structure involving a board of directors, hospital administration and the medical staff. This arrangement was enforced by regulations of the Joint Commission on Accreditation of Healthcare Organizations, and by insurance programs such as Medicare, Medicaid, and Blue Cross. Separate reimbursement systems for physicians in hospitals reinforced separation of physicians and hospital organizational structures.

Within medicine, the dramatic increase in specialty practice and the growth of organized group practice added to the complexity of the medical care system and the organizational arrangements required to provide care. In the 1970s the surge in medical school graduates and the growth of medical technology combined to increase the number of physicians employed or contracting with hospitals and other health care organizations.

There has been rapid development of managed care systems in the past 20 years in which the process of care and the process of insuring the benefits has been integrated in the form of health maintenance organizations and preferred provider organizations. These systems of managed care are designed to assure government, industry, and other third party payers that the cost of care can be controlled. These changes have led to a dramatic increase in the management of medical practice in hospitals, nursing homes, and in the ambulatory care setting involving group practices. In response to greater regulation and economic opportunity, industry and entrepreneurial health care systems have been created which need physicians in key leadership roles.

HOSPITAL OPPORTUNITIES

Hospitals have shifted from being "the doctor's workshop" to being the center of health care for communities. In these settings, the professions, the capital equipment, and the technical support to provide the full range of health care services for a community are assembled. The organization of hospitals to provide these services is required to be responsive to external expectations as well as to competition from other hospitals and other organizations.

These pressures have mandated that physicians cooperate or coordinate their services with the hospital resources. Hospitals are seeking ways of having that integration of effort occur in a systematic way. Physicians can contribute significantly to the effectiveness of that effort because of their understanding of the clinical implications of management decisions. Physicians' opportunities in hospital management range from serving as the chief executive officer, the management of clinical activities, directing major departments, such as radiology, pathology, anesthesiology, and emergency medical services, through the coordination of educational programs, quality assurance activities, and the conduct of clinical research. In particular, larger hospitals with major teaching activities and joint ventures with their practicing physicians use physicians in their key administrative positions.

A physician chief executive officer may be valuable in major teaching hospitals because of the large number of full-time physician staff employed by the hospital or related medical school. Effective planning, allocation of resources, communication of programs, and monitoring of practice is required in these settings. Frequently physicians are called upon to serve in these roles because of their ability to relate to the direct medical practice that is conducted through the hospital organization. These individuals frequently are required to be superb clinicians with excellent clinical skills and reputations. These individuals are managing multimillion-dollar business enterprises which also require well-developed skills in various areas of health administration.

Hospitals require consistent and effective medical staff leadership. Many hospitals employ physicians in the role of vice president for medical affairs or medical director serving as the interface between hospital administration and the medical staff. Many intermediate-sized community hospitals and most larger hospitals will identify a full-time or part-time physician executive who relates to the various clinical department chiefs and unit clinical directors to assure coordination of patient care efforts and development of programs. These individuals will guide senior hospital administrators and the board of directors in making resource allocation decisions involving capital equipment, expansion or contraction of services, and conduct of appropriate quality assurance and educational programs. These individuals will also assure integration of effort between the hospital and the medical staff in relating to the formal activities of the organized medical staff.

DEPARTMENT CHIEFS

Most hospitals will employ individuals to head various hospital-based departments, such as pathology, radiology, anesthesiology, emergency medical services, rehabilitation, and others, depending on the size and scope of services offered. These physicians may be full-time employees of the hospital or have contractual relationships that effectively integrate them into the hospital organization. These physicians serve as senior middle managers of crucial hospital resources. They are often responsible for multimillion-dollar budgets and the direction of various physicians, various technical professionals, and the control of major portions of hospital high technology investment. The use of these resources and the integration of effort between these departments and the other members of the medical staff are key to the success of the hospitals. In addition, many of these physicians are responsible for the conduct of key clinical programs that reach into the community, the marketing of hospital services, and the support for the clinical programs being conducted by the private medical staff. The interests of the hospitals and the clinical departments are best served if these individuals are thoroughly prepared to serve their administrative function, as well as their clinical responsibilities.

QUALITY ASSURANCE AND UTILIZATION REVIEW

The Joint Commission on Accreditation of Health Care Organizations, many third party payers, and professional review organizations require that hospitals maintain an ongoing program of surveillance of quality of care and utilization of hospital resources. This key function must be integrated between the medical staff providing care to individual patients, and the hospital's admissions, utilization review, medical records, and quality assurance departments. A physician is frequently identified to conduct these important programs that require certain skills of communication, negotiation, analysis, planning, and implementation. An individual prepared in these areas of hospital administration can be a major asset to a large hospital.

The quality assurance and utilization review functions are developing into the most important elements of a hospital care program. Marketing techniques demand that the product being marketed be of high quality. Third party payers and regulators are analyzing and comparing institutional performance in specific services. Every institution must demonstrate to itself and to its consumers that services are of high quality. Concurrent financial review is required to demonstrate that services being provided are generating sufficient income to meet expense. The pattern of utilization, resource allocation, and income potential must be continuously analyzed and monitored. These functions are essential to the practice of medicine and the effectiveness of institutional planning and performance.

NURSING HOMES AND LONG-TERM CARE

Medical services are a key component of the organizations created to provide the full range of services to the aging population. Nursing home chains require systems to assure quality of care, relations with local physicians, and intervention when deficiencies or improvement opportunities are identified. Physicians in the role of medical director are required, both for the conduct of care as well as the monitoring and control of quality of care. They should be prepared to understand the importance of appropriate investment and effective systems of providing services. An individual with training and experience in geriatrics, as well as health administration, is the ideal candidate for this role.

MANAGED CARE SYSTEMS

The growth of group practice has been dramatic in the past 30 years with physicians moving to group practice in growing numbers. The most significant growth of group practice has involved managed care through health maintenance organizations (HMOs) and preferred provider organizations. After many years of resistance, health maintenance organizations have been widely accepted. We estimate that 25 percent of the American population may be served by HMOs by the year 1990.

Key to the success of managed care is a focus on the physician practice patterns, particularly in the utilization of hospital resources. Physicians have a crucial role to play in working with other medical practitioners in planning services, developing systems to monitor care, conducting the monitoring, and intervening to alter patterns of practice where indicated. Opportunities to expand managed care systems are largely influenced by the relationship of physicians and hospitals. Physicians can play an important role in this marketing process. A physician executive is valuable to intervene with the organized medical staff in contractual hospitals.

GROUP PRACTICE

Many group practices are not involved in managed care. However, when a large number of physicians join together to enjoy the advantages of shared time and shared capital investment, the resulting organizational structure is highly complex. Many group practices with more than 25 physicians identify a physician to play a key role in providing management activities for their practice. This individual must be prepared to administer multimillion-dollar practice contracts with hospitals and industry and develop marketing programs to maintain a patient flow and other sources of revenue. Key decisions about technology investment, marketing, planning and practice expansion require consistent physician participation. In addition, this physician must provide leadership and coordination among physicians who are often resistant to being managed. The individual(s) with these responsibilities may do this part time or full time depending on the size or organization and the institutional arrangements.

PUBLIC HEALTH

Governmental health care services are based in public health. Services provided through provincial, state, county, and city public health departments include a spectrum of preventive services—environmental control, maternal and child health, immunizations, communicable disease control, health planning, and services to the disadvantaged. Some state departments administer Medicaid programs. Physicians are required to participate in the design of government policy with an understanding of its impact on medical practice, hospital organizational structure, private insurance, and on industry. Many physicians have prepared for careers in government medicine through studying public health administration. Physicians in public health administration may be board certified in preventive medicine by obtaining a master's degree in public health. Health administration is one component of the MPH curriculum. Increasingly, physicians choose to concentrate on health services administration in their training by seeking the master's degree in health administration, an M.B.A in health administration, or equivalent from a recognized health administration program.

THE INSURANCE INDUSTRY

Insurance programs have enormous effect on the quality of care and the cost of services. Because indemnity insurance must now compete with managed care systems, most insurers utilize systems to control utilization and their level of payment for various services. Physicians are needed to assess the cost and necessity of care. Involvement in insurance investment decisions and the monitoring and control of medical and hospital practice are major opportunities for physicians.

INDUSTRY

Industry has recognized that the best opportunity for restraining health care costs and assuring a capable work force is to invest in the prevention of illness and injury. Occupational medicine has been a traditional means of focusing on injury and environmental control in industry. In recent years industry has begun to employ health administrators to design health benefit packages to control the use of benefits and to work with the private sector to assure minimum cost, high quality services for employees. Industry investments made in screening and health promotion programs require thorough analysis and understanding of the health risks of the population and the benefits to be achieved. Prevention may not always be the least expensive alternative for industry. The organization and design of the optimum health strategy for industry provides major opportunities for physicians trained in occupational medicine and in health administration.

TECHNOLOGY ASSESSMENT

The health care system is being driven by the rapid advances in medical technology. The application of new technology is enormously expensive and complex. Great individual benefit may be derived; however, much technology is applied without demonstrating its cost effectiveness. Many organizations, including government, industry, and health care systems are developing mechanisms for assessing technology and its implications for the care of individuals and its costs. Involvement in the administration and assessment of technology is becoming a growing opportunity for physician administrators with solid management skills.

ACADEMIC ADMINISTRATION

The United States has 127 schools of medicine most of which are in academic health centers which also include other health science schools and teaching hospitals. The leadership of these organizations has traditionally been dominated by physicians. Most of these institutions involve large hospitals with very complex related physician practices. The administration of academic programs involves deans, associate deans, department chairmen and other individuals providing leadership in research, teaching, and patient care activities. These organizations are the focus of the development and application of new technologies and deliver the most sophisticated medical care practiced in the world. More than 60,000 physicians are employed as members of the faculties. There is obvious need for an opportunity for effective physician management of these major medical and educational organizations.

CONCLUSIONS

The physician is generally a well educated and highly motivated individual who is concerned about the care of individuals and the success of organizations in which that care is provided. Few physicians have specific training in management decision making and quantitative analysis. Preparation in finance, accounting, economics, and organizational theory are a major deficit in the education of many physician executives. The impact of the law, government, politics, and regulation must be understood in order to manage successfully complex, large health care organizations. Specific training programs exist to facilitate physicians in obtaining the training required to increase their opportunity for success in health services administration. In the past many physicians entered their management role with a minimum of formal training in management. If physicians recognize that a significant part, or all, of their careers will be devoted to health administration, they will be well served to obtain the specific training required. This training, with emphasis on addressing the health care needs of populations, can be obtained on a part-time or full-time basis through health care administration programs. The return on this investment will be a more qualified and more competent physician executive capable of providing leadership. The reward for this investment is largely in the satisfaction of seeing an organized response to a major need in health care in a community. Inadequate leadership in these areas leads to conflict, inadequate care, and frustrated individuals. Superb medical administration results in a harmonious approach to providing needed services, a community with pride and confidence in the quality of care being provided, and satisfaction for the organizations and individuals responsible for paying for care.

The individual physicians making this investment can expect to be reasonably rewarded for their time with salaries that are competitive with physicians in private practice. The greatest reward for effective medical administration is found in planning and implementing health care services in organizations that effectively serve the health care needs of communities.

The opportunity and need for effective medical administration can be demonstrated in every sector of the health care system. Physicians properly prepared and motivated to provide leadership to physicians and to the hospitals and to other organizations make a difference in the quality of life in their communities. This form of service to the community is ultimately rewarding, although it is perhaps not as immediately satisfying as private medical practice. The individual willing to look to the long run can expect a rewarding career serving as a physician executive.

REFERENCE

1. Starr, P. *The Social Transformation of Medicine.* New York: Basic Books, 1982, 178–79.

19

NURSES IN HEALTH ADMINISTRATION: FROM BEDSIDE TO BOARDROOM

ELLEN W. GUTSTADT

The American Hospital Association's Council on Nursing and the American Organization of Nurse Executives conjointly define a nurse administrator as a

> registered nurse on the hospital executive management team who is responsible for the management of the nursing organization (nursing department, nursing division, etc.) and for the clinical practice of nursing throughout the institution. ... The nurse executive is mutually responsible for the provision of high quality and cost effective patient care ... [and] is accountable for establishing productive working relationships with the medical staff and support departments, and for being responsive to community needs [1].

The Joint Commission on Accreditation of Healthcare Organizations (JCAHO) defines a director of nurses in their accreditation manual as "the administrator of the nursing department/service is a qualified registered nurse with appropriate education, experience, and licensure and with demonstrated ability in nursing practice and administration" [2].

Both definitions are broad, but they agree that a nurse administrator must

---

Ellen W. Gutstadt is assistant director of Hospital Nursing Services at Kaiser Permanente Medical Center in Hayward, CA. She earned M.P.H. and B.A. degrees from the University of California at Berkeley, and also holds a Master of Science (nursing) from the University of California–San Francisco and a B.S.N. from California State University–Hayward.

be a professional registered nurse (RN) who understands the practice of nursing and is the spokesperson for maintaining professional standards. According to one source, in 1985, 94.5 percent of nurse administrators were female [3].

The job of nurse administrators is complex. On the one hand, they are expected to be the conscience of the hospital, the patient advocate. On the other hand, they are usually responsible for the greatest number of personnel, the largest budget, and the coordination of many projects and departments. The traditional caring role of the nurse is juxtaposed with the productivity-oriented role of a business person.

The nurse administrator needs to be able to understand all aspects of patient care—literally, from birth to death. It is important to be able to predict where all types of nursing practice are headed. We therefore need to examine the daily activities of a nurse administrator when considering how to prepare for the role.

PRIMARY RESPONSIBILITIES

PATIENT CARE DELIVERY

Although it seems obvious, one is reminded that hospitals exist to provide nursing and medical care to patients. The need for professional nursing care is the critical indicator for acute care hospitalization; if the patient does not need nursing care, the patient will be sent home. Patients once routinely admitted for postoperative care (for example, following cataract or hernia surgeries) are now discharged home to recover. The issue of delivering nursing care, therefore, is a primary focus of a nurse administrator.

The nurse administrator must understand the many specialty nursing services that the hospital provides. The technical knowledge within each area may be complex. The nurse administrator must be able to understand the level of care provided at the hospital and the community standard for that service. Maternal nursing is a good example.

Obstetrics is one of the most competitive fields among hospitals, and it is a litigious area of practice. Nurse administrators are challenged to create an environment in which babies can be delivered to the consumer-patients' satisfaction while practicing defensive care. Most women do not like medical intervention, yet fetal monitoring (a record of the labor that is extremely important in a legal action) enables the physicians and nurses to make better decisions. Another important issue is the role the nurse can undertake. What is acceptable practice for the nurse? Knowledge of how other nurses in the community are functioning is vital.

Because there are so many areas of practice, and no one nurse can possess complete knowledge of them all, nurse administrators must rely on the clinical expertise of their managers.

Nurse administrators are responsible for the care provided to patients. A major issue is determining whether the care is good. Two components of the assessment are quality assurance and patient feedback.

QUALITY ASSURANCE

The measurement of quality assurance is undergoing frequent changes influenced by community, JCAHO, and professional practice standards.

In the past, patient care was examined retrospectively, after the patient was discharged. The medical record was reviewed by several people, who looked for a logical sequence of events. For example, was the surgical consent signed—a legal requirement? Was there a postoperative nurse's note? Were the medical orders carried out?

Today, the focus is changing. Standards are written for different areas of practice and more specific information is gathered. An advantage of this change is that standards can be reviewed concurrently, while the patient is still hospitalized. Another difference is the shift of focus to the outcome of the care given.

Indicators of quality care other than adherence to standards and outcome are nosocomial (hospital-acquired) infection rates, legal actions, incident reports (which describe unusual occurrences such as medication errors or patient falls), patient compliments and complaints, readmission rates, and other identified problems.

PATIENT FEEDBACK

Patients' compliments and complaints are important. Feedback from patients reveals their expectations of care. The new health care environment is intensely competitive, characterized by advertisements for hospitals, special services (sports care orthopedic units, women's centers, and school vacation specials), gifts, bonuses, and unique payment plans. Patients are being treated as consumers and it is important to understand what they want. Information regarding patients' experiences can be compiled from surveys, discharge phone calls, and interviews during hospitalization. Nurse administrators must have a thorough understanding of the patient population being served.

HUMAN RESOURCE MANAGEMENT

Human resources occupy a major amount of nurse administrators' time. Three areas are worthy of note—the development of nurse managers, recruitment and retention of nurses, and labor relations.

Nurse Managers

Depending on organizational structure, nurse managers may or may not report directly to a nurse administrator. In many hospitals, they report to an assistant (for example, assistant director of nurses or patient care coordinator). A nurse manager has 24-hour responsibility for a particular department, including accountability for patient care, staffing, budget, and supplies. Usually, a nurse manager is a staff nurse who was promoted to a management position after demonstrating strong clinical skills, leadership abilities, and an aptitude for management. Many nurse managers have associate degrees in nursing. As the complexity of the unit increases, a higher educational level may be required. Because increased academic preparation may have a clinical focus, the nurse administrator must assess management abilities and guide managers in developing their effectiveness.

A nurse manager must be able to motivate and develop staff, to analyze and maintain the quality of care given in the unit, to establish unit-specific goals within those of the entire hospital to keep abreast of changes in practice, to maintain multiple interdepartmental relationships, to establish and monitor the budget, and to set productivity standards. The responsibilities are challenging whatever the educational background and nurse managers likely have little formal education. It is obviously important for nurse administrators developing effective managers to support attendance at seminars, management training programs, and conferences relating to clinical practice, and to encourage seeking at minimum, a baccalaureate degree. As nursing becomes more complex and more patients are acutely ill, additional education is a must for nurse managers.

Recruitment and Retention

Without an adequate supply of RNs, hospitals cannot function. A nurse administrator is responsible for hiring and retaining nurses—a difficult task because the supply of nurses fluctuates. Schools of nursing graduate RNs to meet the demand of hospitals. When the demand is met the field is less attractive to students and fewer nurses are graduated. This cyclic phenomenon is becoming worse as many students choose other careers. Nurses are predominantly women, and many women are now choosing nontraditional careers. The challenge of staffing a hospital can only increase in the future. In a highly competitive area, the nurse administrator must know how to recruit nurses and also how to create a satisfying work environment that will retain them.

RECRUITMENT. Marketing, a field once reserved for the sale of consumer goods, is expanding into health care. It is necessary for the nurse administrator to understand principles of marketing, not only to market the hospital services to consumers but in order to market the hospital to potential nursing staff.

There are many reasons why an RN may choose to work at a specific hospital—salary, benefits, location, scheduling, and professional growth or several of these. It is necessary for nurse administrators to understand why nurses choose to work in their hospital.

A marketing plan should be developed to define and locate the targeted RN population and attract applicants.

Recruitment is a function of both the nursing and personnel departments. With good support from personnel, a nurse recruiter, a reputable advertising agency, and the planning or marketing department, nurse administrators' recruitment efforts can be significantly eased. These support services, however, vary dramatically from hospital to hospital.

RETENTION. Retention is the key to maintaining a qualified permanent staff. Two major studies have indicated reasons why nurses stay at their jobs. In 1980, the National Commission on Nursing was established. The American Hospital Association, Hospital Research and Educational Trust, and American Hospital Supply Corporation sponsored this Commission with the purpose of studying nursing-related problems in the U.S. health care system.

The study identified five major factors which affect nursing: the status and image of nursing, nursing education, the effective management of nursing resources, relationships among nursing and other health care professionals and development of nursing as a profession. Then, in the fall of 1981, the American Academy of Nursing Task Force on Nursing Practice in Hospitals initiated a study to look at "magnet hospitals"—those hospitals that exemplify professional nursing—and to identify the factors that seem to be associated with their success [4]. Both studies gave similar results: nurses want to work in a supportive environment that allows them to practice professional nursing and compensates them fairly for their work. The magnet hospital study listed the issues as management style, personnel policies and programs, professional practice, and professional development.

The issue of retention affects all aspects of both the management and practice of nursing. As nursing changes, nurse administrators must ask themselves if their nursing departments are right for today's environment. If they do not examine this question periodically, it will be answered by an increase in the nursing turnover rate at the hospital.

Leading and Listening

A major frustration for RNs is their lack of participation in the decision-making process. Nurses make many decisions daily about the care their patients receive but are often excluded from making important policy decisions. The traditional hierarchical and often autocratic management style should no longer apply to nursing.

Nurses want nurse administrators to be visible and approachable. The business style advocated by Tom Peters and John Waterman of "management by walking around" is desirable for nurse administrators [5].

At the same time, nurses want nurse administrators who are leaders, resources for them, experts, and outspoken supporters of the nursing profession. Nurses want to see a commitment by nurse administrators to high-level patient care. These can be difficult expectations to meet. Nurse administrators traditionally have done rounds in their nursing departments. Nurses support this approach and want to use this time to communicate with the nurse administrators.

PLANNING

Nurse administrators must be expert planners. Constant demands on time make analysis of nursing department priorities necessary.

Nurse administrators are the voice of nursing. They represent a large group of professionals and must have an understanding of trends and projections in nursing. This vision or futuristic look will help guide planning decisions. Moreover, with this vision, nurse educators can begin to prepare curricula that will meet the needs of hospitals.

The nurse administrator's vision must look to these issues: what services to offer, discontinue, and develop; what skills the staff should have in order to provide these services; what projects are expected (that is, new phone system, computerization); what patients want, expect, and need; what plans the medical staff have for future changes; and what other hospitals are doing.

The planning goals of the nursing department support the goals of the hospital and guide the work of the nurse managers. Again, it is easier if qualified planners help identify a nursing department's planning goals. A hospital planner can provide background information on the patient-consumer population and on other hospital services in the community.

The planning cycle must precede the budgeting cycle so anticipated or new services can be provided for. There must be constant evaluation and reevaluation of the plan, as any changes alter it. For example, if a new pediatric surgeon plans to join the medical staff, a training program for nurses must be developed and new equipment ordered. If the physician decides not to join the staff, these plans must be canceled. Planning is a vital component of a nurse administrator's job.

FINANCIAL MANAGEMENT

Nurse administrators need a solid understanding of financial management. Many factors influence the financial outlook of the hospital and there are three distinct budgets—personnel, nonpayroll or supplies, and capital (large-cost items).

The personnel or payroll budget for nursing is likely to be the largest in the hospital. Many nursing staffs today include a high percentage of RNs, and they are paid some of the highest salaries in the hospital. The use of RNs, therefore, becomes a major issue. How many RNs are there or are needed on each unit? It is difficult to evaluate the costs of using RNs in relation to the quality of care delivered to patients. Sometimes the number of RNs is determined by state law or Joint Commission.

Both California law and the Joint Commission state that staff numbers shall be based on the level of care necessary for the patient [6, 7]. The Joint Commission manual states that a sufficient number of qualified RNs will be on duty at all times to give patients any nursing care requiring their judgment and specialized skills.

A work standard or measure is essential for deciding how many RNs are required. Whether the system measures how sick patients are (a patient acuity system) or how many tasks or procedures the nurse performs for them (a work load measurement system), it is necessary to develop standards to monitor the adequacy and appropriateness of the staffing level.

Once the staff numbers are determined, then the mix (RN to other nursing personnel) must be considered. The budgeter must examine the hospital's past use of staff, types of patients, length of stay, and occupancy rates. Nurse administrators are only now trying to evaluate in detail the costs of nursing care. Traditionally, nursing costs were charged to the patient through the daily room charge. This is an inequitable system, because patients require varying levels of nursing care.

Supply budgets can be determined by past usage information and by the type of patient on the unit. Since Medicare's implementation of the diagnostic-related-group payment system, many hospitals calculate supply costs by diagnostic category.

Expensive equipment necessary to run a hospital must be carefully planned for and money designated. When decisions are made to offer a new service, it may be necessary to purchase equipment to support the service. A good example is the lithotripsy machine, which can help a patient avoid surgery by breaking up kidney stones. The machine is extremely expensive. Understanding the principles of cost-benefit analysis on services provided by the hospital is therefore an important budgetary skill.

Nurse administrators are beginning to hire financial analysts who develop and monitor the nursing budget. The ideal candidate might be an RN with a master's degree in business administration capable of suggesting realistic budget changes based on nursing experience. With multimillion-dollar budgets, more help with the budget is desirable to ease the task and sharpen the skills of the nurse administrator.

Another aspect of both budgeting and planning is construction management. As hospital occupancy rates decline, so does new construction and more hospitals are remodeling existing areas. Understanding architectural blueprints and anticipating future space needs are necessary skills for nurse administrators.

BUILDING STAFF RELATIONSHIPS

Nurse administrators interact with many different people. As administrators of many nursing units, they are often seen as coordinators. When issues touch many units, they will often be brought to nurse administrators instead of to several nurse managers. The nurse administrators need to possess good interpersonal skills and a great deal of patience.

In an article on orienting a new nurse administrator, Vicki Schofield [8] surveyed 100 nurse administrators and identified 19 personnel categories important to the nurse administrator. At the top of the list were the chiefs of the medical staff, followed by the chief executive officer (CEO), nurse managers, the fiscal manager, the personnel manager, and nursing department staff educators. Nurse administrators' relationships with the medical staff are vital to success. It is difficult for the nurse administrators to work well with physicians because nursing staff often interpret the relationship as physicians dominating or managing nursing. Nurse administrators must develop nurse-physician relationships to dispel this feeling.

Nurse administrators must build trusting relationships with staff and labor unions. By interacting with staff regularly, by maintaining fair and consistent policies, and by keeping communications open, nurse administrators will develop positive working relationships with staff and unions.

Nurse administrators are members of many hospital committees (sometimes too many). Two of the most important are the hospital's executive committee and the ethics committee. It is necessary for nurse administrators to report on nursing regularly, in order to keep others informed about nursing issues and projects.

The days of sitting in the nursing office or administrative suite and communicating among several individuals are over. Nurse administrators must be able and willing to communicate well with many people.

Nurse administrators must be able to interpret many documents such as professional and Joint Commission standards, state hospital regulations, nurse practice acts, labor laws, and union contracts.

Hospital attorneys, personnel managers, and the staff of professional associations can make nurse administrators' jobs easier, but they must understand what can and cannot be done. Intricate legal questions can arise, sometimes on a daily basis. Some examples are: Can a pregnant woman in labor refuse a caesarean section? Can an employee waive overtime? Can a nurse be fired for incompetence without progressive discipline?

Knowledge of labor law is essential to nurse administrators' ability to function effectively.

PROFESSIONAL DEVELOPMENT

Nursing is stressful and physically demanding work. It is important to create an environment where nurses can develop professionally. Continuing education programs, upgrade programs (licensed vocational nurse to RN, RN with associate degree or diploma to baccalaureate degree, tuition reimbursement, inservice education, cross-training programs (intensive care nurse to recovery room or emergency room nurse), and a clinical ladder (advancement through clinical excellence), are examples of ways to help nurses grow.

As nurses become more scarce, nurse administrators take on the role of educators. Programs may be offered to new RNs to bridge the gap between education and practice; to RNs seeking reentry to clinical practice; and to RNs wanting to change areas of clinical practice (for example, from medicine to obstetrics).

JOB OPPORTUNITIES

The number of nurse administrator positions seems to fluctuate with the supply of nurses. At times when nurses are in short supply, the demand for nurse administrators seems to rise.

When there is little turnover, it is difficult to get a nurse administrator position because there is only one position per hospital. There are usually more opportunities at the assistant or associate level that are easier to obtain. A nurse administrator can make a lateral move to hospital assistant administrator, or move up to chief executive officer (also limited to one per hospital). A move from nurse administrator to CEO seems logical. After all, the nurse administrator has the largest number of employees and a correspondingly large budget, numerous projects, and responsibility for providing quality patient care. Yet, this is not the usual progression. In reality, the nurse administrator is often passed over in favor of a less experienced assistant administrator.

Nurse administrators must chart careers carefully to attain the chief executive level by designing projects broader in scope than nursing; developing power bases that include board members and vice presidents, who influence decisions; and achieving educations equal to or better than assistant administrators' (that is, master's degrees in health services administration, public health, or business administration from respected programs).

There are, however, many other possible career moves. Nurse administrators may become consultants, educators, ambulatory care managers, or move to the public sector, perhaps to a state health department.

Nurse administrators can switch to other nonnursing roles within hospitals, such as clinic management, but more often they move to a different type of setting—from a nonteaching hospital to a university facility or from a nonprofit medical center to a county hospital. Nurse administrators tend to stay in fairly similar roles because job opportunities exist and the responsibilities and salaries are difficult to match.

Salaries of nurse administrators range from less than $30,000 to more than $65,000 per year. Based on 1985 data, the average salary range is between $40,000 and $50,000 [9].

Mary Alice Huser, RN, a senior associate at Witt Associates, Inc., in a study of 94 nurse administrators found that they are very satisfied in their jobs. Ms. Huser concluded that "the study indicates that nurses are being allowed to manage; that they believe they are making a difference to the well-being of patients, staff, and their institutions, and that their jobs offer variety [10].

OBLIGATIONS

Nurse administrators are busy. The pace is fast and the environment is changing. It is, therefore, extremely important for them to keep current in many areas; to belong to professional organizations, such as the American Organization for Nurse Executives or state organizations for nurse administrators. Many local nurse administrator groups meet regularly. It is necessary to keep a network of colleagues and to work together to solve problems. Issues current at one hospital may have already been solved at other hospitals (for example, how to decrease staff).

As a member of the hospital's administrative team, it is also important to belong to hospital organizations. Nurse administrators can then observe trends in health care and in hospitals in general.

By becoming officers in professional organizations, nurse administrators can gain additional, varied experience, helping them grow and promoting recognition for both them and their hospitals.

Nurse administrators must attend conferences, continuing education seminars, and college courses to keep current, to be credible leaders, and to function as resources.

Nurse administrators can keep current in two additional ways—by reading a variety of journals covering all aspects of nursing, medicine, and management and by being mentors for administrative residents who have up-to-date training and a willingness to look at old problems with a fresh approach.

Nurse administrators must understand today's world and beyond. Their decisions today may influence the care given in five or ten years. Remodeling of a labor and delivery area may be a good example of practice that can be influenced by the physical environment.

The work of nurse administrators is complex. We will consider what type of education makes a good foundation for the job.

HIGHER EDUCATION

An RN going back to school should consider three choices: whether to stay in practice as a clinical specialist or nurse practitioner, to become an educator, or to go into administration. The majority of nurses in master's level programs choose a clinical focus and the rest divide approximately equally between the choices of education and nursing administration. The emphasis in nursing graduate schools has been on developing clinical expertise. Most nurses who become educators study in schools of education and those interested in management attend graduate schools in business, health services administration, public health, or public administration.

In a 1985 study, Cynthia Freund found that 73.1 percent of nurse administrators had a master's degree or higher, a 15.1 percent increase [11]. She found that nurse administrators held the following degrees: diploma or associate, 3.5 percent; bachelor's (nursing), 4.1 percent; bachelor's (other), 7.6 percent; master's (nursing), 60.2 percent; master's (business or health services administration), 8.2 percent; doctoral 4.7 percent; other 11.7 percent. A position statement on graduate education in nursing administration by the American Association of Colleges of Nursing and American Organization of Nurse Executives, stated that "graduate education in nursing administration must be comprehensive, relevant, appropriate, and responsive to present and future health care environments and nursing practice settings" [12].

One appropriate academic setting would be collegiate schools of nursing offering specialized graduate programs in nursing administration. The program that future nurse administrators attend must (1) prepare them for the role they will undertake, (2) provide them with appropriate credentials to increase credibility with coworkers and to pursue expanded job opportunities (that is, through CEO), and (3) encompass a generalist approach. A master's degree in nursing is not likely to prepare a nurse administrator adequately for the role. The scope may be limited to nursing topics and the breadth may be too narrow.

In a 1984 study, Sylvia Price found that graduate schools of nursing did not meet the educational needs of the nurse administrator [13]. She concluded that the nursing administration curriculum should encompass administration and management, financial management and budgeting, organizational theory, labor relations and human relations, economic and political aspects of management, research, and a generalist approach to clinical subject matter. Price's curriculum would be compatible with the actual responsibilities of the nurse administrator. It is important for students contemplating nursing administration to find a master's level program that fulfills these requirements.

When examining educational preparation, it is important to remember who hires nurse administrators: in most cases, the administrator-CEO. According to Freund, 81.6 percent of CEOs have master's degrees [14]. Academic preparation on a par with administrators' increases nurse administrators' acceptability as colleagues.

In a study by Butts, Berger, and Brooten, 46 percent of nurse administrator jobs required (and 35 percent preferred) a master's degree [15]. Graduate education is a necessity to prepare properly for nursing administration.

CONCLUDING THOUGHTS

The role of the nurse administrator is broad and complex. Adequate educational preparation is essential to provide a framework for the nurse administrator to build upon. Nursing administration requires enthusiastic, energetic individuals.

The work of nursing administration is totally consuming. Nurse administrators must question values; weigh patient care against the budget; be public figures; be leaders, mentors, and teachers to the staff; stand being attacked and praised in the same day. Projects will go on and on and the paper flow will be unending. With all of this, it is an exciting, dynamic, and challenging career.

REFERENCES

1. American Hospital Association. Role and Functions of the Hospital Nurse Executive [Guidelines]. Chicago: The Association, 1985.
2. Nursing Services. In Joint Commission on Accreditation of Healthcare Organizations. *Accreditation Manual for Hospitals*, 139–48. Chicago: The Commission, 1986.
3. Nurse Executives Most Often Picked from Hospital Staff. *Hospitals* 60 November 5: 91, 1986.
4. American Nurses' Association and American Academy of Nursing. Task Force on Nursing Practice in Hospitals. *Magnet Hospitals: Attraction and Retention of Professional Nurses*. Kansas City, Mo: The Association.
5. Peters, J., and Waterman, R. H. *In Search of Excellence*. New York: Warner Books, 1982.
6. California Administrative Code, Title 22: Social Security, published by the Office of Administrative Hearings, State of California (Documents Section).
7. Joint Commission on Accreditation of Health Care Organizations. *Accreditation Manual for Hospitals*.
8. Schofield, V. M. Orientation of Nurse Executives. *Journal of Nursing Administration* 16: 13–17, 1986.
9. Hospitals, see number 3.
10. Nurse Executives Surprisingly Happy in Their New Roles. *Hospitals* 60 April 5: 92, 1986.
11. Freud, C. M. Director of Nursing Effectiveness: DON and CEO Perspectives and Implications for Education. *Journal of Nursing Administration* 15: 25–30, 1985.
12. American Association of Colleges of Nursing and American Organization of Nurse Executives. Position Statement on Graduate Education in Nursing Administration. *Journal of Professional Nursing* 2:263, 1986.
13. Price, S. A. Master's Programs Preparing Nursing Administrators: What Are the Essential Components? *Journal of Nursing Administration* 14: 11–17, 1984.
14. Freund, C. M. See 8.
15. Butts, P. A., B. A. Berger, and D. A. Brooten. Tracking Down the Right Degree for the Job. *Nursing Health Care* 7:91-5, 1986.

20

CAREER ENTRY AND CAREER DEVELOPMENT

JOHN S. LLOYD

You may read this book when you are preparing for your first career or your second or third. Unlike previous generations, when a person's education and training were supposed to carry that person through a lifetime occupation, many people today will embark several times on a new career path. The information explosion has caused us to reassess our careers every 20 years or so, as a matter of course.

A health services administration career combines two important elements of life—hard work that is meaningful, that can help save or change a life. There is the challenge of working in one of the best health care delivery systems in the world while you seek to improve it. You will be trying to slow the rapid rate of cost escalation while keeping care within the reach of all people, to manage new technological miracles while attending to the ethical concerns of quality of life and dignity in death.

This chapter focuses on *getting a job*. Professional education will help you examine issues, expand your understanding and lay a foundation for your later growth and work. Your education is less likely to include the nuts-and-bolts information contained here. This is intended to help you identify and then get a job that will allow you to reach your life's goals.

Maybe you are thinking of the job search as a "someday" activity. If you delay your consideration of the job market until later, perhaps until your

John S. Lloyd is president of Witt Associates Inc., consultants to health care management, in Oak Brook, IL. He holds an M.B.A./M.S.P.H. degree in health care management and finance and a B.S. degree in business administration from the University of Missouri.

final term, you are not likely to have much success in accomplishing your objectives. Your job search can and should begin in your senior year of college or on the first day of graduate school—or even earlier. Orientations and other hospitality events often punctuate the new school year in major universities, and these can be your starting points.

As a principal in a national executive search firm that has specialized in the health care industry for 20 years, I can tell you that you will never have greater job-finding resources than in your undergraduate or graduate school environment. Take full advantage of them.

The alumni, your faculty, guest lecturers, residencies, field work and externships are great opportunities, if you approach them properly. Many of you will have invitations to attend gatherings sponsored by your program's alumni. Perhaps a speaker has been arranged, or it may be simply a social get-together. These invitations are as good as gold and should never be ignored. At these meetings, introduce yourself to anyone and everyone—they are there to meet you and to let you meet them. The program's alumni understand the value of these contacts. They stood in your shoes, not so long ago, and were glad when more senior people gave them time and attention.

Health care is probably less competitive in this regard than other industries. It is a tradition in our field that those who have already achieved some success help along those who are just getting started. For the tradition to be carried on, you have to do *your* part. Look for opportunities to meet practicing administrators and boldly shake the hands of alumni. As a student, you can ask them almost anything and expect to get a thoughtful response. Pick their brains, challenge them, seek their advice and counsel—they have already indicated a willingness to provide assistance, and they will be pleased by your interest.

Some alumni gatherings are held at major national and regional health care meetings. If your budget permits, try to attend some, but never overlook your school's alumni programs. Do not waste these opportunities by standing around and chatting with fellow students. Take the initiative and extend yourself; the rewards will be substantial.

You will establish relationships that can stand you in good stead throughout your professional career, but that are especially important at the outset. This is the foundation of your professional network. It is only the first step in career development, however.

Consider becoming a student affiliate of one or more of the national organizations that hold regular meetings in your area—WHEN (Women's Health Executive Network) or your local YAG (young administrators' group) are two examples. As a student member, you will have access to the senior people who attend their sessions, and you may be able to participate on a committee or task force to work on some specific topic or concern. This type of exposure can be invaluable as you begin to define your job goals.

The members of your program faculty are far more than instructors; they can be guides to the real world. Many faculty members have had experience in the industry and have exceptional insights and ideas to share. You may have the impression that they are "just teachers." Find out more about them by looking beyond the school's catalog into some of the sources in the library—*Who's Who* for example. You may be surprised to learn the scope of their experience and contacts. Give faculty members a chance to take you under their wing, and they will do so. The clinical/medical model for this mentor philosophy is still very strong, even though the formal process may be in decline. Clinical faculty and guest speakers from practice are in an excellent position to get to know you and to be able to measure your qualities over an extended period of time. They may encourage you to pursue specific lines of research, or suggest that you consider acquiring specific management development experiences. Listen to their advice and take it when you can.

Internships, residencies and fellowships are obviously very important resources for your career planning and development. Placement in an internship/residency or fellowship can influence the choices you will make for several years to follow. Many people use the terms "internship," "externship" and "residency" fairly interchangeably. Each one has a different structure, but all have the objective of providing a structured learning/working experience.

If you think your focus should be on managed care, seek a placement in that segment of the industry. If you really think that you will prefer a career in association work, look for opportunities in that area. If you want to understand the acute-care sector, look for a role there. If you want to know whether you might have a career in long-term care, or biotechnology, or whatever—make it your goal to have a working experience in that area. Your program faculty should be responsive to your specific interest.

Even if you later choose to pursue another avenue, the contacts and experiences you gain will be invaluable. You will at least know what many people do not, which is *what they do not want*.

The mistakes you make as a resident or fellow are usually viewed as the inevitable cost of learning. Do not be afraid to make a mistake. Do not be reluctant to *try* something, even though you are not sure it will work out well for you. Remember that your options are probably greater now than they will be later in your working life, so it is appropriate to take chances, to "go for it" and to fail, if necessary. It will not be held against you by those who will evaluate your performance in the future.

Keep informed and up-to-date. It sounds simple until you are in the middle of a research project and your reading list has gathered dust from disuse. Read *The Wall Street Journal, Hospitals, Dimensions in Healthcare Services, Modern Healthcare, Health Affairs, Business Week, Maclean's, Fortune, Modern Maturity, People,* the Sunday *Times* or whatever other periodicals will help to nourish the "big picture" side of you. These resources provide information on what is happening in the world that will indirectly or directly affect your life and options.

If you do not keep up, and maintain only your academic reading, you will miss an important key to professional growth and leadership. You should be alert to developments in a new market segment, and be watching for the signals that indicate when a tradition is dying or a new trend is coming along. By working hard at being broadly well-informed, you will be in a good position to make the best career decisions.

All these avenues have one general purpose—to expand your career and job choices. The intent is to build and strengthen your network of people. One idea is to keep a list of key people with whom to keep in contact. Send a note or call when there has been a promotion or "just to stay in touch." It is possible to do this without appearing to fawn. It is ultimately *your* network—grow it and cultivate it however you feel most comfortable.

Another thought is to develop a "Fortune 100" list of the top organizations in your targeted industry segment, complete with the names of the CEO and human resources director for each organization. Select two or three organizations each week and write letters to these key people, introducing yourself, describing your interest in the field and in them as an employer. Mention graduation dates and ask for corporate brochures. Always be sincere (they are experts in recognizing b.s.), be accurate (they are industry leaders for a reason), and be brief (their time is valuable).

It is a matter of impact and exposure. The more often your name crosses their desks, the more likely they are to remember you. Follow-up is essential. Six to eight months before you graduate, send out the second round of letters—an effective, low-cost marketing tool. Some day, you will be shaking hands at a conference or seminar and hear, "Oh, yes, you are the one who keeps sending me letters. Let's talk."

The most important step in starting your job search is setting your own priorities. Here are five priority areas that you will consider when you are seeking your first job.

PRIORITIES—FIRST JOB

No. 1—The industry segment
No. 2—The individuals and/or organization you will be working with
No. 3—The location

No. 4—The function you will perform
No. 5—The salary you will earn

These are the issues that you should address, and the *order* in which you should consider them. Let us look at each in more detail, and some of my thinking on these priorities will become more apparent.

THE INDUSTRY SEGMENT

After reading this book and doing all of your other homework, it should be clear that there are one or more segments of the health care industry for which you are best suited. It may be because of your interest or skills, or because your personal style is more apt to fit, or because you are attracted to it. You will have listened to the advice of your faculty advisers, you will have consulted with your alumni contacts, and you will have talked it over with your fellow students, family and friends who work in other industries.

Hopefully, you will have focused on a segment of health services administration that is right for your abilities and your interests. Then the most important thing is *to find a job in that industry segment*. It may not be easy. It could be a tight job market when you are ready to look actively. Should you compromise? Should you look for a job in another industry segment (i.e., acute care instead of managed care)?

Absolutely not! For your first job, stick with it, even to the point of *volunteering*, taking on a project for no salary, if need be, to gain some experience in your chosen field. Is this risky advice? If you starved in the interim, you could say it was risky. But your chances of perishing are slight. It would be far more risky, in my view, to move on to an industry segment where you are less likely to be successful.

Remember the joke: A man sees a fellow at the circus who walks behind the parade, cleaning up after the elephants with a pushbroom and a pail. He has a sour look on his face, as though the odors are really offending him. Our observer asks: "Why don't you quit that job and get something you really *like?*"

"What?" replies the circus worker, "and get out of show business?"

Do not let any obstacle stand in the way of your own personal choice for your professional career.

THE ORGANIZATION AND PEOPLE

I have already noted how different health care is from many other industries; we have a tradition that senior administrators work with young administrators to help develop them as managers. This tradition is one reason that the organization—or the specific individual with whom you work—should rank in second priority in your first job specifications.

The work style and habits developed in your first job are vitally connected to the career opportunities you will have for the rest of your professional life. If you take a first job with a second-rate outfit, you may develop second-rate skills and you will be long associated with its indifferent reputation. Remember what Mr. Shakespeare said: "Who steals my purse steals trash ... but he that filches from me my good name ... makes me poor indeed." In health care administration, a "good name" is essential to fundamental career development.

But the organization is only part of what you must consider ... the *people* with whom you work are equally important. This is the time to look for a mentor, someone who is committed to developing future administrators. Choose wisely. Look for someone who has achieved success in your areas of interest, and who is willing and able to give you time and attention as your career begins.

You probably will want to draw upon the judgment of your first employer in the same way you have relied on the advice of teachers and preceptors in your university years. Work at being a good listener and try to probe their experience. These individuals have the insight to see a little farther and a little more clearly than you will, at least at the outset of your career.

LOCATION

Geography is the next priority for your consideration. Although it may move up to first place later, location is accorded a low ranking for your first job. It *is* important, of course, but it is not as critical as the industry and the organization.

Though you may want to be in California eventually, it may make sense to take your first position elsewhere—if the industry niche and the organization are just right. The geographic question is always a complicated one, especially since family considerations will enter into the decision-making process. But try not to let geography limit your options. There will be future opportunities in your preferred location, so do not give it much consideration at this point.

YOUR ASSIGNMENT

It's about time, you are probably thinking, to consider the job itself, the work you want to do! If this priority order seems topsy-turvy to you—trust me. *What* you will be doing in your first job is of lesser importance than the other priority issues we have already considered. You will have other, better opportunities to demonstrate what you can do. In any event, you are more likely to have a staff than a line position in your first job, and your scope of responsibilities will be limited.

There are many good books on how to make yourself visible, how to network, how to make a lot out of a little. Consult your local library and book stores—good new titles appear constantly. Read and use some of them for the advice they can provide, *if* it fits your situation. Never act out a part—be yourself in this first job, and all your life.

SALARY

Last on the list of priority considerations for your first job is salary. If all of the other elements are right, your salary should be less important. Not *unimportant*, just subordinate to the other priorities. Be particularly resistant to competition with your classmates on the basis of salary. If you have thought through the other priority issues, you are on firm ground. Be content for a year or two with a modest wage—greater rewards will come later.

It is worth noting that only in the past few years have the rewards even been there. Until very recently, most senior health care executives were seriously underpaid when compared to those in other industries. One result of a more competitive health care environment is more appreciation for the contribution of the excellent executive. Health care administrators' salaries, bonuses and other forms of compensation have begun to reflect that. But it is a fact that, in health care administration, you may have to "pay your dues" in entry-level positions, and part of that payment may be lower salary.

Your first job in health care administration should be approached as a completion of your formal education. It is true that an employee receives far more benefit than does the employer in this first "real" job. What you want to hear at the end of your first two years is, "We thought you would be good when we hired you, but you have pleased us beyond our expectations." But your *own* expectations are even more important. Set your standards high. Always perform quality work, act in an ethical manner and keep the "customer" uppermost in your mind at all times.

After a year or two, you will know when it is time to move on. You will be thinking about your second job, and the priorities are very likely to have rearranged themselves. Look at how the same issues are ranked compared with your first position:

PRIORITIES—SECOND JOB

No. 1—Industry segment
No. 2—Function

No. 3—Salary
No. 4—Organization and/or individual you work with
No. 5—Geography

One of the reasons why these priorities change is that you can expect to be in this position much longer—two to seven years, on average. You will really grow in this job, and have the opportunity to show what you can do. This may be the last time geography can be so low on the list. By the time you change jobs again, you are likely to have a family, with a spouse and children whose own needs and wishes must be taken into consideration.

The segment of the industry you have selected—hospitals, nursing homes, managed care, occupational health or health care products—is still your highest priority in selecting a job, because building a track record in a special area is important. A second consideration is the work you will do, followed by salary. Less important now is the individual or organization with whom you work—you can expect to have learned enough to want to spread your wings and fly. Geography, which is primarily a lifestyle issue, gets low billing.

HOW TO LOOK FOR A SECOND JOB

When looking for a second job, the sources you used the first time will be helpful, but you will also need to expand your horizons. You can turn to your university program for suggestions on opportunities, and you can expect to hear suggestions from your network or contacts in the field. But it is vital to enlarge your base by approaching new organizations and new people. You may be just what they are looking for, so give them the chance to meet you.

Your resume will be a major factor in your job search at this point. Invest considerable effort to make it a dynamic document—without stretching the truth in any way. This is not the time just to update your old resume. Claim your share of the credit when it is due for projects and programs, but do not forget to position yourself as a team member. It is unlikely that your major achievements were strictly solo accomplishments, and the people who interview you know that.

The cover letter that accompanies your resume is really important. It allows you to emphasize your interests and nonprofessional achievements that may be significant. Use the cover letter to reach out to the reader. The resume is a rather cool piece of information and your cover letter can warm it up. Always present yourself as you are, not as you wish to be or as you hope to be in a few years. *Never* lie about your education or accomplishments. You can expect your resume to be verified by conscientious executive recruiters and prospective employers throughout your working life, so be sure it is accurate.

Interviewing is a very serious process. Develop, through reading, seminars, and experience, a set of strong interviewing skills. Work on your shyness or modesty. Have a wardrobe consultant help you to develop an executive appearance and style, if you think you need guidance in this area. Second opinions are often helpful. Accept interviews whenever you can— practice is essential.

Be aware that some of the traditional concepts no longer hold: Loyalty no longer requires that you stay in a position for years and years, for example. You will not be considered untrustworthy or unstable if you have changed jobs every few years early in your career. Once this was considered to be a red flag that indicated a "jumper" who could not be counted on. Also, you need not have *completed* every assignment to be ready to leave; you may have done all you can and need new challenges.

NEW CAREERS

The futurists have told us that we will have three, four, five careers in our lifetime, and we are already seeing the evidence that bears out their predictions. Not jobs, but *careers*. This means that employers are much more understanding of time you have spent in an unrelated field. They rarely expect you to have concentrated solely on a single career track or path. In a reversal of the old pattern, the time may be coming when an employer will view individuals with only one job or one organization with suspicion.

Some of the key job growth opportunities I see are these:

— Care and management of lifestyle of our aging society. Read Ken Dychtwald's many articles to get a better perspective on this.

— Focus on quality management. Our firm has developed a national quality award which is presented annually to an organization with excellent quality systems in place, and these require managers. Read articles by Don Berwick, George Lebovitz, Bill Gantz, and others, for example, to get more focus on this vital topic.

— Pharmaceuticals and biotechnology. Our world is changing so rapidly and the breakthroughs are coming so fast, it is clear that excellent managers are needed in these areas. *The Wall Street Journal* may be your best source of information on these areas.

— International health care. Our delivery systems and quality standards in the U.S. and Canada are the envy of the world. Some large hospitals and systems in foreign countries seek individuals who can assist their organizations to provide superior health services in a consulting role. Read international business publications for ideas on what other countries are doing, and travel as widely as possible, so that you are comfortable in a variety of settings.

WORKING WITH A SEARCH FIRM

After you have been in your second job for a few years, you can expect to hear from executive search firms. It is unlikely that the firms would be able to match you with a client's position earlier in your career. Clients turn to search firms to identify senior level administrators, often with specific experience and always with proven skills. If you have achieved professional visibility and real accomplishments, you will be of interest to the recruiter who has a client needing your skills.

But what if they don't call?

Then it is perfectly appropriate for you to send your resume with a covering letter to executive search firms. In your letter, indicate how interested you are in moving now or later, so the search firm will know how to work with you. If you are truly not interested in moving, do not send a resume, of course.

It is important to understand the difference between an ethical *executive search firm*, a *contingency firm* and an *agency*. Both executive search and contingency firms are paid by the client to identify and attract a key executive. An agency is paid by the individual who is seeking a position.

But the differences go beyond the mechanisms of payment. A contingency firm will "float" resumes to clients, with little attention perhaps to the nuances of the situation. Your own boss could find *your* resume in a batch from a contingency firm—it has happened!

Remember that you should be treated well throughout the process. Are you truly interviewed, or are you simply asked a few basic questions? If that does not seem to matter much, consider how unhappy you would feel if you moved across the country for a job, only to find in a short time that it was not a good match for you.

In addition, pay attention to how much the person who works with you knows about the position and the client organization. A simple test will help you to distinguish among these various forms of recruitment: Notice how much the person who calls you knows about both the organization and the position. A search firm's consultants will have detailed knowledge and will use the call as a "selling" opportunity for the position if there seems to be a good match. The contingency representative may be much cagier on the phone, as he or she may know very little about the specifics of the job or the organization. If you are fortunate, you will develop some friendships with search consultants as part of your continuing network efforts. These people know where the jobs are—and are in the best position to evaluate your qualifications compared with those of many others.

SOME FINAL THOUGHTS

As you enter upon your career in health care administration, you could hardly have picked a more exciting or challenging time; if anything, the pace is going to quicken in the coming months and years.

Health care truly has become a place for the "best and brightest" in our society, and the salaries and status are beginning to reflect a new awareness of the industry's critical role in our economy.

Your commitment to humanity, expressed in your career choice, should be a source of pride for you and your family. In service to your fellow men and women, you will find deep satisfaction.

Good luck in your health services administration career!